The Physiology and Pathophysiology of the Skin

The Physiology and Pathophysiology of the Skin

Edited by

A. JARRETT

*Department of Dermatology,
University College Hospital
Medical School,
London, England*

Volume 8

The Photobiology of the Skin
Lasers and the Skin

1984

ACADEMIC PRESS

(Harcourt Brace Jovanovich, Publishers)

London   Orlando   San Diego   San Francisco   New York
Toronto   Montreal   Sydney   Tokyo   São Paulo

ACADEMIC PRESS INC. (LONDON) LTD
24–28 Oval Road,
London NW1 7DX

United States Edition published by
ACADEMIC PRESS INC.
(Harcourt Brace Jovanovich, Inc.)
Orlando, Florida 32887

British Library Cataloguing in Publication Data

The Physiology and pathophysiology of the skin.—
Vol. 8
1. Skin
612′.79′05   QP88.5

ISBN 0–12–380608–9
LCCCN 72–7711

FILMSET IN MONOPHOTO BASKERVILLE BY
LATIMER TREND & COMPANY LTD, PLYMOUTH
PRINTED IN GREAT BRITAIN BY
THOMSON LITHO LTD, EAST KILBRIDE

Contributors

VOLUME 1   The Epidermis

A. JARRETT, M.B., D.Sc., F.I.Biol., F.R.C.Path., F.R.C.P.Ed.

Director, Department of Dermatology, University College Hospital Medical School, London; Reader in Dermatological Histology, University of London; Hon. Consultant, University College Hospital, London, England.

VOLUME 2   The Nerves and Blood Vessels

D. C. SINCLAIR, M.A., M.D., D.Sc., F.R.C.S.Ed.

Regius Professor of Anatomy, University of Aberdeen, Aberdeen, Scotland; Late Professor of Anatomy, University of Western Australia

T. J. RYAN, B.M., M.R.C.P.

Consultant Dermatologist, Slade Hospital, Oxford; Late Senior Lecturer in Dermatology, St. John's Hospital for Diseases of the Skin; Editor of the Proceedings of the British Microcirculation Society; Hon. Consultant in Dermatology, Royal Postgraduate Medical School, London

VOLUME 3   The Dermis and the Dendrocytes

A. JARRETT, M.B., D.Sc., F.I.Biol., F.R.C.Path., F.R.C.P.Ed.

P. A. RILEY, M.B., Ph.D.

Reader in Biochemical Pathology, University College Hospital Medical School, London

T. J. RYAN, B.M., M.R.C.P.

R. I. C. SPEARMAN, B.Sc., Ph.D., F.I.Biol.

Senior Lecturer, Department of Dermatology, University College Hospital Medical School, London

VOLUME 4   The Hair Follicle

A. JARRETT, M.B., D.Sc., F.I.Biol., F.R.C.Path., F.R.C.P.Ed.

ELIZABETH JOHNSON, B.Sc., Ph.D.

Senior Lecturer in Zoology, University of Reading, London Road, Reading, England.

R. I. C. SPEARMAN, B.Sc., Ph.D., F.I.Biol.

VOLUME 5   The Sweat Glands; Skin Permeation; Lymphatics; The Nails

K. HASHIMOTO, M.D.

Professor and Head of Dermatology Section, Veterans Administration Center, 4100 West Third Street, Dayton, Ohio 45428, U.S.A.
Late of the Division of Dermatology, Department of Medicine, The University of Tennessee, Memphis, Tennessee, U.S.A.

A. JARRETT, M.B., D.Sc., F.I.Biol., F.R.C.Path., F.R.C.P.Ed.

T. MORIMOTO, M.D.

Professor of Physiology, Department of Physiology, Kyoto Prefectural University of Medicine, Kyoto, Japan.

T. J. RYAN, B.M., F.R.C.P.

R. J. SCHEUPLEIN, Ph.D.

Chief, Dermal Toxicology Branch, Food and Drug Administration, 200 'C' Street, S.W., Washington, D.C., U.S.A.
Late Principal Associate in Biophysics, Department of Dermatology, Harvard Medical School, Massachusetts General Hospital.

R. I. C. SPEARMAN, B.Sc., Ph.D., F.I.Biol.

VOLUME 6   The Mucus Membranes; The Action of Vitamin A on the Skin and Mucus Membranes; Transepidermal Water Loss

K. A. GRICE, M.D.

Consultant Dermatologist, Watford General and Hemel Hempstead Hospitals, Hertfordshire, England.

A. JARRETT, M.B., D.Sc., F.I.Biol., F.R.C.Path., F.R.C.P. Ed.

C. M. RIDLEY, M.A., B.M., F.R.C.P.
Consultant Dermatologist, Elizabeth Garrett Anderson, Royal Northern and Whittington Hospitals, London, England.

R. I. C. SPEARMAN, B.Sc., Ph.D., F.I.Biol.

VOLUME 7   Hormonal Control of Pigmentation; The Biology of Malignant Melanoma; The Pharmacology of Histamine: The Subcutaneous Tissue

J. J. H. GILKES, M.D., M.R.C.P.
Consultant Dermatologist, University College Hospital, London; Senior Lecturer, Department of Dermatology, University College Hospital Medical School, London.

M. W. GREAVES, M.D., Ph.D., F.R.C.P.
Professor of Dermatology, Institute of Dermatology, University of London; Director, Skin Pharmacology Laboratories, Institute of Dermatology; Hon. Senior Lecturer in Pharmacology, University College, London; Consultant Dermatologist, St. John's Hospital for Diseases of the Skin, London.

R. M. MacKIE, M.D., F.R.C.P.(Glasg.), M.R.C.Path.
Professor of Dermatology, University of Glasgow, Scotland; Hon. Consultant, Western Infirmary, Glasgow.

R. I. C. SPEARMAN, B.Sc., Ph.D., F.I.Biol.

B. WEATHERHEAD, M.A., Ph.D., M.I.Biol.
Lecturer, Department of Anatomy, School of Medicine, University of Leeds, Leeds, England.

VOLUME 8   The Photobiology of the Skin; Lasers and the Skin

B. E. JOHNSON, B.Sc., Ph.D.
Senior Lecturer in Photobiology, Department of Dermatology, University of Dundee, Ninewells Hospital, Dundee, Scotland.

J. A. COTTERILL, B.Sc., M.D., F.R.C.P.
The General Infirmary at Leeds, Great George Street, Leeds, England.

To Harold Blum

who did so much to set out a solid foundation for
modern dermatological photobiology

Preface

The major section of this volume on the photobiology of the skin is written by Brian Johnson who is an experienced scientist in this particular aspect of dermatological research.

The first two chapters are devoted to the basic scientific aspects of natural and artificial radiation of the skin, and the reactions of normal skin to these radiations.

Chapter 81 deals with the abnormal reactions encountered in disordered skin, and in this chapter Dr Johnson has had the invaluable help of Dr W. Frain-Bell who has also helped with the following chapter dealing with light sensitivity engendered by drugs and other chemicals applied either topically or systemically.

Chapter 83 discusses the use of photo-chemotherapy for psoriasis with special reference to the mechanisms involved. The next chapter is concerned with the complications of this form of treatment, and also its therapeutic value for skin disorders other than psoriasis.

The last section written by John Cotterill is related to the relatively new field of laser radiation of the skin. Dr Cotterill has considerable personal experience in the use of this form of radiation for the treatment of skin disorders. He deals with the physics of their generation, and also with their biostimulative, and other biological effects. The various types of laser beams and the particular use of each of these different radiations for the treatment of particular skin disorders are dealt with in some detail. The value of the new "tuneable" laser is also mentioned.

It is hoped that this volume will be of use and interest to dermatologists and scientists involved in the photobiology of the skin both from experimental and clinical aspects. The section on laser radiation should be of interest to all dermatologists, and it also gives valuable background information for those who themselves contemplate using this new form of therapy for the treatment of skin lesions.

A. JARRETT   *February 1984*

Acknowledgements

Thanks are due to Dr A. Jarrett and Dr W. Frain-Bell for their continued encouragement during the writing of this manuscript. In particular, I should like to acknowledge the major intellectual influences in the field over the last 25 years, I. A. Magnus, Farrington Daniels, Jr, and J. C. van der Leun.

B. E. JOHNSON   *February 1984*

Contents

81 Abnormal Reactions Associated with Skin Disorders
B. E. JOHNSON

82 Light Sensitivity Associated with Drugs and Chemicals
B. E. JOHNSON

83 Phototherapy
B. E. JOHNSON

84 Photochemotherapy and its Complications
B. E. JOHNSON

85 Lasers and the Skin
J. A. COTTERILL

Contents of Volume 1
The Epidermis

Contents of Volume 2
The Nerves and Blood Vessels

Contents of Volume 3
The Dermis and the Dendrocytes

Contents of Volume 4
The Hair Follicle

Contents of Volume 5

The Sweat Glands
Skin Permeation
Lymphatics
The Nails

Contents of Volume 6
The Mucus Membranes
The Action of Vitamin A on the Skin and Mucus Membranes
Transepidermal Water Loss

Contents of Volume 7

Hormonal Control of Pigmentation
The Biology of Malignant Melanoma
The Pharmacology of Histamine
The Subcutaneous Tissue

Natural and Artificial Radiation of the Skin

79

B. E. JOHNSON

Department of Dermatology, University of Dundee, Ninewells Hospital, Dundee, Scotland

I. INTRODUCTION

Photobiology is defined as the study of the action of light on living things. As such it involves disciplines as diverse as those of atomic physics and anthropology.[1,2,3,4] Strictly speaking "light" indicates radiation that can be seen by the human eye and therefore should be correctly restricted to wavelengths from within the range of approximately 380–700 nm (Fig. 1). However, common usage allows for inclusion of the UV wavelengths (290–380 nm) whose biological action is of such fundamental importance. Visible radiation which is the major component of sunlight, is absorbed by specialized molecular structures which are involved in vision

1. McElroy, W. D. and Glass, B. (1961). Eds. 'Light and Life'. The John Hopkins Press, Baltimore, Maryland.
2. Seliger, H. H. and McElroy, W. D. (1965). 'Light: Physical and Biological Action'. Academic Press, London, Orlando and New York.
3. Giese, A. C. (1976). 'Living with our Sun's Ultraviolet Rays'. Plenum Press, New York and London.
4. Smith, K. C. (1977). Editor, 'The Science of Photobiology'. Plenum Press, New York and London.

PHYSIOL. PATHOPHYSIOL. OF SKIN Vol. 8
ISBN 0 12 380608 9

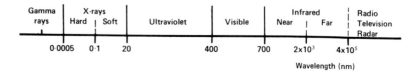

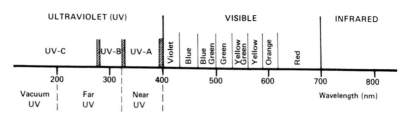

Fig. 1. Top: The major regions of the electromagnetic spectrum. Bottom: The ultraviolet, visible, and near infrared regions of the spectrum relevant to photodermatology.

and photosynthesis. The biomolecular building blocks of the earliest forms of life were derived in part from high energy UVR induced photochemical reactions involving certain simple elements. In the basic photobiological reaction of photosynthesis, the chlorophyl-dependent utilization of visible solar energy leads both to a supply of energy for animal life as well as to the creation of the oxygen atmosphere. Oxygen is essential for the aerobic respiration of the various forms of higher life as well as for the development of the ozone layer in the upper atmosphere which acts as a shield against the otherwise lethal effects of the shorter wavelength UVR produced by the sun. This ozone layer provides a cut-off at around 290 nm which then becomes the short wavelength limit of terrestrial solar radiation. As a result investigative studies making use of wavelengths below 290 nm will require artificial sources for the provision of such radiation. Also, most wavelengths below 200 nm are strongly absorbed by air and their effects therefore can only be studied *in vacuo*. The effects of infra-red radiation appear to be those of local heat production and although properly falling within the terms of our definition, consideration of this form of radiation will be confined to those situations where it can be shown to modify the effect of other parts of the solar spectrum. Similarly, consideration of other forms of non-ionizing radiation such as microwaves and ultrasonic radiation will be omitted since different mechanisms appear to be involved here which are outside the scope of the present text. Also, radiation at the extreme short wavelength end of the spectrum such as the effects of ionizing beta, gamma and X-rays are properly left to the field of radiobiology. Therefore for the purpose of this text photobiology will be defined as the study of the interaction between biological material and radiation from within the electromagnetic spectrum between approximately 200 and 700 nm.

Photobiology of the skin[1,2,3,4,5] is the study of the normal and abnormal reactions of human skin to "sunlight" (terrestrial solar radiation) which varies both quantitatively and qualitatively with geographical location as well as with time of day and year. A brief discussion of these variations and their relevance to the various skin reactions is dealt with later (see pages 2379–2384).

Although the majority of the reactions of the skin result from exposure to solar radiation, exposure to environmental artificial sources of radiation (see page 2385) may play a part particularly when the reaction is abnormal.

The reaction of the skin to either solar or artificial sources of radiation can be classified as normal as seen in the acute response of sunburn and in the age changes following prolonged exposure. The abnormal reactions, often called "the photodermatoses", can be subdivided into those which are idiopathic such as polymorphic light eruption, and solar urticaria; those in which a non-light sensitive dermatosis such as psoriasis is adversely affected by light; those in which a photoactive substance (chemical photosensitivity) is present which may be either a metabolic product (porphyria), a parenterally administered therapeutic drug, or a substance absorbed into the skin following direct external contact. Reactions produced by such photosensitizers may result from direct damage to various cellular components in which case the term "phototoxicity" is used, or an immunological mechanism may be inferred, and the reactions are then classed as "photoallergy". Lastly, those where there is some disturbance of the skin's ability to protect against the damage resulting from exposure to UVR. On the one hand

1. Kimmig, J. and Wiskemann, A. (1959). Lichtbiologie und Lichttherapie. *In* 'Handbuch der Haut and Geschlechtskrankheiten. Erganzungswerk'. (Eds, Marchionini, A. and Schirren, C. G.) **II**, 1021. Springer, Berlin.
2. Urbach, F. (1969). Ed. 'The Biologic Effects of Ultraviolet Radiation (with emphasis on the skin)'. Pergamon Press, Oxford.
3. Fitzpatrick, T. B. (1974). Ed. 'Sunlight and Man. Normal and Abnormal Photobiologic Responses'. University of Tokyo Press, Tokyo.
4. Magnus, I. A. (1976). 'Dermatological Photobiology. Clinical and Experimental Aspects'. Blackwell Scientific Publications, Oxford.
5. Parrish, J. A., White, H. A. D. and Pathak, M. A. (1979). Photomedicine. *In* 'Dermatology in General Medicine'. (Eds, Fitzpatrick, T. B., Eisen, A. Z., Wolff, K., Freedberg, I. M. and Austen, K. F.), pp. 942–994. McGraw-Hill Book Company, New York.

this may be impairment of melanin pigmentation as in vitiligo, or on the other an enzyme defect such as is present in xeroderma pigmentosum, as a result of which damaged cellular DNA is inadequately repaired leading to premature malignant changes in the skin. In addition, there are a number of genetic abnormalities such as Bloom's syndrome, in which changes in the skin follow exposure to light are a feature of a multi-system disease.

Certain terminology is used for preference, either because it has a great familiarity or because of international convention. Units of wavelength are used for UV and visible radiation since it is simpler to think in terms of direct linear measure. The units conventionally accepted are nanometers (nm); $1\,\mathrm{nm} = 10^{-9}$ metres. These wavelength units had previously been called millimicrons (mμ), and ångströms, equivalent to $0\cdot 1$ nm, have also been used in the past.

The UVR spectrum has been subdivided in a number of different ways. In one, wavelengths from 200–290 nm are known as "far UV". The long wavelength limit is set at 290 nm because this is the shortest wavelength commonly detected at the earth's surface while wavelengths shorter than 200 nm, known as the "vacuum UV", are absorbed by air. The "near UV" extends from 290 nm to the visible around 390–400 nm. In skin photobiology, however, it now appears usual to speak of UV-B, 280–320 nm; UV-A, 320–400 nm; and UV-C, 200–280 nm. The latter divisions are based on those defined in 1932 by the use of selected filters for the standardization of UVR sources used in medicine.[1] At that time wavelengths shorter than 280 nm were designated as UV-C, the approximate spectral band between 280 and 315 nm as UV-B, and between 315 and 400 nm as UV-A. Slight changes in the boundaries between the spectral regions classified in this way have occurred from time to time and different texts present the spectral bands with slightly different wavelength limitations. However, since there is no sharp cut-off of the radiation by the filters used, or any biological effect of this radiation at the designated boundaries, these minimal variations in the definition of UV-C, UV-B and UV-A are of little importance. The classification remains useful however for dividing the UV spectrum into broad bands of particular interest. UV-A is present in terrestrial solar radiation, but it is considered to be relatively harmless to biological systems for all practical purposes. UV-B is the biologically damaging UVR component of sunlight and UV-C, although not present in sunlight, is produced by artificial sources and has a high potential for damage to biological material.

1. Coblentz, W. W. (1932). The Copenhagen meeting of the Second International Congress on Light. *Science* **76**, 412.

For such a heterogeneous target tissue as skin, the use of radiological terminology for photobiological reactions complicates matters. Thus, the term "fluence" used to describe radiation energy entering a small area is sometimes used in photobiological literature to indicate the radiation dose at the surface of the irradiated material. Where this irradiated material is skin the term "exposure dose" is better. International convention (SI units) does not recognize the centimetre although this unit remains in use in dermatological photobiology, where the exposure dose is expressed as millijoules cm^{-2} (mJ/cm^2) or Joules cm^{-2} (J/cm^2), although in general photobiology J/m^2 is preferred. However, the inter-conversion of these various units is not difficult. The "exposure dose" is calculated by multiplying the amount of radiation reaching the skin by the time in seconds of the duration of the irradiation. The exposure dose rate, known as the irradiance, is measured by calibrated thermopiles or photocells, or by chemical actinometry. The units or irradiance meas-ured at the irradiated surface are given as watts or milliwatts per cm^2. The expression of the exposure dose as J/cm^2 or mJ/cm^2 is simply derived from the fact that 1 watt equals 1 joule per second. The erg, equal to 10^{-7} joules is no longer in general use but features in much of the earlier literature. The output from any irradiation system may vary from instant to instant so that it is essential that the exposure dose should be expressed in these calculated energy terms, rather than as exposure times. For a more detailed discussion of terminology and the units involved, the reader is recommended to consult "Dermatological Photobiology" by Magnus[1] and Parrish et al.[2]

II. THE SUN AND ITS RADIATION[3, 4]

The sun is a middle order, yellow star of spectral class G. In the dense gaseous mass of its centre, thermonuclear reactions result in the transformation of hydrogen to helium with the concomitant release of high energy gamma radiation. It is the interaction of this gamma radiation with the various gaseous constituents of the more peripheral

1. Magnus, I. A. (1976). 'Dermatological Photobiology, Clinical and Experimental Aspects'. Blackwell Scientific Publications, Oxford.
2. Parrish, J. A., Anderson, R. R., Urbach, F. and Pitts, D. (1978). 'UV-A Biological Effects of Ultraviolet Radiation with Emphasis on Human Responses to Longwave Ultraviolet'. John Wiley and Sons, New York.
3. Sanderson, J. A. and Hulbert, E. O. (1955). Sunlight as a source of radiation. In 'Radiation Biology', Vol. II. (Ed., Hollaender, A.), p. 95. McGraw-Hill, New York.
4. Henderson, S. T. (1970). 'Daylight and Its Spectrum'. Hilger, London.

regions of the sun which gives rise to the mainly visible radiation emission characteristic of the G class stars.

Measurement outside the earth's atmosphere, some 150 million kilometres (93 million miles) from the surface of the sun, have provided what is known as the extraterrestrial spectrum (Fig. 2). It is, for the most part, a continuum with a peak around 500 nm and shows a marked decrease in intensity with decreasing wavelength down to about 160 nm in the far UV. At this point emission lines, particularly characteristic of hydrogen and helium at 121·6 nm, 58·4 nm, and 30·4 nm are super-imposed on the continuum and a band of X-radiation, with a maximum intensity between 1 and 10 nm, extends beyond the UV. The details of this short wavelength high energy radiation are of indirect importance in the context of skin photobiology, since although radiation from the sun of wavelengths below 200 nm amounts to less than 0·05% of the total, life as we know it would not be tenable in its presence. The earth's atmosphere must therefore act as a radiation shield and indeed measurements of terrestrial sunlight even with the most advantageous conditions of latitude and altitude have failed to detect wavelengths below 286 nm.

Between approximately 85 and 250 km above the earth's surface, oxygen and nitrogen absorb X-rays and short wavelength UV radiation,

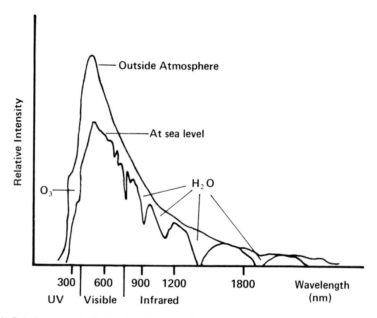

Fig. 2. Relative spectral distribution of solar radiation outside the atmosphere and at sea level, illustrating the effects of absorption by water and ozone.

oxygen absorbing up to approximately 243 nm with a peak at about 150 nm. In this way, an initial cut-off is established. However, molecular dissociation of the oxygen occurs, some of the so-formed atoms diffusing to lower levels of the atmosphere where they may interact with other oxygen molecules to form ozone (i). Alternatively, excited state, molecular oxygen may itself react with ground state molecules, again forming ozone (ii).

$$\text{(i)} \quad O + O_2 + O_2 \rightarrow O_3 + O_2$$
$$\text{(ii)} \quad O_2 + O_2 \rightarrow O_3 + O$$

These reactions take place between 15 and 35 km above the earth's surface to form the so-called ozone layer.

The maximum concentration of ozone, found at 25 km, is some 10 parts per million. The total thickness of the ozone layer calculated at standard temperature and pressure is approximately 3 mm, a remarkably flimsy shield to exert so profound an effect in biological terms. This may vary with time of day, with weather conditions, particularly high level storms, and with both latitude and season. Ozone absorbs UV radiation between 200 and 350 nm with a peak at 255 nm; the absorption beyond 290 nm is weak, but a distinct second peak is present at 310 nm. It is this layer therefore which effectively blocks the high energy radiation between 240 and 286 nm, and reduces the levels of possibly damaging short wavelengths up to above 300 nm. In the process of absorbing short wavelength UVR, ozone is itself decomposed. Moreover, the nitrogen cycle of biological activity on Earth results in diffusion of nitrogen oxides into the stratosphere where ozone levels are further reduced by reactions with nitric oxide. The ozone layer is therefore in a state of dynamic equilibrium which is maintained in the face of various natural forces such as sun spot cycle effects, and high level atmospheric storms. In recent years it has become evident that the by-products of the industrialized world may also pose a threat to this equilibrium. Intensified agriculture with increasing use of nitrate fertilizers has added to the nitrogen oxide load of the atmosphere. The exhaust emission from supersonic aircraft may also have a similar effect. Chlorine, photochemically released from the chlorofluoromethane (freon) aerosol propellant, after it had diffused into the stratosphere, would also lead to decomposition of ozone, pushing the equilibrium to a lower ozone level. A minor effect of decreased ozone in the stratosphere would be an increase in human skin cancer incidence, but were a significant decrease in the equilibrium level of ozone to occur, it could lead to great changes in the ecology of food chain systems which would be serious, if not catastrophic, for man. Ozone also absorbs minimally in the infra-red but the major modification of the solar spectrum in this region is due to water vapour in the lower atmosphere. Some slight effect is also exerted by atmospheric carbon dioxide, but as the infra-red has little relevance to skin photobiology, a more detailed discussion here would be inappropriate.

Of the solar radiation incident upon the surface of the earth's atmosphere, some 15–30% may be directly absorbed. Further attenuation occurs through reflection from the outer surface of clouds and by scattering. Gaseous atoms and molecules throughout the atmosphere cause a Rayleigh type scattering in which the degree of scatter is inversely proportional to the fourth power of the wavelength. This relationship depends on the particle size being of much smaller dimension than that of the incident radiation and results in much greater scattering at the blue end of the visible spectrum, and of the UVR. Aerosol scattering, due to larger particles found in the first 5 km above the earth's surface and giving rise to haze conditions, is not wavelength dependent but constitutes a minor overall contribution to the total attenuation, except where it is in the form of industrial smog, in which case it causes an additional 20% decrease in transmittance throughout the UVR range.

The effects of cloud cover have been evaluated in terms of varying degrees of different heights of cloud and total hemisphere covered, there being little apparent effect with light cloud. However, it is evident that although such conditions may even tend to increase the relative UVR content of the spectrum by scattering, particularly at high altitudes, closed layers of thick clouds cause a much reduced intensity of all regions in the spectrum.

It is obvious that in terms of skin photobiology, the major attenuation of radiation in the atmosphere occurs with the UVR and the shorter the wavelength the greater the attenuation. This is so when the incident radiation is thought of as being at right angles to the earth's surface, i.e. when the sun is directly overhead at a zenith angle of $0°$. Because of the scatter functions of the atmosphere, even under these circumstances, the UVR reaching the earth's surface is made up of two components, direct solar and scattered sky UVR. As the zenith angle increases, either with time of day from midday or with latitude, so that pathlength through the atmosphere increases (Fig. 3). Attenuation due to both absorption by ozone and the scattering functions is therefore also increased. However, a relationship between zenith angle and attenuation is very complex as illustrated by the fact that a change from $0°$ to $60°$ increases the pathlength by a factor of 2 but decreases the intensity of 300 nm radiation by a factor of 10. Shorter wavelengths are decreased by a greater factor, while little effect is evident at the red end of the visible spectrum.

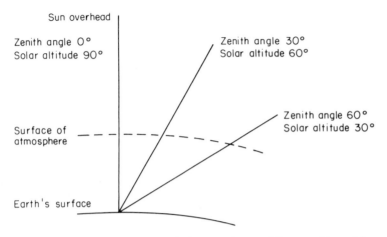

Fig. 3. The pathway of sunlight through the atmosphere at different positions of the sun.

Calculated values of direct and sky scatter UVR indicate that the decrease is principally in the direct component of UV-B. Although a similar relative decrease exists with longer wavelengths, the overall decrease is less and therefore, with UV-A and visible radiation, at any zenith angle, the relative contribution of direct radiation is greater. A zenith angle of 60° is approximately that found in equatorial latitudes in the early morning and in the evening. In latitudes of the UK and northern Europe, it may be found at midday in spring and autumn, but the relationship is complicated by seasonal changes in ozone concentration, the latter being maximal in spring and minimal in autumn in these latitudes.

Tables of daily UVR values at sea level for clear sky conditions at monthly intervals and for 1 nm wavelength bands at 5 nm intervals from 285 nm to 340 nm and at 5° intervals of latitude from 0° to 65° have been computed from data such as solar irradiance, zenith angle, atmospheric ozone content with the inclusion of an average correction for cloudiness.[1] The values obtained have been shown to be useful in estimating exposures required for normal human erythema production, and may also be used for other biologic effects.[2,3] Moreover, it is obvious

1. Green, A. E. S., Samada, T. and Shettle, E. P. (1974). The middle ultraviolet reaching the ground. *Photochem. Photobiol.* **19**, 251.
2. Green, A. E. S., Mo, T. and Miller, J. H. (1974). A study of solar erythema radiation doses. *Photochem. Photobiol.* **20**, 473.
3. Mo, T. and Green, A. E. S. (1974). A climatology of solar erythema dose. *Photochem. Photobiol.* **20**, 483.

tables could be extended to include data for longer wavelength radiation. In general, measurements of solar radiation at the earth's surface have used complex apparatus and yielded masses of data for individual sites.[1, 2] With the increased interest in UVR carcinogenesis, simple compact recording instruments have been set up at numerous locations which have provided comparative data on UV-B levels over a number of years. The sensitivity of these instruments is weighted with respect to the longer wavelengths of the UV-B; nevertheless a calibration in sunburn units has appeared satisfactory.[3, 4, 5]

An even simpler device, a polysulphone-film, badge detector, has also been used to measure UV-B radiation. This device has proved particularly useful in that it has also provided data on topographical, anatomical and habitual variations to UV-B exposure in individuals.[6, 7, 8] The long wavelength weighting with this detector is slightly greater than that for the sunburn meter, but if this is taken into account, the simplicity and versatility of this method has much to recommend it.

It is apparent that a great deal is known concerning the radiation environment of the Earth, but detailed studies of the variations, particularly of the highly biologically active UV-B region, are still required. It is this region of the spectrum which is subject to the greatest variations due to season, latitude, altitude, time of day, and atmospheric pollution. Moreover, changes in the constituents of the slowly circulating stratosphere, particularly the ozone layer, would appear to give rise to disproportionate changes in this range, with their consequent disquieting biological consequences.

1. Henderson, S. T. (1970). 'Daylight and its spectrum'. Hilger, London.
2. Bener, P. (1964). Tages- und Jahresang der spektralen Intensitut der ultravioletten Global und Himmelsstrahlung bei wolkenfreiem Himmin in Davos (1590m/m). *Strahlentherapie* **123**, 306.
3. Robertson, D. F. (1969). Long-term field measurements of erythemally effective natural ultraviolet radiation. *In* 'The biologic effects of ultraviolet radiation'. (Ed., Urbach, F.), p. 433. Pergamon Press, Oxford.
4. Berger, D. S. (1976). The sunburning ultraviolet meter; design performance. *Photochem. Photobiol.* **24**, 587.
5. Frain-Bell, W. (1979). What is that thing called light? Dowling Oration 1978. *Clin. exp. Dermatol.* **4**, 1.
6. Davis, A., Deane, G. M. W., Gordon, D., Howell, G. V. and Ledbury, K. J. (1976). A worldwide program for the continuous monitoring of solar UV radiation using Poly (phenylene oxide) film and a consideration of results. *J. appl. Poly. Sci.* **20**, 1165.
7. Diffey, B. L., Tata, T. J. and Davis, A. (1979). Solar dosimetry of the face: the relationship of natural ultraviolet radiation exposure to basal cell carcinoma. *Physics Med. Biol.* **24**, 931.
8. Challoner, A. V. J., Corless, D., Davies, D., Deane, G. M. W., Diffey, G. L., Gupta, S. P. and Magnus, J. A. (1976). Personal monitoring of exposure to ultraviolet radiation. *Clin. Exp. Dermatol.* **1**, 175.

III. THE ARTIFICIAL RADIATION ENVIRONMENT[1, 2]

The natural radiation environment is predominantly visible radiation, but it includes ultraviolet radiation and both vary with latitude, time of day, time of year, altitude and weather conditions. The artificial radiation environment began with the introduction of window glass which acts as a cut-off filter at about 320 nm, and thereby significantly reduces the damaging effects of sunlight.

Electric lighting, either in the domestic or working environment, is the major component of artificially produced radiation. Tungsten has the highest melting point (3370°C) of commonly available metals, and when heated sufficiently emits a continuum of visible radiation. When tungsten filaments are heated by the passage of an electric current, the incandescent light emission is relatively homogeneous although there is a bias towards the red end of the spectrum. Enclosed in a quartz envelope and operating very near the melting point temperature, just below 3100°C, as in a 1500 watt projection lamp, some 0·2% of the output is in the UV. However, this is a very inefficient source for this region of the spectrum as the operating lifetime of the lamp is very short. The normal domestic tungsten light bulbs consist of glass envelopes which are opaque to UVR below 320 nm, and operate at relatively low wattage so that the UVR content of the emission is low. The inclusion of halides within the bulb does not change the wavelength characteristics of the tungsten emission but it does extend the effective lifetime of the lamp by preventing both the loss of tungsten from the surface of the filament and the deposition of metal film on the glass envelope.

Fluorescent tube lighting is based upon the simple low pressure mercury arc lamp. When an electric current is passed through mercury vapour at low pressure, the excitation energy is released mainly in the 254 nm resonance line. Although emission at 185 nm may be 10% of the total production within the lamp envelope, most low pressure mercury lamp envelopes are transparant to the 254 nm line, but opaque to 185 nm. Using a quartz envelope which is transparent to short wavelengths, low pressure mercury arcs are employed as germicidal lamps for sterilization plants and in tissue culture cabinets (Fig. 4). Thus, UV-C may in this context become a part of the human skin radiation environment. However, when the lamp envelope is constructed of glass and the interior is coated with a "phosphor" of appropriate fluorescent characteristics, the emitted UV-C, particularly the 254 nm line, is

1. Sumner, W. (1962). 'Ultraviolet and Infrared Engineering'. Pitman, London.
2. Koller, L. R. (1952). 'Ultraviolet radiation'. John Wiley and Sons, New York.

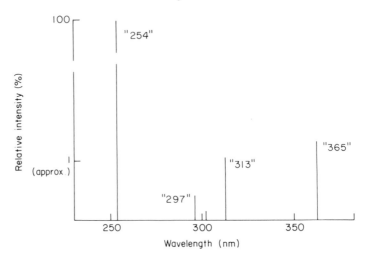

Fig. 4. The emission spectrum of a cold quartz, low pressure mercury arc. Almost all the output is in the 254 nm line. (N.B. the vertical scale is broken.)

absorbed in the phosphor and a visible spectrum is emitted from the lamp. The phosphors are commonly silicate, borate, or phosphate salts of alkaline earth metals such as barium. Slight variations in the composition allow variations in the colour content of the visible emission, giving rise to type descriptions such as "warm white", which has a high red component, and "northlight" in which the emission is spread more evenly over the spectrum, the blue component being increased at the expense of the red (Fig. 5). Even though the source is essentially a low pressure mercury arc, it should be emphasized here that the mercury lines more characteristic of medium or high pressure arcs, are present in the emission and that some UV-B, particularly in the 313 nm region, may be present.

Special function fluorescent tubes may be obtained in which the phosphors have been selected to produce one particular part of the spectrum. A red emitter is used in experimental horticulture and blue fluorescent tubes serve both as insect attractants, for hygiene purposes, and also in phototherapy for hyperbilirubinaemia.

When UV-B therapy is required "sunlamp" fluorescent tubes having an emission of approximately 280–340 nm, with a peak at around 310 nm, are used (Fig. 6), the phosphor usually being calcium zinc thallium phosphate. Sources of UV-A generally produce an emission approximately ranging from 310 to 390 nm, peaking at either 355 or

a.

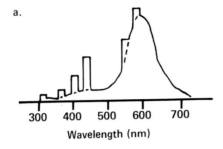

Wavelength (nm)

b.

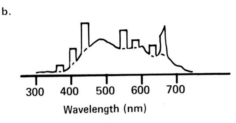

Wavelength (nm)

Fig. 5. The emission spectra of domestic fluorescent lighting. a. Warm white; relatively high red component. b. North light; more even distribution through the visible. (N.B. the minimal but significant emission in the UV-B.)

365 nm (Fig. 6). When these lamp envelopes contain nickel or cobalt, they are dark purple in colour and are known as "blacklights". They are commonly used in theatre and discotheque lighting since the emission produces striking fluorescent effects on human skin and fluorochromed clothing materials. The various sources of UV are used in therapeutic

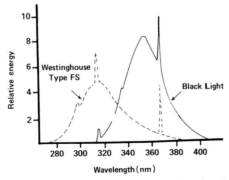

Fig. 6. The emission spectra of a typical UV-B (Westinghouse FS type) and a typical UV-A (Black light) fluorescent source.

procedures in which psoralens may also be employed as photosensitizing chemicals, particularly in the photochemotherapy of psoriasis. As with all forms of fluorescent tube lighting, the emission may be increased in intensity by the construction within the tube of a reflecting surface which coats one half. Since the output efficiency of fluorescent tubes decreases with increase in temperature, and since there is evidence that an internal reflector tends to increase this temperature effect more rapidly, it is not clear whether the increased directional output of these lamps is an advantage.

While "sunlamp" fluorescent tubes can be used, the more usual form of home sunlamp, either for therapy or for cosmetic "sun-tan" purposes, is a medium or high pressure mercury arc. When an electric current is passed through mercury vapour under pressure, the original resonance lines at 185 nm and 254 nm become quenched by secondary atomic collision and a complex of emission lines associated with the mercury molecule predominate.

With quartz or vitreous silica envelope, particularly strong emission lines at 297, 302, 313 and 365 nm make up the major UV emission so that UV-B effects may be easily elicited (Fig. 7). With higher pressures, a low intensity continuum of emission occurs upon which the major mercury lines are superimposed, thus effects of any part of the spectrum may be obtained. Although these lamps are not used for illumination, developments in lamp technology have resulted in the production of high

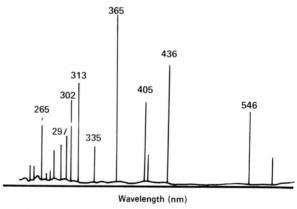

Fig. 7. The emission spectrum of a medium pressure mercury arc.

intensity, metal halide, mercury lamps having a wide spectrum for such uses as industrial photoprocessing.

When intense sources of visible radiation are required, such as in floodlighting or cinematograph projection, then Xenon discharge arc lamps are used. Since these lamps operate at high pressures and temperatures, normal glass is unsuitable as an envelope and quartz is used. The construction may be in tubular form, typically the 6 kW, water-cooled long arc lamp, or in compact bulb form, with a short arc path across large tungsten electrodes. The emission characteristics are the same for both and they give a continuum from about 200 nm through the UV, visible, and infra-red ranges. When UVR below 290 nm is cut off with an appropriate filter, the spectrum closely resembles that of terrestrial solar radiation in the UVR and visible ranges. The excess infra-red may also be excluded by suitable filtering and the resultant spectrum is as close as is presently possible to natural sunlight. In normal use, these lamps have accessory filtering to exclude the UVR below 320 nm. However, the low power lamps, 100 to 150 W, are used without filters in spectrophotometers where they provide a source of UVR essential for analytical procedures. Without adequate screening these lamps could represent a radiation hazard. Without adequate ventilation, the build-up of photochemically formed ozone could also be a health hazard.

Two further examples of artificial radiation environment should be mentioned. First, in electric arc welding, intense visible and UV radiation emission occurs and elaborate protection rules have been laid down in Safety at Work Codes of Practice. Secondly, laser beam technology has been developed for use, not only in endoscopic and microsurgery, but also for cytological analysis. Moreover, the use of low intensity devices has provided photodynamic therapy for relatively deep-seated tumours. Laser emission is not only of high intensity, it is also monochromatic, and tuned lasers are available which can provide high intensity UV-A. Future developments should also give rise to UV-B devices, thus allowing sunburn-type reactions to be elicited with exposures lasting only fractions of a second.[1]

---

1. Anderson, R. R. and Parrish, J. A. (1980). A survey of the acute effects of UV lasers on human and animal skin. *In* 'Lasers in Photomedicine and Photobiology'. (Eds, Pratesi, R. and Sacchi, C. A.), p. 109. Springer-Verlag, Berlin.

IV. ARTIFICIAL RADIATION IN THE STUDY OF
SKIN REACTIONS[1, 2, 3]

Where possible studies of skin reactions due to solar radiation should ideally be carried out with the sun as the radiation source. However, if carefully controlled studies are intended, then this practice is not always satisfactory since even in geographic locations where there is little cloud cover, the irradiance at the earth's surface is constantly changing. Thus, a number of artificial radiation sources have been utilized to provide the required radiation for controlled studies of skin reactions. Some have been constructed to simulate terrestrial solar radiation as closely as possible; others have been selected for their particular emission characteristics in a given part of the spectrum. In the first category, carbon arcs were originally used as they provided a continuum of emission in the ultraviolet. Although differing from sunlight in wavelength contribution, they did nevertheless approximate to the UV component of sunlight. By using various metal cores in the carbon rods, the nature of the spectrum could be adjusted. However, the use of such a lamp system was difficult and required continual monitoring of the electrode gap. Of the mercury arc lamps available, some use could be made of the medium pressure arc's considerable, albeit line spectrum, UV component. The high pressure mercury arcs, in which some continuum is emitted together with a superimposed spectrum, do provide a closer simulation to sunlight. However, it is with the xenon arcs that a real simulation of the solar spectrum is obtained.[4, 5] As with the other sources, there is a short wavelength UV component, below 290 nm, which must be filtered out to give a simulation of solar UV (Fig. 8). In addition, the infra-red is in excess of that in the solar spectrum at the earth's surface. The infra-red can be removed by the use of a cold mirror type of filter (Dichroic mirror) in which the UV component is reflected at right angles while the visible and infra-red are transmitted and lost to the main beam. A short

1. Harber, L. C., Bickers, D. R., Epstein, J. H., Pathak, M. A. and Urbach, F. (1974). Light sources used in photopatch testing. *In* 'Sunlight and Man'. (Ed., Fitzpatrick, T. B.), p. 559. University of Tokyo Press, Tokyo.
2. Magnus, I. A. (1976). 'Dermatological Photobiology, Clinical and Experimental Aspects'. Blackwell Scientific Publications, Oxford.
3. Diffy, B. L. (1982). 'Ultra-violet Radiation in Medicine. Medical Physics Handbook II'. Adams Hilger, Bristol, UK.
4. Wiskemann, A. and Wulf, K. (1959). Untersuchungen uber den auslosenden Spektralbereich und die direkte Lichtpigmentierung bis chronischen und akuten Lichtausschlagen. *Arch. klin. exp. Derm.* **209**, 443.
5. Berger, D. S. (1969). Specification and design of solar ultraviolet simulators. *J. Invest. Derm.* **53**, 192.

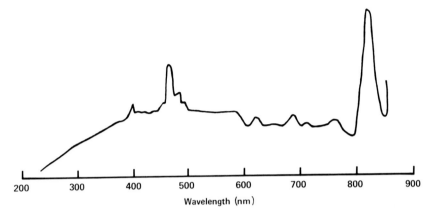

Fig. 8. The emission spectrum of a high pressure Xenon arc lamp. There is a continuum of infrared emission some way beyond 900 nm.

wavelength cut-off filter then removes the unwanted UV-C. This kind of instrument produces an emission which closely resembles the ultraviolet component of terrestrial solar radiation. However, the dichroic mirror does not reflect the visible radiation and thus the simulation of sunlight is deficient. A closer simulation may be obtained by using a single heat filter, designed specifically to cut off most of the infra-red.

To investigate the contributions of various wavelength regions to any particular response induced by the simulated solar radiation, additional optical filters can be employed. These may be either cut-off filters, the shorter wavelengths of radiation being removed from the spectrum, waveband by waveband, until no reaction is obtained.[1,2] Alternatively with a sufficiently high intensity solar simulator interference filters may be used to isolate a particular waveband. A more sophisticated examination of wavelength dependence for the various skin reactions may be undertaken by using an irradiation monochromator. Here again, the best source is a xenon arc, the emission being focussed through a dispersion instrument such as a quartz prism or grating monochromator, which allows the linear dispersion of the spectrum. This can then be sampled in sections of the spectrum either by moving a slit along the plane of spectrum or moving the spectrum past a fixed slit. By adjusting the optics of the instrument, the width of the waveband related to its central

1. Pluis, A. H. G. (1969). Observations with a 6000 watt xenon-arc lamp for diagnostic purposes in light dermatoses. *Dermatologica* **138**, 328.
2. Turnbull, B. C., Frain-Bell, W. and Mackenzie, L. A. (1967). The development of xenon arc lamp equipment for the assessment of photosensitivity. *Br. J. Derm.* **79**, 32.

wavelength may be varied. When a reactive skin is being examined, a waveband of only 1 or 2 nm can thus be obtained and the responsible wavelengths exactly defined.[1, 2, 3, 4, 5, 6] In this context, however, it should be remembered that scattering of radiation within these instruments themselves may produce contamination of the selected waveband. This problem may be lessened by using as narrow a waveband as possible and maintaining absolute cleanliness of the optics. Obviously, if an active short wavelength radiation contaminates a genuine non-active radiation band, a false positive will be obtained. This same problem can also be brought about by secondary harmonic diffraction. Filters can be used to cut-off this short wavelength contamination.

When individual regions of the spectrum are required for the study, the low pressure mercury arc is particularly useful. On its own, it provides an almost monochromatic source of highly active 254 nm radiation. Other spectral regions may be obtained with the incorporation of different phosphors into the lining of the lamp envelopes. Where sunburn reactions or other skin responses to UV-B wavelengths are the subject of study, the special sunlamps with emission from 280–340 nm may be used. "Black light" or simpler long-wave UV lamps are available with emission from 315–400 nm for the study of UV-A effects, especially the photosensitized skin reactions. With different phosphors, different regions of the visible spectrum may also be provided. Although the chemical composition of the phosphor determines the major emission characteristics of these fluorescent sources, the major mercury lines may still be present and some UV-B may be detected, even in the visible radiation sources. To ensure that this UV-B does not produce a false positive reaction in studies with UV-A or visible sources, filters should be used and for this purpose, window glass is usually adequate as for practical purposes it removes all radiation below 320 nm.

1. Magnus, I. A., Porter, A. D., McRee, K. G., Moreland, J. D. and Wright, W. D. A. (1959). A monochromator. An apparatus for the investigation of the response of the skin to ultraviolet, visible and infrared radiation. *Br. J. Derm.* **71**, 261.
2. Sayre, R. M., Straka, E., Anglin, J., Jr and Everett, M. A. (1965). A high intensity ultraviolet light monochromator. *J. invest. Derm.* **45**, 190.
3. Knox, J. M., Warshawsky, J., Lichodziejewski, W. and Freeman, R. G. (1967). *Archs Derm.* **95**, 319.
4. Berger, D., Magnus, I. A., Rottier, P. B., Sayre, R. M. and Freeman, R. G. (1969). Design and construction of high-intensity monochromators. *In* 'The Biologic Effects of Ultraviolet Radiation'. (Ed., Urbach, F.), p. 125. Pergamon Press, Oxford.
5. Cripps, D. J. and Ramsay, C. A. (1970). Ultraviolet action spectrum with a prism-grating monochromator. *Br. J. Derm.* **82**, 584.
6. Mackenzie, L. A. and Frain-Bell, W. (1973). The construction and development of a grating monochromator and its application to the study of the reaction of the skin to light. *Br. J. Derm.* **89**, 251.

V. BASIC PHOTOCHEMICAL ASPECTS OF SKIN PHOTOBIOLOGY

For radiation to have a biological effect it must be absorbed. This statement of the apparently obvious is at times overlooked when wavelengths which are totally reflected from, or totally transmitted through, a system are investigated for their role in photobiological reactions due to broad band radiation. The principle is fundamental to photochemistry and is known as the Grotthus–Draper Law (sometimes known as the First Law of Photochemistry) which states that only absorbed radiation can produce chemical change. This is not to say that chemical change inevitably follows the absorption of radiation, whether in a simple chemical solution or in a complex biochemical system such as skin. The absorbed energy may simply be dissipated harmlessly as heat, or it may be re-emitted as luminescence. This latter term includes the more familiar phenomena of fluorescence, both short lived and delayed, and the longer lifetime emission known as phosphorescence. When chemical change occurs it may take various forms. Turro and Lamola[1] classify photochemical reactions in two ways, first as overall photoreactions, and secondly the earlier events preceding them. The most common of the latter are called "inherently uni-molecular overall photoreactions" as illustrated in the following examples. A simple break in molecular bonding may occur as in the photolysis of hydrogen iodide, when molecular hydrogen and iodine are formed (Fig. 9). This type of

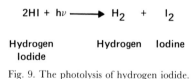

$$2HI + h\nu \longrightarrow H_2 + I_2$$

Hydrogen   Hydrogen   Iodine
Iodide

Fig. 9. The photolysis of hydrogen iodide.

reaction is classified as a "fragmentation", following what is termed a simple homolytic bond cleavage. It is not restricted to inorganic biatomic molecules and may take place in larger important biomolecules, as well as in complex chemicals such as phenothiazines and halogenated salicylanilides which lose halogen atoms on exposure to UVR. The bond cleavage proceeds through the formation of highly reactive intermediates.

Another example of bond disruption is the UV-induced breakage of disulphide bonds leading to the inactivation of certain enzymes, which

1. Turro, N. J. and Lamola, A. A. (1977). Photochemistry. In 'The Science of Photobiology'. (Ed., Smith, K. C.), p. 63. Plenum Press, New York.

B. E. JOHNSON

appears more closely related to the molecular bond rearrangement class of reaction than bond cleavage mentioned above. This is typified by the UV-induced opening of the second benzene ring in 7-dehydrochloesterol to produce pre-vitamin D_3 (Fig. 10). In skin this would appear to be a useful rather than a damaging effect of UVR.

A third class of reaction which is useful rather than destructive is the cis-trans isomerization in which the absorbed energy induces a change in

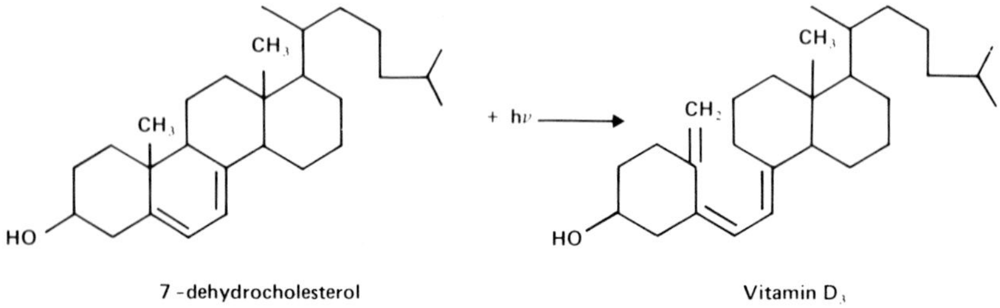

Fig. 10. The photosynthesis of pre-vitamin D from 7-dehydrocholesterol.

the spatial alignment of the molecule. It is illustrated by the change from a 11-cis to all-trans form of the retinal component of visual pigment. A similar reaction but involving a trans to cis photo-isomerization is encountered when the histidine derivative, urocanic acid, is exposed to UV-B (Fig. 11), and this may play a part in the skin's natural protection against solar UVR damage.

The bimolecular class of reactions is more complex, but may have greater relevance for photobiology. The participation of molecular oxygen is characteristic of these photosensitization reactions. However, the formation of radicals in the simple homolytic cleavage type of

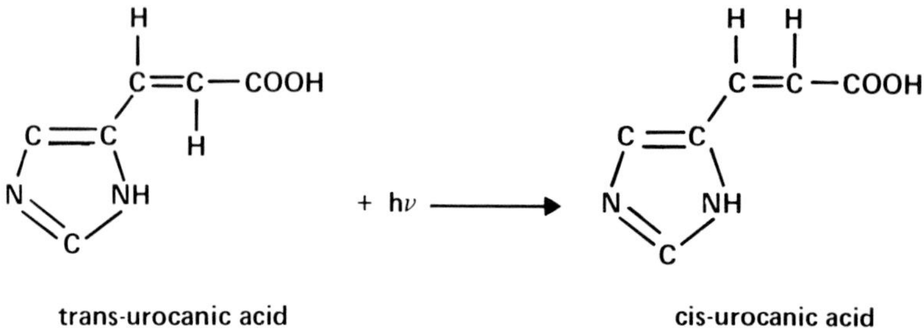

Fig. 11. Photo-isomerization of urocanic acid.

photoreaction may lead to oxidation reactions through the interaction of these radicals with molecular oxygen.[1] An example of this is given by the UV-induced lipid peroxides in unsaturated fatty acids and thereby in the complex lipoprotein of cellular membranes. Cyclic addition reactions such as the formation of cyclobutyl type dimers of pyrimidines like thymine (Fig. 12), and the covalent binding of psoralens with pyrimidines, are of the same class. So also are linear addition reactions, illustrated by the UV-induced binding of cysteine to uracil, and by the binding of cysteine to thymine. These reactions are thought to occur in protein–DNA binding. Just as in the unimolecular reactions, the primary step may involve the formation of excited intermediates which may then proceed by such pathways as hydrogen abstraction or electron transfer. Specific photo-oxidation, by a sensitizer, is included in the bimolecular class of reactions: the protoporphyrin photosensitization of cholesterol being cited as a typical example (Fig. 13).

For more details of these reactions the reader is referred to such modern photochemistry texts as W. M. Horspool's "Aspects of Organic Photochemistry" (1976), Turro's "Modern Molecular Photochemistry" (1977), Benjamin, San Francisco. The electron physics, quantum

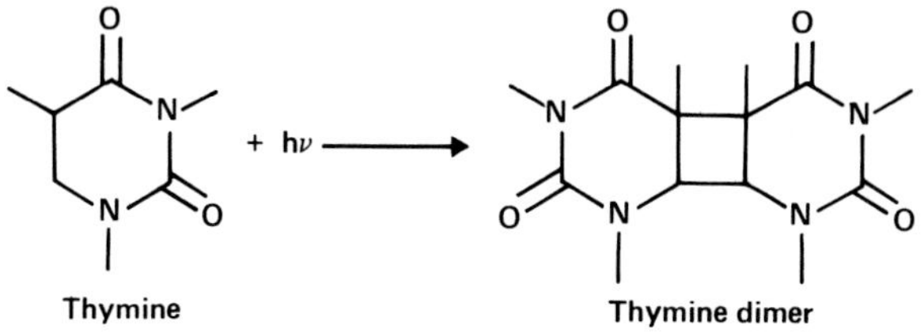

Fig. 12. UV-induced thymine dimer formation.

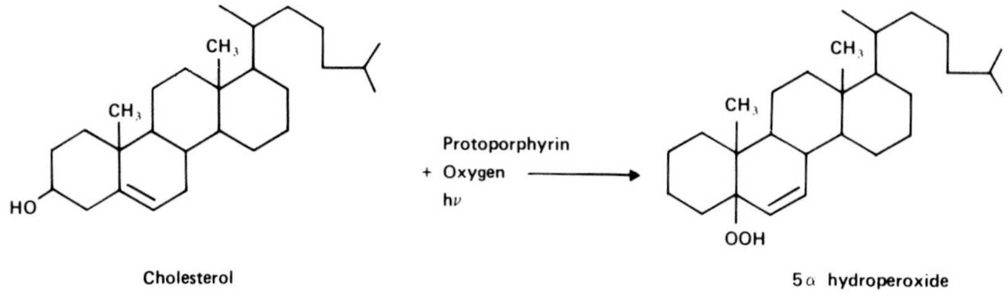

Fig. 13. Protoporphyrin photosensitized oxidation of cholesterol.

1. Slater, T. F. (1972). 'Free Radical Mechanisms in Tissue Injury'. Pion, London.

mechanics and molecular mechanisms involved in the interaction of non-ionizing radiation and matter are also dealt with in these texts. Also, Seliger and McElroy (1965) "Light: Physical and Biological Action", Academic Press, presents a useful introduction as does Lamola's chapter in "Sunlight and Man", ed. Fitzpatrick, T. B., Tokyo University Press (1974) pp. 17–567. A more simple and easily understood introduction to the complexities of the subject are to be found in Jagger's "Introduction to Research in Ultraviolet Photobiology" (1967), Prentice Hall; "Light and Living Matter" by Clayton (McGraw-Hill, 1970), and in "Dermatological Photobiology" by Magnus (Blackwell, 1976).

A. Atomic and Molecular Considerations

The initial step is to consider an atom in terms of the original Bohr model in which a central, positively charged nucleus is surrounded by negatively charged electrons. The electrons are distributed in successive shells, the orbits of which represent discrete energy values. In the majority of atoms, the normal condition is one in which the electrons occupy the lowest energy levels possible for the system and is known as the "ground state". If an external source of energy is applied, as for instance an electric discharge in a low pressure mercury arc, the electron distribution in the atom changes with a shift to the higher energy level orbits, and an excited state of the atom results. This excited state is inherently unstable with a half-life of about 10^{-9} s, the electrons returning to the ground state orbits and the excess energy being emitted as radiation. It is at this point that the essential particulate nature of radiation is emphasized and the concept of the quantum most appropriately introduced. The emitted radiation is in the form of quanta or particles of energy, the magnitude of which is directly related to the difference of energy levels between the excited and the ground states. The quantum energy is in turn related to the wavelength of the emitted radiation by the equation $e = hc/\lambda$ where h is Planck's constant $(6\cdot6 \times 10^{-27}$ erg/s), c is the speed of light in a vacuum $(3 \times 10^{-10}$ cm/s) and λ is the wavelength of the emitted radiation in cm. As frequency and wavelength are related by the speed of light, this equation is often expressed in the form $e = h\nu$, where ν is the frequency. It may be seen that on appropriate stimulation each atomic species with its unique electron content and distribution, will emit radiation in a specific wavelength pattern.

The absorption of radiation depends in the same way on the energy level differences available within the irradiated atom. Only that wavelength of radiation whose quantum energy matches the available energy level difference of the electron orbits will be absorbed. Each atomic species, having different and specific electron distributions, will therefore have different absorption characteristics. This is the basis of the wavelength dependency for both absorption spectroscopy by which a chemical may be identified, and action spectroscopy by which the wavelengths involved in photochemical or photobiological reactions may be defined. With atoms, the changes in electron distribution are relatively simple in that they are single step transitions between discrete energy levels. Each of these steps is therefore represented by the absorption of a single wavelength, and the whole spectrum is made up of a series of sharply defined lines representing the total absorbed wavelengths specific for the particular atom involved (Fig. 14).

Photobiology is concerned with molecular, rather than atomic, interactions with radiation. The basic principles already outlined apply, but as molecular structure is more complex than atomic structure, so the molecular interactions are more involved. The major difference is that whereas the atom has clearly defined ground and excited electronic

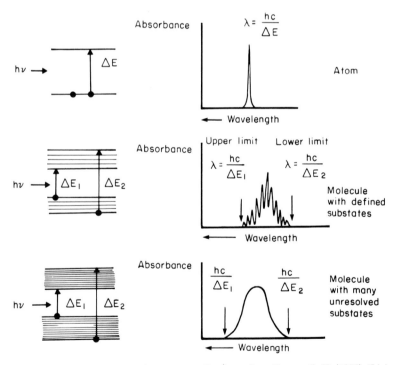

Fig. 14. The derivation of an absorption spectrum. Re-drawn from Clayton, R. K. (1970). 'Light and Living Matter, Vol. 1. The Physical Part'. McGraw-Hill Book Company.

states, molecules have a number of substates derived from the different modes of vibration and rotation of atomic nuclei and groups of nuclei in the molecule. The relation to each other and to the surrounding environment also complicates the situation. Therefore, the single step transition from ground to excited state characteristic of an atom is replaced in the molecule by a range of possible steps (see Fig. 14). The close spacing of the spectral lines resulting from these steps, plus the interactions between a molecule and its surroundings, leads to the formation of a broad absorption band (see Fig. 14). It is in this way that the absorption spectra are derived which enable simple molecules to be characterized. Complex biomolecules such as nucleic acids, proteins, and porphyrins, have sufficiently different molecular structure to produce different absorption spectra for each group of compounds. The wavelength dependency for a photochemical reaction, presented as an action spectrum, is essentially dependent on the absorption spectrum of the primary photochemical reactant or chromophore. The likelihood of a given compound being involved in a direct light induced reaction, or acting as a photosensitizer, may be partly deduced from the absorption spectrum of that compound.

The division of major electronic states of a molecule into substates also explains why the fluorescence of an irradiated substance is always of a longer wavelength than that of the exciting radiation. The electrons of a molecule in the ground state usually occupy the lowest available energy substate. On excitation, the most usual transition is to an intermediate level of the possible excited substates. The electron then undergoes a relaxation process to the lowest of the excited substates before returning to an intermediate level of the ground state. Finally, a second relaxation takes the electron back to the lowest level ground state and in both relaxation processes, energy is given up as heat. The quantum energy in the secondary radiation is therefore less than the energy absorbed from the exciting radiation. Since the quantum energy is inversely related to wavelength, the emitted radiation will be of longer wavelength than that absorbed. This process is known as Stokels shift (Fig. 15).

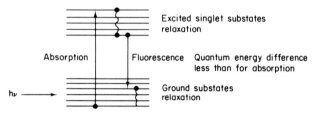

Fig. 15. Diagrammatic representation of the derivation of fluorescence.

In the ground state, each electronic orbit contains a pair of electrons, spinning on their axes in opposing directions to give a net electron spin of zero in what is called the "singlet state". With appropriate irradiation, one electron from a pair is raised to a higher energy orbital; the excited state. The spin direction is retained in this initial change and the irradiated molecule is then said to be in the "excited singlet state". However, it is possible for the spin direction to be reversed, the net electron spin then being equal to 1, and the resulting excited state is known as the triplet state (Fig. 16). The complex electron inter-relationships within a molecule are such that the energy level occupied in the triplet state is always lower than that of the excited singlet. However,

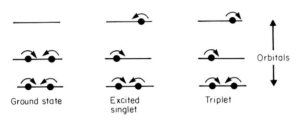

Fig. 16. Diagram of change in electron distribution and spin with transition from ground to excited singlet and triplet states.

the reversal of electron spin direction cannot be directly induced by absorbed energy, as the transition from the ground singlet to the excited triplet state does not occur. However, what is known as an intersystem cross transition in which an excited singlet transforms to a triplet state commonly occurs. While the excited singlet is short lived, existing for some 10^{-9} s, the triplet state is "metastable" having a lifetime of from 10^{-3} to, in rare cases, over 100 s. It is the transition of electrons from the triplet state directly back to the ground state that gives rise to the relatively long lifetime light emission known as phosphorescence. In certain instances, the absorbed energy is sufficient to remove an electron completely from an atom, rather than just raising it to a higher energy level. When this occurs, the unbalanced, and often highly reactive molecule which remains is in a free radical state.

Fluorescence or phosphorescence may be the only result of energy absorption by a chemical and the analysis of the light emission may be useful in identifying the chemical involved and may also give some information concerning the possible mechanisms for photochemical change. However, under suitable conditions photochemical reactions will occur (see Fig. 17), the absorbed energy leading to the rearrangement of the molecular structure, the dissociation of existing chemical bonds, or the formation of new ones, and the production of free radicals with subsequent chemical change (see page 2393).

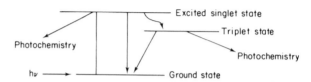

Fig. 17. Pathways for electron excitation and relaxation which give rise to photochemistry or fluorescence.

We have seen that the quantum energy of radiation may be related to its wavelength by the equation, $e = hc/\lambda$. The quantum energy of 300 nm radiation may therefore be determined as

$$e = \frac{(6 \cdot 6 \times 10^{-27}\ \text{erg/s})(3 \times 10^{10}\ \text{cm/s})}{3 \times 10^{-5}\ \text{cm}} = 6 \cdot 6 \times 10^{-12}\ \text{ergs}$$

Since 1 erg $= 10^{-7}$ J, the use of accepted units produces the minute value for 300 nm of approximately 7×10^{-19} J. This may be converted to molar terminology using Avogardro's number. Just as one mole of a chemical equals 6×10^{23} molecules, so one mole equivalent of radiation equals 6×10^{23} quanta, known as 1 einstein. For 300 nm radiation, therefore, 1 einstein may be equated to 4×10^5 J. This value may be related to electron bond energy values in terms of kilocalories per mole. From this kind of calculation, it is possible to obtain some idea of which chemical structures might be affected by different wavelengths of UV and visible radiation. Table I shows how wavelength, quantum energy and various chemical bonds are related.

In complex chemical compounds such as proteins, lipids and nucleic acids, as well as other biomolecules, the energy level changes required for absorption may be present within the molecule but there appears to be little absorption. It seems that the molecular organization is important in such absorption. Visible radiation, of relatively low quantum energy when compared with the UVR, produces photochemical change with great efficiency as illustrated by photosynthesis, visual stimulation of the retina and photographic effects. It is obvious that biological change can

Table 1

Relationships between wavelength, quantum energy of the radiation and chemical bond energy

Wavelength (nm)	Part of spectrum	Energy (kcal/mole)	Chemical bond type (bond energy)
200	UV-C	140	C=O (145)
250	UV-C	110	O—H (118)
			C=C (102)
300	UV-B	90	C—H (94)
350	UV-A	80	S—H (87)
400	Violet	70	C—O (69)
			S—S (63)
450	Blue	62	C—C (58)
500	Green	54	
550	Yellow	50	
600	Red	48	
650	Red		
1000	Infra-red	29	

The energy values are necessarily approximate but the relationship between the quantum energies of the different wavelength regions and the energy values associated with various common chemical bond types is clearly illustrated.

be brought about by relatively low energy radiation and that the significant biological effects of UV radiation are due to the nature of the biomolecules which absorb the UVR, rather than by the quantum energy of the radiation. None the less, at the other end of the wavelength scale, it is clear that the quantum energy of the infra-red wavelengths is only sufficient to change the vibration or rotation characteristics of a molecule rather than induce electron excitation. It is possible that infra-red radiation may influence a photochemical reaction but it does not, on its own, initiate such a reaction.

The Stark–Einstein law of equivalence states that the absorption of a single photon results in a photochemical change in one molecule only. This simple relationship gives rise to the concept of the quantum yield or efficiency of photochemical reactions. This is an important concept in photochemistry because it reveals the importance of the initial photochemical event in a general photochemical reaction. It may be set down as a ratio of the number of molecules changed per number of photons absorbed as follows:

$$\Phi = \frac{\text{number of molecules of photoproduct formed}}{\text{number of photons absorbed by the chemical}}$$

There are other ways of expressing this ratio, but as pointed out by Magnus,[1] its application to photodermatology is not practical since the chemical involved is not known in many cases. Neither is the photoproduct known, nor the quantity of radiation actually absorbed. However, it is possible to derive a useful ratio which Magnus calls the "Photobiological Efficiency". This is defined as:

$$\frac{\text{Degree of observed response}}{\text{Number of photons delivered at unit area of skin surface}} = \frac{R}{D}$$

This is a most useful concept because the dose D can be adjusted to give a standard response R, which may be minimal as in the determination of threshold doses in the case of minimal erythema dose. Alternatively D may be varied to obtain a dose response curve from the observed variations of the skin response R.

In a simple photochemical reaction, if the intensity of the irradiation is low, a long exposure time will be required. If the intensity is increased, the exposure time required to bring about the same degree of chemical change will be reduced. This inverse relationship between exposure time and irradiance is known as the Bunsen–Roscoe Law of Reciprocity. The demonstration of reciprocity in a photobiological reaction could give some indication of the relative importance of the initial photochemical reaction and the subsequent, secondary reactions. In ideal conditions, the demonstration of reciprocity is required for the definition of action spectra but this is not appropriate for the complex situation involved in skin reactions. None the less, with monochromatic radiation, reciprocity is seen to hold good over a wide range of UV-induced erythema[2] despite the fact that a biological system might change during prolonged exposure times. The maximum time for skin appears to be around $1\frac{1}{2}$–2 h but with polychromatic radiation such as sunlight, the relationship does not hold.

VI. BIOPHYSICS OF THE SKIN IN RELATION TO UV AND VISIBLE RADIATION

The understanding of the mechanisms involved in skin reactions in solar radiation would be easier if the precise anatomical site of the initial photochemical reaction (the target site) could be ascertained. Although

1. Magnus, I. A. (1976). 'Dermatological Photobiology', pp. 26–28. Blackwell Scientific Publications, Oxford.
2. Blum, H. F. and Terus, W. S. (1946). The erythemal threshold for sunburn. *Am. J. Physiol.* **146**, 97.

there is sometimes evidence for this being in the epidermis, in others only the dermis appears to be affected. A consideration of the optical properties of skin and its constituents helps to provide an insight into this problem. For instance, if it can be shown that radiation of a particular wavelength is totally reflected at the skin's surface, then it is obvious that this radiation can have no effect. Also, if the wavelength is completely transmitted through the epidermis, then it can have no effect on this tissue.

Scheuplein[1] and Tregear[2] have presented concise discussions of skin optics and the problems of measuring such physical functions as reflection, light scattering, and transmittance. Daniels[3] has summarized the available data with particular regard to its application relating to UV erythema and other solar skin reactions.

Just as solar radiation is attenuated by the atmosphere, so any incident radiation is reflected, scattered or absorbed by the skin. This heterogeneous medium has great optical complexity in purely physical terms, as illustrated by the examination of its various constituent parts, particularly the epidermis.

A. Effects of Keratin and Melanin on Incident Radiation

The thickness of the horny layer varies greatly over the surface of the body, and even though it is thought that keratin provides a good protection against solar radiation it is relatively thin over exposed areas such as the face. A single value for horny layer thickness is of little value and in any event it is not easily measured because of difficulties in its histological preparation. Also the degree of hydration of this keratinized tissue greatly alters its thickness, as keratin is a highly hygroscopic material (see p. 1511, Vol. 4).

The fixed and processed cells of the stratum corneum have cell membranes 12·5 nm thick when measured under the electron microscope. They contain keratin filaments 10 nm in diameter, embedded in an electron dense cement, which lie horizontally to the surface and show birefringence under the polarizing microscope. Electron microscopy demonstrates that intercellular spaces observed with the light microscope in fixed sections are, in fact, filled with a non-homogenous substance having moderate opacity and containing fine, opaque filaments and

1. Scheuplein, R. J. (1964). A survey of some fundamental aspects of the absorption and reflection of light by tissue. *J. Soc. cosmet. Chem.* **15**, 111.
2. Tregear, R. T. (1966). 'Physical Functions of Skin'. Academic Press, London, Orlando and New York.
3. Daniels, F., Jr. (1969). Optics of the skin as related to ultraviolet radiation. *In* 'The Biologic Effects of Ultraviolet Radiation'. (Ed., Urbach, F.), p. 151. Pergamon Press, Oxford.

granules of different shapes, sizes and ultrastructure. Whether the dense mat of birefringent fibres in the cells acts as some kind of specific optical barrier is not known, but it is probable that optically varying interfaces are present in high number in this superficial layer.

Current dermatological literature concerning racial pigmentation divides Man into four major groups. The first includes Europeans, Asians and certain North African types of varying degrees of pigmentation (Caucasoids). The second consists of African negroes (Negroid). Orientals, including American Indians, make up the third (Mongoloid), while the fourth is restricted to the aboriginal inhabitants of Australia (Australoids).

Melanin may be present in Caucasoid, even lightly pigmented horny layer. In negro epidermis, the melanin granules are larger, more numerous, and more densely clustered. Older descriptions of a decrease in melanin in the stratum corneum are partly artefacts based upon the spreading out of the cells as they become flattened; the polymer itself is not destroyed although its histological observation is clearly made only when it is in association with the protein matrix of the melanosome. This matrix is reduced by enzyme action in the viable epidermis. Thomson separated stratum corneum from white and negro subjects and demonstrated that negro stratum corneum is a better ultraviolet filter than white because of its melanin content, not because of any difference in thickness.[1] However, for a given measured thickness from similar anatomical locations, negroid horny layer contains more cell layers and the increased numbers of optical surfaces implied may give greater degrees of optical filtering.[2] The size of melanin granules and particles varies between 0·1 and 1·2 microns. Particles of this size may exert a Mie scattering effect on incident radiation in the wavelength range concerned. A high degree of forward scattering arises with this effect, and this is well illustrated by the appearance of granules as bright spots in dark field microscopic examination. Melanin therefore adds an unexpected further dimension to the problem of radiation attenuation in the stratum corneum.

The reflection and scattering components of attenuation are obviously complex. Especially for the ultraviolet radiation region of the spectrum, the wavelength specific absorption of the biochemical constituents of the skin add to the complexity of the radiation attenuation. The chemical constitution of the stratum corneum has not been fully analysed.

1. Thomson, M. L. (1955). Relative efficiency of pigment and horny layer thickness in protecting the skin of Europeans and Africans against solar ultraviolet radiation. *J. Physiol.* **127**, 236.
2. Wiegand, D. A., Haygood, C. and Gaylor, J. R. (1974). Cell layers and density of Negro and Caucasian Stratum corneum. *J. invest. Derm.* **62**, 563.

However, the proteinaceous keratin has specific absorption in the 280 nm wavelength region. Melanin absorbs in this wavelength, and certainly contributes to the attenuation in this filtering effect of the keratin.

In the living keratinocytes of the epidermis, the cells might be considered in terms of protein, ribonucleic and deoxyribonucleic acid, vertically orientated birefringent fibrils, melanin granules, and lipoprotein membraneous organelles such as mitochondria, as well as the nucleus. Melanosomes are also present, and they influence the incident radiation. They are present in their highest concentration in the basal layer. Hair, with or without pigment, is a highly efficient radiation filter acting by both absorption and scattering.

B. Reflectance

The presence of so many diverse optical interfaces within the superficial layers of the skin leads to considerable scattering of both UV and visible radiation which penetrates these layers. This scattering may lead to a pathway for the radiation which is longer than the thickness of the tissue itself. Moreover, some of the scattering leads to an actual reversal of the direction of the radiation, and this might be termed "reflection from depth" (Fig. 18). Although this leads to a complex reflectance pattern made up of surface, epidermal and dermal components, its measurement is one of the simplest that can be made on skin. Such measurements are made with a recording reflectance spectrophotometer having an

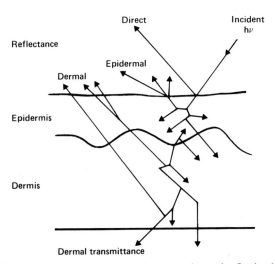

Fig. 18. Optical pathways of transmission, scattering and reflection in skin.

integrating sphere to ensure complete collection of the reflected radiation. The data so obtained are not only concerned with the absorbed radiation but may also indicate the molecular nature of the absorbing substances within the skin. Spectral reflectance curves have been obtained for the wavelength range from 250 nm through the visible spectrum.[1−8]

Most of the figures for reflectance measurements agree fairly well, except in one study which reports an approximately 20% reflection in the wavelength region 250–320 nm[2]. However, at least 20% of the radiation measured in this wavelength region is in fact fluorescence from excited skin components, and these could vary from site to site. Although there is some indication of specific absorption in the waveband, 250–290 nm, small variations in reflectance in this wavelength region are difficult to evaluate. In the sunburn region there is little or no difference between white and negro skin.

The effect of pigmentation is more clearly seen when the visible spectrum is considered. Lightly pigmented skin reflects some 30–40% of the total incident light while the value for a dark negroid skin is only about 16%. Analysis of the reflectance spectrum of fair skin shows a maximum at 700 nm with the curve falling towards the ultraviolet and interrupted by characteristic troughs which mainly represent the absorption peaks of haemoglobin: these being most prominent at 417, 548 and 578 nm. A slight trough between wavelengths 455 and 485 is thought to represent carotene.[2] The steep decline in reflectance in the UV represents an increased absorbance rather than transmittance, due mainly to the concentrated accumulation of aromatic amino acids such as

1. Edwards, E. A. and Duntley, S. Q. (1939). The pigments and colour of living human skin. *A. J. Anat.* **65**, 1.

2. Edwards, E. A., Finkelstein, N. A. and Duntley, S. Q. (1951). Spectrophotometry of living human skin. *J. invest. Derm.* **16**, 311.

3. Jacquez, J. A., Kuppenheim, H. F., Dimitroff, J. M., McKeehan, W. and Huss, J. (1955). Spectral reflectance of human skin in the region 235–700 nm. *J. appl. Physiol.* **8**, 212.

4. Hardy, J. D., Hammel, H. T. and Murgatroyd, D. (1956). Spectral transmittance and reflectance of excised human skin. *J. appl. Physiol.* **9**, 257.

5. Daniels, F., Jr and Imbrie, J. D. (1958). Comparison between visual grading and reflectance measurements of erythema produced by sunlight. *J. invest. Derm.* **30**, 295.

6. Johnson, B. E., Daniels, F., Jr and Magnus, I. A. (1968). Response of human skin to ultraviolet light. *In* 'Photophysiology', Vol. IV (Ed., Giese, A. C.), p. 139. Academic Press, London, Orlando and New York.

7. Feather, J. W., Dawson, J. B., Barker, D. J. and Cotterill, J. A. (1981). A theoretical and experimental study of the optical properties of *in vivo* skin. *In* 'Bioengineering and the Skin'. (Eds, Mark, R. and Payne, P. A.), p. 275. MTP Press, Lancaster.

8. Anderson, R. R., Hu, J. and Parrish, J. A. (1981). Optical radiation transfer in human skin and applications in *in vivo* remittance spectroscopy. *In* 'Bioengineering and the Skin'. (Eds, Marks, R. and Payne, P. A.), p. 253. MTP Press, Lancaster.

tryptophan and tyrosine in the keratinized horny layer. The characteristics of the reflectance spectrum of fair skin are lost with the development of a tan, the result being akin to that of a negro skin (Fig. 19).

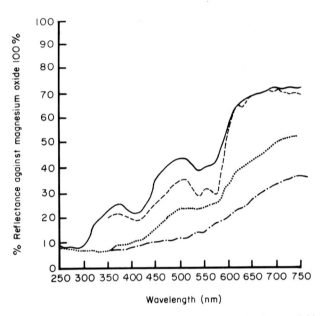

Fig. 19. Reflectance spectroscopy of human skin. ———— Normal lightly pigmented skin. — — — — Lightly pigmented skin with a 24-hour sunburn erythema. ·········· Sun-tanned skin. —·—·—·—· Negro skin. (Redrawn from Johnson, B. E., Daniels, F., Jr and Magnus, I. A. (1968). Response of human skin to ultraviolet light. *In* 'Photophysiology, Current Topics', Vol. IV (Ed., Giese, A. C.), p. 139. Academic Press, London, Orlando and New York.

C. Transmission

Spectral transmission through the various skin layers is more difficult to measure, but it would be of value for the determination of the target sites for solar radiation.

Red light penetrates considerable thickness of biologic material, particularly skin. It is detected through closed eyelids and it is also visible through full thickness of cheek skin when the buccal cavity is illuminated, whereas the transmittance of shorter wavelength radiation is greatly reduced.

Hasselbach,[1] using corpse skin, a quartz spectrograph, and photographic recording, compared the transmission of the emission lines from a medium pressure mercury arc through full thickness skin and also through the separated epidermis. Disregarding the difficulties of measuring skin thickness and the lack of correction for scatter and induced fluorescence, the values obtained (Table 2) indicate a general pattern for UV absorption in the skin. Critically analysed, the absolute values were shown to be low by a factor of 1·5 to 30 times for wavelengths from 404 to 289 nm respectively.[2] Living rabbit skin 1·2 nm thick showed considerable transmission at 280 nm.[3] With a monochromator as source and

Table 2

Biophysics of the skin

Wavelength (nm)	Transmittance as a percentage
289	0·01
297	2
302	8
313	30
404	55

Transmittance of medium pressure mercury arc lines through 0·1 mm thickness of skin (after Hasselbach).

correcting for fluorescence which had previously given false high results, a 6–10% transmission for wavelengths between 250 and 300 nm was found.[4] However, despite the skin having an apparently adequate blood supply, it became increasingly opaque to the shorter wavelengths the longer it was maintained as an open flap. It is not known how this observation affects results obtained with dead skin, with separated epidermis or with isolated stratum corneum, but little attention has been paid to this observation in later work.

Stratum corneum, epidermis, corium, and subcutaneous layers, separated by blister formation or microtome section and examined by

1. Hasselbach, K. A. (1911). Quantitative Untersuchungen uber die Absorption der menschlichen Haut von ultravioletten Strahlen. *Scand. Arch. Physiol.* **25**, 55.
2. Lucas, N. S. (1931). The permeability of human epidermis to ultraviolet radiation. *Biochem. J.* **25**, 57.
3. Macht, D. I., Anderson, W. T. and Bell, F. K. (1928). The penetration of ultraviolet rays into live animal tissues. *J. Am. Med. Ass.* **90**, 161.
4. Anderson, W. T. and Macht, D. I. (1928). Penetration of ultraviolet rays into live animal tissue. *Am. J. Physiol.* **86**, 320.

photographic and photoelectric cell methods produced equivocal results; different methods of measurement gave different results because of differences in the recording of pure absorption, scattering and fluorescence. However, it was apparent that penetration by the wavelengths causing sunburn are greater than previously thought. Also, the different layers of the skin exhibited different absorption characteristics.[1] Frozen sections of plantar skin placed over the slit of a spectrograph confirmed an earlier finding that the skin is so heterogeneous that, because of reflection and fluorescence, thicker specimens gave lower absorption coefficients than thinner ones.[2] The findings of Bachem and his co-workers were tabulated: reflection and absorbed radiation were given for the stratum corneum, and absorption and transmission for the other layers.[3] Transmittance was calculated in terms of defined thickness of the different layers, as indicated in Table 3. The specimens were from the flexor surface of presumably white arm skin. The dimensions used by this worker are not far removed from those reported by Kligman[4] and Van

Table 3

Biophysics of the skin

	Corneum 0·03 mm	Epidermis 0·05 mm	+ Papillary dermis 0·5 mm	+ Dermis 2 mm
260	18	8	0	0
280	20	12	0	0
300	26	18	0	0
320	50	23	1	0
340	68	38	2	0
360	72	48	3	0
380	76	54	4	0
400	80	58	5	1
500	87	76	22	4
600	86	75	38	10
700	80	68	38	20

Percentage transmittance of different skin thicknesses at various wavelengths in the UV and visible spectrum.

1. Bachem, A. (1929). Transparency of live and dead animal tissue to ultraviolet light. *Am. J. Physiol.* **90**, 600.
2. Bachem, A. (1930). The ultraviolet transparency of the various layers of human skin. *Am. J. Physiol.* **91**, 58.
3. Bachem, A. (1931). Die Lichtdurchdringung der menschlichen Haut. *Strahlentherapie* **39**, 30.
4. Kligman, A. M. (1964). The biology of the stratum corneum. *In* 'The Epidermis'. (Eds, Montagna, W. and Lobitz, W. C., Jr), p. 387. Academic Press, London, Orlando and New York.

der Leun.[1] The problem of scatter was thought to be insignificant in these recordings using a photoelectric instrument, as the incident beam and the tissue specimen were small in comparison with the sensitive surface.[2]

Lucas[3] repeated the work of Hasselbach using parallel incident radiation, and demonstrated conclusively the importance of scattering in the epidermis, particularly the stratum corneum. After applying corrections, his results were similar to those of Bachem.

Further studies have been carried out since this time. Miescher[4] exposed skin through various thicknesses of isolated horny layer to establish the degree of the protection in terms of increased minimal erythema. He showed that the results could be described by an exponential extinction with a half-value of 9μ. Later Mitchell[5] measured the transmission of stratum corneum and his results differed little from those of Bachem.

More recent studies, using horizontal freezing microtome sections[6] or chemicals, such as catharidin,[7] to separate the stratum corneum, and also chemical and physical methods to produce isolated epidermis have added valuable data, but the results differ little from those of Bachem's group.

Pathak and Epstein[8] have assembled a diagrammatic presentation of 250–400 nm radiation transmittance through the stratum corneum of lightly pigmented skin from different body sites. There is little difference above 300 nm, but below this wavelength, body sites with thicker corneum show a lower transmittance.

Lucas[3] showed that if epidermis was "cleared" in glycerol or acetic acid to decrease scattering by the stratum corneum, the measured transmittance for wavelengths between 250 and 440 nm was increased.

1. Van der Leun, J. C. (1966). Ultraviolet erythema. A study of diffusion processes in human skin. Thesis, Utrecht.
2. Bachem, A. and Reed, C. I. (1931). The penetration of ultraviolet radiation through human skin. *Am. J. Physiol.* **97**, 86.
3. Lucas, N. S. (1931). The permeability of human epidermis to ultraviolet irradiation. *Biochem. J.* **25**, 57.
4. Miescher, G. (1931). Die Schutzfunktionen der Haut gegenuber Lichstrahlen. *Strahlentherapie* **39**, 601.
5. Mitchell, J. S. (1938). The origin of the erythema curve and the pharmacological action of ultraviolet radiation. *Proc. R. Soc. B.* **126**, 241.
6. Tronnier, H. and Merten, W. (1956). Uber die Durchlassigkeit der menschlichen Haut fur ultraviolette Strahlen verschiedener Wellenlange. *Zeit. f. Haut u. Geschlechtskrankheiten* **21**, 157.
7. Everett, M. A., Yeargers, E., Sayre, R. M. and Olson, R. L. (1966). Penetration of epidermis by ultraviolet rays. *Photochem. Photobiol.* **5**, 533.
8. Pathak, M. A. and Epstein, J. H. (1971). Normal and abnormal reactions of man to light. *In* 'Dermatology in General Medicine', 1st Edition. (Eds, Fitzpatrick, T. B. *et al.*), p. 977. McGraw-Hill, New York.

Water was used as the control for the isolated epidermis in these experiments. Solan and Laden[1] in a recent study of the transmission characteristics of isolated stratum corneum, measured the transmittance of dried horny layer in air, and compared the results with those obtained with horny layer exposed to increasing amounts of water vapour up to full saturation, and also to a number of organic solutions of increasing refractive index. Increased relative humidity (r.h. 90%) increased the transmittance slightly, but the wavelength dependence for this change showed a clear peak between 290 and 320 nm. When the keratin was saturated with water, a marked increase in transmission was demonstrated throughout the wavelength range 280 to 450 nm. At 300 nm there was about a threefold increase but there was little difference in the increased transmittance produced by saturation with water, ethanol, propylene, glycol, or silicone fluid.

At longer wavelengths, however, increased transmittance obtained was greater according to the refractive index of the solution used. Although saturation with water may lead to a doubling of the actual thickness in the stratum corneum, this thickened layer will nevertheless transmit more radiation to the deeper layers than a relatively dry stratum corneum. For 300 nm radiation this increase may be in the order of three times, while for 260 nm the transmittance may be doubled. Changes such as these have obvious application in considering the effect of solar radiation on human skin exposed to varying environmental humidities.

The specific effect of pigmentation on transmission has attracted the attention of many workers. Hansen reported that there was no transmission of 330 nm radiation through the outer 0·3 mm of "moderately" pigmented skin. "Slightly" pigmented skin showed about 2% transmission, while that for "very faintly" pigmented skin was approximately 5%.[2] Kirby-Smith and his colleagues found that 300 nm transmission through variously tanned epidermis varied inversely with the degree of pigmentation within the range 1–10%.[3] A more recent survey of stratum corneum and whole epidermis produced similar results.[4] Thomson's finding that the transmission of 290–320 nm radiation through negro stratum corneum was about 2·5 times less than through lightly pigmented

1. Solan, J. L. and Laden, K. (1977). Factors affecting the penetration of light through stratum corneum. *J. Soc. Cosmet. Chem.* **28**, 125.
2. Hansen, K. G. (1948). On the transmission through skin of visible and ultraviolet radiation. *Acta Radiologica Suppl.* **71**.
3. Kirby-Smith, J. S., Blum, H. F. and Grady, H. G. (1942). Penetration of ultraviolet radiation into skin as a factor in carcinogenesis. *J. natn. Cancer Inst.* **2**, 403.
4. Pathak, M. A. and Fitzpatrick, T. B. (1974). The role of natural photoprotective agents in human skin. *In* 'Sunlight and Man'. (Ed., Fitzpatrick, T. B.), p. 725. University of Tokyo Press, Tokyo.

stratum corneum was attributed to the presence of melanin. However, the differences in transmission through pigmented and apparently non-pigmented stratum corneum may be less than 2·5 times,[1] and melanin in the viable epidermis, rather than the horny layer, is responsible for the considerable difference in transmission of these wavelengths through negroid and lightly pigmented caucasoid epidermis as a whole.

It may be concluded that although most of the radiation in the wavelength region 250–320 nm is absorbed in the epidermis, at least 1% does reach the papillary dermis. However, if the sunburn radiation at ground level is considered (the relevant wavelengths are between 290 and 320 nm) then 10–35% is the probable figure for white skin: with at least 30% reaching the viable layer of the epidermis. These figures are obtained by combining and rounding off the findings of several different workers; in some, fluorescence may have given a false high result, in others, scattering may have led to low results. For negro skin, the figure of around 5% transmission for whole epidermis[2,3] appears reasonable, but it should be remembered that the wavelength region under consideration varies widely in biologic effectiveness and that some of the penetrating radiation is made up of the less damaging longer wavelengths to a large degree.

1. Thomson, M. L. (1955). Relative efficiency of pigment and horny layer thickness in protecting the skin of Europeans and Africans against solar radiation. *J. Physiol.* **127**, 236.
2. Kaidbey, K. H., Poh-Agin, P., Sayre, R. M. and Kligman, A. M. (1979). Photoprotection by melanin—a comparison of black and caucasian skin. *J. Am. Acad. Derm.* **1**, 249.
3. Everett, M. A., Yeargers, E., Sayre, R. M. and Olson, R. L. (1966). Penetration of epidermis by ultraviolet rays. *Photochem. Photobiol.* **5**, 533.

Reactions of Normal Skin to Solar Radiation

80

B. E. JOHNSON

Department of Dermatology, University of Dundee, Ninewells Hospital, Dundee, Scotland

I. INTRODUCTION

The physical manifestations of sunburn are familiar to most lightly pigmented individuals. Even "negroid" types, living in geographical locations where a prolonged winter season limits exposure to sunlight, may experience discomfort after injudicious sunbathing in the early summer. Although there is considerable variation between individuals,

PHYSIOL. PATHOPHYSIOL. OF SKIN Vol. 8
ISBN 0 12 380608 9

the reaction, which is restricted to the exposed areas, is in its mildest form a transient erythema. This may take some hours to develop and usually fades rapidly. With increasing exposure, more intense erythema is produced which may become visible during the exposure.[1] This more intense reaction reaches a peak intensity after about 24 h, and persists for up to 20 days.[2] In individuals with a tendency to tan, pigmentation begins to develop 72 h after exposure. However, an earlier pigmentary change may occur as a result of the immediate pigmentation type of reaction (see page 2491). With longer exposures, erythema may be accompanied by oedema, itching and pain. Blistering may develop, in which case any suntan will be lost in the blistered area. Even with mild sunburn, the outer layers of the stratum corneum tend to be shed as sheets rather than as the normal minute scales. In some instances this shedding may be seen to be initiated by the build-up of sweat in the sweat ducts, the openings of which appear to be blocked by changes induced in the epidermis.

In already tanned skin, in Asian caucasoids, and in the less heavily pigmented negroids, the intensity of the inflammation produced by a given exposure dose is less than that in fair-skinned persons. Even in the latter, slight variations in the degree of pigmentation produce differences in the intensity of reaction to sunlight.[3] Sunburn and tanning were probably the earliest photobiological reactions to be recognized by man. Recorded comment on these reactions is limited, possibly because they were so common. The deification of the sun, a major feature of many religions, was associated with the Greek word "Heliosis", meaning controlled exposure of the body to sunlight for health reasons.[4] A general interest in "heliotherapy" was revived in the late eighteenth century. In particular, the relationship between rickets and a lack of sunlight exposure was noted and this initiated discussions on the relative effects of heat and light on the body.[5] Also, the apparent relationship between sunlight and skin colour attracted the attention of naturalists such as Blumenbach[6] who drew freely from the reports of Humboldt and Cook to compare the tanning of white skin with the natural skin colour of negroes.

1. Langen, D. (1938). Experimentelle Studien über die Erythembildung der Sonnen- und Himmelsstrahlung. Strahlentherapie 63, 142.
2. Breit, R. and Kligman, A. M. (1969). Measurement of erythemal and pigmentary responses to ultraviolet radiation. In 'The Biologic Effects of Ultraviolet Radiation (with emphasis on skin)' (Ed., Urbach, F.), p. 267. Pergamon Press, Oxford.
3. Wucherpfennig, V. (1931). Biologie und praktische Verwendbarkeit der Erythemschwelle des UV. Strahlentherapie 40, 201.
4. Licht, S. (1959). In 'Therapeutic Electricity and Ultraviolet Radiation' (Ed., Licht, S.), p. 179. Licht, New Haven, Connecticut.
5. Bertrand, M. (1799). Essai Touchant l'influence de la Lumière sur Etres Organisés, Paris.
6. Blumenbach, J. F. (1798). In 'Natural History' (Ed., Wood), Vol. 8, p. 405.

Although the discovery of ultraviolet radiation (UVR) was reported as early as 1803,[1] the importance of this region of the electromagnetic spectrum in biological reactions was not realized for many years. However, Cauvin in 1815[2] distinguished between the heat from the sun and other solar energies as a factor in the effects of sunlight. The practice of heliotherapy and the natural history of pigmentation combined to increase the interest in the skin and its reactions to sunlight. In 1821 Home[3] reported his early experiment of applying black paint to his skin, observing that the painted area neither burned nor tanned. He mistakenly concluded that the paint acted exactly as did the pigment in negro skin and tanned white skin, and that the pigment was actually formed on the outer surface. The heating effect of sunlight would still be effective in the presence of the black paint and therefore heat did not cause the reactions of burning and pigmentation. Bostock in 1825[4] located the site of skin pigment as being between the epidermis and the cutis; the part upon which the sun acted could not be ascertained, but it was probably the epidermis, as he observed that a blister removed the tan. Davy[5] stimulated by these works and by his interest in skin colour, carried out the first thorough investigation of sunburn. He observed a severe sunburn reaction at intervals during a 3-week period and noted a transient increase in skin temperature followed by desquamation and, finally, tanning. He went on to show that, although the tan protected against severe effects, erythema was still produced when tanned skin was exposed to sunlight.

The advances in optical physics at this time were rapid, and powerful electric light sources were developed for studying optical physics. Thus, in 1858 Charcot[6] reported the experience of two physicists, Foucault and Despritz, who had been exposed to the unfiltered emission from an electric arc and had suffered what appeared to be typical severe sunburn of the exposed areas. A uranium glass filter placed between the arc and the skin prevented these reactions, thus giving some indication of the causative wavelength. A clear-cut experimental demonstration that UVR was responsible was presented by Widmark,[7] who reported that the

1. Ritter, J. W. (1803). Versuche über das Sonnenlicht. *Ann. Physik.* **12**, 409.
2. Cauvin, J. F. (1815). Des Bienfaits de L'Insolation, Paris.
3. Home, E. (1821). On the black rete mucosum of the negro, being a defence against the scorching effect of the sun's rays. *Phil. Trans. R. Soc. (London)* **111**, 1.
4. Bostock, J. (1825). 'Elementary System of Physiology'. Wells and Lilly, Boston, Massachussetts.
5. Davy, J. (1828). Observations on the effect of the sun's rays on the human body. *Trans. Med. Chir. Soc. Edinburgh* **256**.
6, Charcot, L. (1858). Erythème de la face et ophthalmic produits par l'action de lumière électrique. *Ct. r. soc. biol.* **10**, 63.
7. Widmark, E. J. (1889). Über den Einfluss des Lichtes auf die vorderen Medien des Auges. *Skand. Arch. Physiol.* **1**, 264.

rays from a carbon arc when passed through a window glass filter did not elicit a burning effect like those passed through quartz. It is interesting that although Home's simple experiment a hundred years previously had indicated that the part played by heat in the sunburn reaction was insignificant, popular belief still considered this to be of importance. Thus, the reports by polar explorers[1, 2, 3] that severe sunburn occurred with air temperatures below freezing were received with some surprise. In 1877 Downes and Blunt had shown that bacteria were killed by exposure to sunlight.[4] Niels Finsen received the Nobel Prize in 1903 for his successful ultraviolet lamp treatment of skin tuberculosis. His lamp consisted of a carbon arc with outlet ports for the simultaneous treatment of several patients.[5] At each port the radiation was passed through water to remove the infra-red component, and then through a lens pressed against the skin to improve transmission by excluding the cutaneous blood. Finsen's studies formed the basis of modern photobiology as far as UVR effects are concerned, not only on whole living skin, but also its effects on cells. Early studies of the action of UVR on cells were initiated to elucidate the mechanisms involved in Finsen therapy, and in 1899 Finsen clearly demonstrated that UVR was the active principle in the reaction of normal skin to sunlight. A review of this work may be obtained by consulting the original publications and also the English translation by Sequeira.[5]

Controlled studies of natural sunburn have been few since the pioneering experiments of Davey. Langen[6] and Pfleiderer and Buettner[7] reported studies designed to show the effect of variations in latitude on the degree of the erythema response. The efficacy of anti-sunburn prepara-

1. Peary, R. E. (1907). 'Nearest the Pole', pp. 113, 230. Doubleday, New York.
2. Peary, R. E. (1910). 'The North Pole', pp. 310, 315. Stokes, New York.
3. Shackleton. E. H. (1909). 'The Heart of the Antarctic, Washington Square', pp. 10, 11. Philadelphia, Pennsylvania.
4. Downes, A. and Blunt, T. P. (1877). Researches on the effect of light upon bacteria and other organisms. *Proc. R. Soc. London* **26**, 488.
5. Finsen, N. R. (1901). 'Phototherapy', *translated by Sequeira, J. H.* Edward Arnold, London.
6. Langen, D. (1938). Experimentelle Studien über die Erythembildung der Sonnen- und Himmelsstrahlung. *Strahlentherapie* **63**, 142.
7. Pfleiderer, H. and Buettner, K. (1940). *In* 'Handbuch der Bader und Klimaheikungde'. Springer, Berlin.

tions, either oral[1, 2] or topical[3, 4] has been appropriately investigated by using the sun as the light source.

Also the effects of environmental sunscreens have been similarly studied.[5] The Robertson–Berger meter designed to give a measurement of the dose of *sunburn* radiation by integrating the irradiance within the sunburn wavelength range over a given exposure time,[6] or the personal filmbadge dosimeter[7] giving a similar approximation, may be used in such studies. However, it is obvious that even in Texas, Florida, and North East Australia there is a continual variation in the intensity of sunlight, and certainly in Northern Europe sufficiently intense sunlight over long enough periods is rarely available to allow controlled studies.

Artificial sources have therefore been mainly used for the investigation of sunburn. The original "Finsen Light" was a metal cored carbon arc, filtered to cut off the UVR below 290 nm. Many investigators used the medium pressure mercury arc source in which the UV-C was not removed. They realized this was not the same as solar radiation, but they were mainly interested in the skin reaction to UVR itself rather than to total solar radiation.[8] The high pressure mercury arcs may have some advantage, but the high pressure xenon arc, with the UV-C removed as originally used by Wiskemann and Wulf,[9] remains the best artificial source for studying skin reactions to sunlight under controlled conditions.

1. Imbrie, J. D., Daniels, F., Jr, Bergeron, L., Hopkins, C. E. and Fitzpatrick, T. B. (1959). Increased erythema threshold six weeks after a single exposure to sunlight plus oral methoxsalen. *J. invest. Derm.* **32**, 331.

2. Mathews-Rothe, M. M., Pathak, M. A., Parrish, J. A. and Kass, E. H. (1972). A clinical trial of the effects of oral beta-carotene on the responses of human skin to solar radiation. *J. invest. Derm.* **59**, 349.

3. Pathak, M. A., Fitzpatrick, T. B. and Frenk, E. (1969). Evaluation of topical agents that prevent sunburn-superiority of para-amino: benzoic acid and its ester in ethyl alcohol. *New Eng. J. Med.* **280**, 1459.

4. Sayre, R. M., Desrochers, D. L., Marlowe, E. and Urbach, F. (1978). The correlation of indoor solar simulator and natural sunlight, testing of a sunscreen preparation. *Arch. Derm.* **114**, 1649.

5. Urbach, F., Davies, R. E. and Forbes, P. D. (1966). Ultraviolet radiation and skin cancer in man. *In* 'Advances in Biology of Skin' (Eds, Montagna, W. and Dobson, R. L.), Vol. 7, p. 195. Pergamon Press, Oxford.

6. Berger, D. S. (1976). The sunburning ultraviolet meter: design and performance. *Photochem. Photobiol.* **24**, 587.

7. Challoner, A. V. J., Corless, D., Davis, A., Deane, G. H. W., Diffey, B. L., Gupta, S. P. and Magnus, I. A. (1976). Personal monitoring of exposure to ultraviolet radiation. *Clin. exp. Derm.* **1**, 175.

8. Harber, L. C., Bickers, D. R., Epstein, J. H., Pathak, M. A. and Urbach, F. (1974). Light sources used in photopatch testing. *In* 'Sunlight and Man' (Ed., Fitzpatrick, T. B.), p. 559. University of Tokyo Press, Tokyo.

9. Wiskemann, A., and Wulf, K. (1959). Untersuchungen über den auslosenden Spektralbereich und die direkte Lichtpigmentierung bis chronischen und akuten Lichtausschlagen. *Arch. klin. exp. Derm.* **209**, 443.

II. ULTRAVIOLET ERYTHEMA AND ACTION SPECTRA

A. Ultraviolet Erythema

Of the various skin changes resulting from exposure to UVR, erythema is the most obvious and most easily measured, and has therefore received most attention. Erythema may be evaluated in terms of the variation in intensity of response obtained in different subjects, or different skin areas, after a standard exposure dose. Alternatively, a threshold dose level for erythema may be determined by examining the response to varying exposure doses. Usually the threshold chosen is the just perceptible erythema, and the exposure dose required to produce this is termed the minimal erythema dose (MED).[1] Some confusion has arisen in the literature because different definitions of a minimal erythema have been used, and this point is discussed in detail on pages 2422 and 2429.

The studies of Schall and Alius[2, 3, 4, 5] are typical of those in which the skin responses to a standard exposure are compared. Using an unfiltered medium pressure mercury arc and measuring the exposure dose by chemical actinometry, they graded the responses obtained by comparing them with a standard series of red-stained slides. All the subjects studied demonstrated maximum intensity of redness at about 7 h. After this 7-h period, variations in the course of the erythema were observed. In some, the intensity faded gradually over the next 3 days. In other subjects, the maximum response was maintained for 72 h and then faded. In another group a second peak was observed between 24 and 48 h. Both the time course and the intensity of reactions varied among the subjects tested, fair complexioned subjects being generally more sensitive than darker skinned individuals.

This variation in the erythema response between one subject and another has now been "standardized" as a classification of sun-reactive skin types.[6] An extended form of this classification (Table 1) has been

1. Hausser, K. W. (1928). Einfluss der Wellenlange in der Strahlenbiologie. *Strahlentherapie* **28**, 25.
2. Schall, L. and Alius, H. J. (1925). Zur Biologie des Ultraviolettlichts. I. Zur Frage der Dosimetrie des Ultraviolettlichts. *Stahlentherapie* **19**, 559.
3. Schall, L. and Alius, H. J. (1925). Zur Biologie des Ultraviolettlichts. II. Zur Frage der Messung der Hautreaktion. (Ein neuer Erthem- und Pigment messur). *Strahlentherapie* **19**, 796.
4. Schall, L. and Alius, H. J. (1926). Zur Biologie des Ultraviolettlichts. III. Die reaktion der menschlichen Haut auf die Ultraviolettlichtbestrahlung (Erythemablauf). *Strahlentherapie* **23**, 161.
5. Schall, L. and Alius, H. J. (1928). Zur Biologie des Ultraviolettlichts. Zur die Reaktion der menschlichen Haut auf wiederholte Ultraviolettlichtbestrahlung (Lichtschutz). *Strahlentherapie* **27**, 769.
6. Fitzpatrick, T. B. (1976). Topical photoprotection of normal skin. *In* 'Research in Photobiology' (Ed., Castellani, A.), p. 745. Plenum Press, London.

produced as a guide to exposure doses used in phototherapy and photochemotherapy.[1] Classifications such as these are useful but do not cover all the possible variations in the wide range of ethnic skin types (see page 2404). In Type I and II subjects there is a preponderance of light skin colour, blue or green eyes, fair or red hair and freckling. It is not uncommon, however, for dark haired individuals with blue or green eyes to exhibit Type I or II reactions to sunlight.

Table 1

Skin types in respect to their sensitivity to sunlight (for individuals between 12 and 40 years)

Subject type	Reaction
I.	Always burn. Never tan
II.	Always burn. Slight tan
III.	Sometimes burn. Always tan
IV.	Never burn. Always tan
V.	Pigmented; Mediterranean and Indian Caucasoids; Mongoloids
VI.	Deeply pigmented; Negroids; Australoids (see page 2404, Chapter 79)

The intensity of UV-induced reactions varies, not only between individuals but also between body site on the same subject. Schall and Alius[2] showed that the upper chest was most sensitive with a graded decrease towards the extremities, and Wucherpfennig[3] observed a similar trend using MED determinations (Table 2).

When a variation in intensity of reaction to a single dose is being evaluated, a standard method for measuring the redness is required especially for comparisons between results from different centres. Differences in visual interpretation between one observer and another make the comparison of gradations in redness difficult. Because of this, comparative methods of measuring degrees of erythema have been

1. Melski, J., Tanenbaum, L., Parrish, J. A., Fitzpatrick, T. B., Bleich, H. L. and 28 participating investigators (1977). Oral methoxysalen photochemotherapy for the treatment of psoriasis: A co-operative clinical trial. *J. invest. Derm.* **68**, 328.
2. Schall, L. and Alius, H. J. (1926). Zur Biologie des Ultraviolettlichts. III. Die reaktion der menschlichen Haut auf die Ultraviolettlichtbestrahlung (Erythemablauf). *Strahlentherapie* **23**, 161.
3. Wucherpfennig, V. (1931). Biologie und praktische Vorwendbarkeit der Erythemschwelle des UV. *Strahlentherapie* **40**, 201.

Table 2

Variation of skin sensivity to sunburn UVR with body site (back skin expressed as 100%. Figures are approximate)

Body site		Intensity of reaction Schall and Alius (1926)	MED Wucherpfennig (1931)
Abdomen		124	—
Chest		188	—
Back		100	100
Arm	Inner	22	36
	Outer	11	25
Forearm	Inner	11	0
	Outer	0	0
Thigh	Inner	47	21
	Outer	11	26
Leg		0	—

developed, such as the graded series of slides used by Schall and Alius termed an erythemameter by Bachem,[1] or the red cellophane sheet used by Burckhardt.[2] Recording spectrophotometry has produced good results,[3,4] and simpler devices than those requiring an attached integrating sphere have been used with good effect to record reflectance at a number of specific wavelengths.[5]

Tronnier,[6] by using filters (e.g. 550 nm) to ensure maximum readings for haemoglobin absorption obtained adequate measurements. Nevertheless, the problem of interference by melanin in the skin (see spectral reflectance curve for negro skin as compared with that for white skin) is difficult to overcome. Hansen[7] exerted pressure on the skin to obtain a reading which represented melanin alone and then subtracted this from the overall reading to find the true value for erythema. Other workers

1. Bachem, A. (1955). Time factors of erythema and pigmentation produced by ultraviolet rays of different wavelength. *J. invest. Derm.* **25**, 215.
2. Burckhardt, W. (1966). Reported at 'Intern. Congr. Skin Photobiol.', Philadelphia.
3. Jansen, M. T. (1953). A reflection spectrophotometric study of ultraviolet erythema and pigmentation. *J. clin. Invest.* **32**, 1053.
4. Daniels, F., Jr, and Imbrie, J. D. (1958). Comparison between visual grading and reflectance measurements of erythema produced by sunlight. *J. Invest. Derm.* **30**, 295.
5. Tronnier, H. (1969). Evaluation and measurement of ultraviolet erythema. In 'The Biologic Effects of Ultraviolet Radiation (with emphasis on skin)' (Ed., Urbach, F.), p. 255. Pergamon Press, Oxford.
6. Tronnier, H. (1963). Restimmung der Hautfarbe unter besonderer Berücksichtigung der Erythem- und Pigmentmessung. *Strahlentherapie* **121**, 392.
7. Hansen, K. G. (1966). Reported at 'Intern. Congr. Skin Photobiol.', Philadelphia.

have attempted to follow the course of pigmentation by reflectance measurements at wavelengths taken to represent the presence of melanin only.[1, 2, 3] Tronnier concluded that it is not possible to satisfactorily separate the fading erythema and developing pigmentation with techniques presently available.

Some years ago Jarrett and Riley[4] developed a technique for determination of skin colour due to its melanin content. An Evans Electroselenium reflectance photometer was modified by replacing the normal tungsten light source with an overrun projection lamp (Phillips AL-186). The emission from this source was filtered through a Chance 1 mm OX 1 filter, giving a peak transmission around 365 nm.

The lamp housing was also modified so that it could be cooled by air blown from an electric fan. With this apparatus it was possible to compare the degree of melanization of the epidermis with greater accuracy than was previously possible: even slight differences in the degree of pigmentation could be detected.

Readings were taken from 38 patients both from their exposed and unexposed normal skin. The observations extended over a total period of 33 months. Each patient was seen, on an average, at monthly invervals during this period.

Changes recorded on the exposed and unexposed skin through the months of the year are shown in Table 3. It will be seen that there is a darkening of both exposed and unexposed skin during those months with the greatest incidence of solar radiation. The darkening of the exposed skin can readily be accounted for by the direct pigmenting action of the solar radiation, but it was thought that the darkening of the unexposed skin was probably brought about by an optic–pituitary effect due to alteration of the photoperiod.

However, the MED may be determined without the use of either simple or complex erythema measuring instruments. The human eye is capable of distinguishing the presence or absence of even a faint redness on a paler background. The method usually adopted is to expose a series of skin sites to increasing exposure doses and to examine the exposed sites at specific time intervals thereafter. In this way it is possible to determine the dose

1. Jansen, M. T. (1953). A reflection spectrophotometric study of ultraviolet erythema and pigmentation. *J. clin. Invest.* **32**, 1053.
2. Daniels, F., Jr, and Imbrie, J. D. (1958). Comparison between visual grading and reflectance measurements of erythema produced by natural sunlight. *J. invest. Derm.* **30**, 295.
3. Breit, R. and Kligman, A. M. (1969). Measurement of erythemal and pigmentary responses to ultraviolet radiation of different spectral qualities. *In* 'The Biologic Effects of Ultraviolet Radiation (with emphasis on skin)' (Ed., Urbach, F.), p. 267. Pergamon Press, Oxford.
4. Jarrett, A. and Riley, P. Q. (1962). Unpublished data.

Table 3

Seasonal accumulated changes in reflectance

Month	Exposed skin*	Unexposed skin*
January	10·8	15·4
February	9·4	11·4
March	7·3	7·2
April	7·2	8·8
May	7·2	10·6
June	6·5	9·4
July	6·8	8·5
August	1·6	4·5
September	2·0	13·0
October	1·0	11·1
November	2·8	14·7
December	7·0	19·0
January	10·8	15·4

* Trend figures adjusted for slope of zero axis (0·6) on an arbitrary scale. It will be observed that there is a darkening of unexposed skin beginning in March and lasting until August. In September the reflectance readings revert to those of the winter readings. On exposed areas lightening of the skin colour does not occur until December. Jarrett, A. and Riley, P.A. (1962). Unpublished observations.

which produces a minimal erythema compared with a neighbouring exposure site at which an erythematous reaction has not been produced. The use of different criteria for the definition of a minimal erythema has led to confusion over the time course, intensity, and dose requirements for this reaction. The most complete consideration of the MED reaction and its variations was given by Van der Leun.[1] He emphasized that the minimal erythema does not completely fill the total area of skin exposed. It follows from this that reactions which show definite boundaries which match the irradiation slits used for graded exposures are not minimal erythemas, and the dose required to produce these reactions is greater than the MED by a factor of 2 or more. With artificial sources, the reaction obtained with a MED may well have faded 24 h after the exposure. It is therefore advisable to read the test sites earlier, preferably 7 to 8 h after exposure in addition to the usual intervals. The minimal perceptible erythema has the longest latent period and the shortest duration. Doses higher than the MED result in a shorter latent period, a longer duration of the reaction, and an increased intensity.

1.   Van der Leun, J. C. (1966). Ultraviolet Erythema. A study on diffusion processes in human skin. Thesis, Utrecht.

Determinations of threshold erythema responses, whether of MED or greater, have shown that skin previously exposed to UVR is less sensitive than non-exposed skin[1] and that there is a relationship between darkness of complexion and erythema threshold.[1,2] Moreover, seasonal changes in MED have been described, the threshold falling during the summer from a maximum value in the spring.[3,4] In women, there may be an increase in MED during August in Northern Europe, and this is attributed to tolerance induced by continuous exposure of the test site, the forearm. The extensive studies of Bravi produced similar results to those of other authors, although he used an MED determination which selected that does which just failed to produce a reaction at 24 h.[5] In fact, this may well be the "correct" MED as defined by Van der Leun.

The variations between individual responses in any one study are significant. However, there may also be considerable variation in the overall reaction picture presented by different authors. This is not only because different criteria for the assessment of erythema were used, but also because the spectral characteristics of the radiation sources were different. There are variations in the erythemas produced by different regions of the ultraviolet spectrum, and thus different sources tend to give different results.

B. Action Spectra for UV- erythema

An action spectrum is a plot of the relative effectiveness of a given photochemical or photobiological effect against wavelength. It is presented in this form to show the maximally effective wavelength as a peak in a curve and may be plotted by taking the reciprocal of the dose required for the effect. Ideally, the quantum energy should be equal for the different wavelengths, and the reaction should be brought about by the same mechanisms regardless of wavelength. Also, the monochromatic radiation used to obtain an action spectrum should have a constant bandwidth for each of the selected wavebands. For the complex reaction

1. Wuchrpfennig, V. (1931). Biologie und praktische Verendbarkeit der Erythemschwelle des UV. *Strahlentherapie* **40**, 201.
2. Schall, L. and Alius, H. J. (1928). Zur Biologie des Ultraviolettlichts. Zur die Reaktion der menschlichen Haut auf wiederholte Ultraviolettlichtbestrahlung (Lichtschutz). *Strahlentherapie* **27**, 769.
3. Ellinger, F. (1941). 'The Biologic Fundamentals of Radiation Therapy'. Elsevier, Amsterdam.
4. Knudsen, E. A., Christiansen, J. V. and Brodthagen, H. (1961). Seasonal variations in light-sensitivity. *In* 'Progress in Photobiology'. Proceedings of the third international congress on photobiology, Copenhagen, 1960 (Eds, Christensen, B. C. and Buchmann, B.), p. 521. Elsevier, Amsterdam.
5. Bravi, G. (1959). Dell'estinzione energietica della reazione cutanea per UV. *G. ital. Derm.* **100**, 511.

of cutaneous vasodilatation in which the mechanisms for its production are not known, action spectroscopy is far from ideal. Instrumental problems have resulted in different bandwidths being used in the various studies. Nevertheless, these investigations have been useful in establishing safety levels of exposure to artificial light.[1,2,3] They also form a basis for the study of the mechanisms involved in UV-erythema[4,5] and delimit normal skin reactions from those occurring in the photodermatoses.[6,7,8] The data for standard, normal human erythema action spectrum were tabulated in the International Commission on Illumination in Berlin in 1955.[9] This was derived from the initial work by Hausser and Vahle,[10,11] and later studies by Luckeish and his colleagues[2] and Coblentz and his co-workers.[3] The spectrum showed peak of activity between 290 and 300 nm which fell rapidly towards the longer wavelengths, with little apparent action beyond 315 nm. There was a second, smaller peak around 250 nm and a pronounced trough at 280 nm (Fig. 1). However, more recent studies of the erythema action spectrum have produced significantly different results, the most effective wavelengths being around 260 nm with a tendency for a gradual fall-off of activity in the longer wavelengths. The peak around 295 appeared as a plateau in one study,[12] but was very much reduced in others.[6,13] Wavelengths around

1. Hausser, K. W. (1928). Einfluss der Wellenlänge in der Strahlenbiologie. *Strahlentherapie* **28**, 25.
2. Luckeish, M., Holladay, L. S. and Taylor, A. H. (1930). Reaction of untanned human skin to ultraviolet radiation. *J. Opt. Soc. Am.* **20**, 423.
3. Coblentz, W. W., Stair, A. and Hogue, J. M. (1932). The spectral erythemic reaction of the untanned human skin to ultraviolet radiation. *J. Res. Natl. Bur. Standards* **8**, 541.
4. Mitchell, J. S. (1938). The origin of the erythema curve and the pharmacological action of ultraviolet radiation. *Proc. R. Soc. London* **B126**, 241.
5. Van der Leun, J. C. (1972). On the action spectrum of ultraviolet erythema. *In* 'Research Progress in Organic, Biological and Medicinal Chemistry', Vol. 2, part II (Eds, Gallo, U. and Santamaria, L.), p. 711. North Holland Publishing Co., Amsterdam.
6. Magnus, I. A., Porter, A. D., McCree, K. G., Moreland, J. D. and Wright, W. D. A. (1959). A monochromator. An apparatus for the investigation of the response of the skin to ultraviolet, visible and infra-red radiation. *Br. J. Derm.* **71**, 261.
7. MacKenzie, L. A. and Frain-Bell, W. (1973). The construction and development of a grating monochromator and its application to the study of the reaction of the skin to light. *Br. J. Derm.* **89**, 251.
8. Satoh, Y., Irimajiri, T., Okawara, S., Shimao, K. and Seiji, M. (1974). A newly designed monochromator and action spectra of various photodermatoses. *In* 'Sunlight and Man' (Ed., Fitzpatrick, T. B.), p. 575. University of Tokyo Press, Tokyo.
9. International Commission on Illumination, Berlin (1935). *Compt. rend.* **9**, 596.
10. Hausser, K. W. and Vahle, W. (1922). Die Abhängigkeit des Lichterythems und der Pigmentbildung von Schwingungszahl (Wellenlänge) der erregenden Strahlung. *Strahlentherapie* **13**, 41.
11. Hausser, K. W. and Vahle, W. (1927). Sonnenbrand und Sonnenbraunung. *Wiss. Veroff. Siemen-Konzern.* **6**, 101.
12. Everett, M. A., Olson, R. L. and Sayre, R. M. (1965). Ultraviolet erythema. *Arch. Derm.* **92**, 713.
13. Freeman, R. G., Owens, D. W., Knox, J. M. and Hudson, H. T. (1966). Relative energy requirements for an erythemal response of skin to monochromatic wavelengths of ultraviolet present in the solar spectrum. *J. invest. Derm.* **47**, 586.

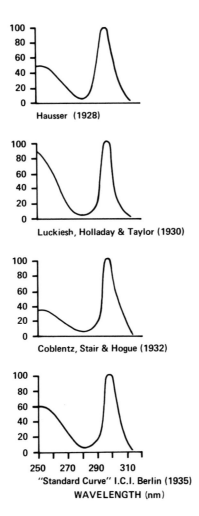

Fig. 1. Early versions of the action spectrum for UV-erythema. Hausser (1928) Forearm skin; medium pressure mercury arc spectral lines dispersed with quartz prism apparatus. Luckiesh, Holladay and Taylor (1930) Back skin; mercury arc lines separated with filters. Coblentz, Stair and Hogue (1932) Forearm skin; mercury arc lines dispersed with quartz prism. Standard Curve; plotted from figures presented at the meeting in Berlin, 1935. For other details and the references, see text.

280 nm were found to be relatively active in these later studies although some form of trough in the action spectrum was found at this wavelength by the majority[1, 2, 3, 4] (Fig. 2).

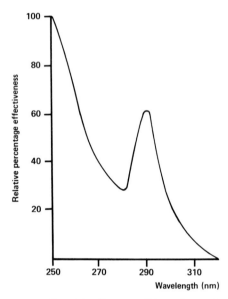

Fig. 2. Typical action spectrum for minimally perceptible erythema obtained with a Xenon arc source and grating monochromator, $\frac{1}{2}$ maximum bandwidth: 5 nm.

It is possible that the loss of definition in later erythema action spectra is partly due to the use of xenon arc with its continuous emission spectrum, rather than the mercury arcs producing line spectra used in the earlier studies. Without careful attention to the optics of the monochromator, active and non-active wavelengths may overlap, and this would

1. Magnus, I. A. (1964). Studies with a monochromator in the common idiopathic photodermatoses. *Br. J. Derm.* **76**, 245.
2. Berger, D., Urbach, F. and Davies, R. E. (1968). The action spectrum of erythema induced by ultraviolet radiation. Preliminary report. *In* 'XIII Congressus Internationalis Dermatologiae' (Eds, Jadassohn, W. and Schirren, C. G.), **2**, 1112. Springer-Verlag, Berlin.
3. Cripps, D. J. and Ramsay, C. A. (1970). Ultraviolet action spectrum with a prism-grating monochromator. *Br. J. Derm.* **82**, 584.
4. Nakayama, Y., Morikawa, F., Fukuda, M., Hamano, M., Toda, K. and Pathak, M. A. (1974). Monochromatic radiation and its application—laboratory studies on the mechanism of erythema and pigmentation induced by psoralen. *In* 'Sunlight and Man' (Ed., Fitzpatrick, T. B.), p. 591. University of Tokyo Press, Tokyo.

result in a flattening of the peaks and troughs in the action spectra.[1] Theoretical analyses of this possibility have, however, suggested this to be an unlikely explanation for the differences between the earlier action spectrum and its more recent versions.[2, 3] It also seems unlikely that the effect of widening the spectral dispersion around the selected wavebands is responsible for the differences although some loss of definition in the action spectrum was obtained when very wide bands of wavelengths were used.[3] The difficulties in accepting in detail the action spectrum formulated in 1935 were foreshadowed by the early work of Hausser and Vahle,[4, 5] who had previously demonstrated significant differences between the erythema due to 254 nm radiation and those obtained with longer wavelengths around 297 nm. In 1931 Adams, Barnes and Forsythe[6] had shown that the action spectrum obtained for a moderately intense erythema appeared similar to the standard; but if minimal erythemas were used, a curve was obtained which more closely resembled the more recently reported action spectra. The greater effectiveness of the 254 nm region of the UV spectrum in eliciting minimal erythema was demonstrated by Blum and Terus[7] using a germicidal mercury lamp which provided an almost monochromatic waveband at 254 nm. This was confirmed later by Rottier who used a mercury arc-quartz spectrograph irradiation system to provide monochromatic radiation at this and other wavelengths.[8] Magnus, using a xenon arc and a water-filled quartz prism also found a greater effect of 260 nm radiation in his erythema action spectrum studies.[9] Later Van der Leun analysed the

1. Diffey, B. L. (1975). Variation of erythema with monochromator bandwidths. *Arch. Derm.* **111**, 1070.

2. Van der Leun, J. C. (1972). On the action spectrum of ultraviolet erythema. In 'Research Progress in Organic, Biological and Medicinal Chemistry', Vol. 3, pt II, p. 711. North Holland, Amsterdam.

3. Johnson, B. E., Herd, Joyce and Mackenzie, L. (1974). Ultraviolet radiation erythema action spectrum; variation with change in $\frac{1}{2}$ bandwidth of monochromatic radiation. In 'Progress in Photobiology', Proceedings of the VI International Congress on Photobiology (Ed., Schenck, G. O.). Deutsche Gesellschaft für Lichtforschung, e.V. Frankfurt.

4. Hausser, K. W. and Vahle, W. (1927). Sonnenbrand und Sonnenbraunung. *Wiss. Veroff. Siemen-Konzern.* **6**, 101.

5. Hausser, K. W. and Vahle, W. Translation by Urbach, F. (1969). Sunburn and suntanning. In 'The biologic effects of ultraviolet radiation (with emphasis on the skin)' (Ed., Urbach, F.), p. 3. Pergamon Press, Oxford.

6. Adams, E. Q., Barnes, B. T. and Forsythe, W. E. (1931). Erythema due to ultraviolet radiation. *J. opt. Soc. Am.* **21**, 207.

7. Blum, H. F. and Terus, W. S. (1946). The erythemal threshold for sunburn. *Am. J. Physiol.* **146**, 107.

8. Rottier, P. B. (1953). The erythematogenous action of ultraviolet light on human skin. I. Some measurements of the spectral response with continuous and intermittent light. *J. clin. Invest.* **32**, 681.

9. Magnus, I. A. (1964). Studies with a monochromator in the common idiopathic photodermatoses. *Br. J. Derm.* **76**, 245.

various factors which influenced the shape of the erythema action spectrum, especially with respect to the 250 nm and 300 nm regions.[1] The minimal erythema due to 250 nm develops quite rapidly, appearing before 6 h and reaching its maximum intensity by 7 to 8 h: it fades before 24 h following exposure. The 300 nm minimal erythema develops more slowly and may not be present for 7 to 8 h after exposure, but it is usually apparent by 24 h. It follows that while a reading after 24 h may give the true MED for 300 nm erythemas, a 250 nm erythema which persists for as long as 24 h requires an exposure dose greater than the MED. Therefore, as suggested by Everett and his colleagues[2] and by Urbach and his co-workers,[3] if the action spectrum is plotted from the results of 24 h post-irradiation readings alone, the 250 nm region will appear less effective than it is in fact. Conversely, if readings are only taken at 7–8 h, the effect of the longer wavelength radiation will appear diminished. This may partly explain the difference between the earlier action spectrum based mainly on 24 h readings, and more recent versions where greater attention is paid to the time of reading. Nevertheless, this may only be part of the explanation since the relationship is not clear cut and, as shown in the table given by Van der Leun,[4] the true MED differs at readings taken at 7 to 8 h and 24 h for both 300 and 260 nm regions (see Table 4).

The second factor which has an effect on the shape of the erythema action spectrum is the intensity of the erythema chosen as the threshold. With wavelengths around 250 nm, increasing exposures result in minimally increasing degrees of redness. With wavelengths around 300 nm, the intensity of redness increases rapidly with increasing exposure dose (see Fig. 3).[3, 5] It follows that if the end point for the determination of the erythema action spectrum is taken as a degree of redness greater than that of a minimally perceptible erythema, the 250 nm region will require much higher exposure doses, relative to the MED, than will the 300 nm region. Therefore, the 250 nm region will appear less effective in the plot of an action spectrum. Using the dose levels required to produce the

1. Van der Leun, J. C. (1972). On the action spectrum of ultraviolet erythema. *In* 'Research Progress in Organic, Biological and Medicinal Chemistry' (Eds, Gallo, U. and Santamaria, L.), Vol. 3, pt II. North-Holland (American Elsevier).
2. Everett, M. A., Olson, R. L. and Sayre, R. M. (1965). Ultraviolet erythema. *Arch. Derm.* **92**, 713.
3. Berger, D., Urbach, F. and Davies, R. E. (1968). The action spectrum of erythema induced by ultraviolet radiation. Preliminary report. *In* 'XIII Congressus Internationalis Dermatologiae' (Eds, Jadassohn, W. and Schirren, C. G.), Vol. 2, p. 1112. Springer, Berlin.
4. Van der Leun, J. C. (1966). Ultraviolet erythema. A study of diffusion processes in human skin. Thesis. Utrecht.
5. Hausser, K. W. and Vahle, W. (1927). Sonnenbrand und Sonnenbraunung. *Wiss. Veroff. Siemen-Konzern.* **6**, 101.

Table 4

Variation in true value of erythema with different criteria for the
definition of MED

Time of observation	260 nm Erythema		300 nm Erythema	
	Just perceptible	Defined boundaries	Just perceptible	Defined boundaries
7 h	1·2	2·5	1·3	2·5
24 h	2·4	5·0	1·9	3·6
Series of observations	1·0	2·4	1·0	2·0

These figures are presented to illustrate the possible variation in MED determination. They were obtained by determining the exposure dose required to produce the degree of erythema stated at the given time of observation and expressing this as the ratio of the actual MED. This was determined as the exposure dose required to produce a minimally perceptible erythema as observed with a series of readings (about 8 at time intervals between 6 and 13 h post-irradiation). They indicate that a 260 nm erythema observed with defined boundaries at 7 h after the exposure is actually 2·5 times the minimal erythema. The dose given to obtain this is 2·5 times the true MED. Similarly, a 300 nm erythema which is just perceptible at 7 h after the exposure is the result of a dose 1·3 times the true MED. These figures are an approximation and are presented to illustrate the possible variation in MED determinations.

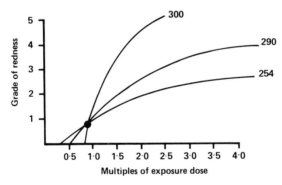

Fig. 3. Variation in degree of redness obtained with different multiples of the MED at different wavelengths.

intense erythema associated with a natural sunburn, the curve obtained shows a single peak around 295 nm with no apparent erythemal activity below 280 nm. A similar action spectrum is obtained if dose levels are used which produce an erythema lasting for 8 days.[1]

1. Hausser and Vahle (1927). Sonnenbrand und Sonnenbraunung. *Wiss. Veroff. Siemen-Konzern.* **6**, 101.

Another factor which may influence the shape of the erythema action spectrum is the anatomical site. It has already been mentioned that the skin's sensitivity to UVR decreases towards the extremities. Olson and his colleagues illustrated this in some detail with respect to 300 nm radiation (Table 5).[1] They also demonstrated that there was a greater change for both 260 nm and 280 nm than for 300 nm. They considered this to be due to the greater thickness of the horny layer of the skin on the forearm and leg. This increase in the keratin layer would lead to an increase in the specific protein absorption band at 280 nm and would therefore tend to produce an exaggerated fall in the effectiveness of this wavelength to cause erythema. This in turn would exaggerate the trough at 280 nm in

Table 5

Variation in sensitivity to monochromatic UVR with body site[1]

	MED mJ cm^{-2} (approximate figures)		
	300 nm	280 nm	260 nm
Abdomen	21	20	10
Chest	21		
Back	23		
Inner arm	36		
Outer arm	37		
Inner forearm	44	82	32
Outer forearm	48		
Leg	80	100	64
Face	22		

1. Olson, R. L., Sayre, R. M. and Everett, M.A. (1966). Effect of anatomic location and time on ultraviolet erythema. *Archs Derm.* **93,** 211.

an action spectrum obtained with forearm skin compared with that of back skin. The value of about 20 mJ cm^{-2} for the 300 nm MED on trunk skin, appears to be reasonable according to Magnus,[2] although in his own studies he reports a range from 9 to 120 mJ cm^{-2}. In tests on 35 normal subjects we have found that a narrow range of only 15–39 mJ cm^{-2} was required for the MED of monochromatic 300 nm radiation (half

1. Olson, R. L., Sayre, R. M. and Everett, M. A. (1966). Effect of anatomic location and time on ultraviolet erythema. *Arch. Derm.* **93**, 211.
2. Magnus, I. A. (1964). Studies with a monochromator in the common idiopathic photodermatoses. *Br. J. Derm.* **76**, 245.

maximum bandwidth; 5 nm) on the back, but it is probable that with a larger and more heterogeneous population a greater range would have been obtained.

Although the details of the action spectrum published by different authors vary in the wavelength region below 295 nm, there is general agreement concerning the rapid fall in erythemagenic activity with increasing wavelength so that, beyond 320 nm, the relative erythemal effectiveness requires to be plotted on a logarithmic scale. When this is done (Fig. 4) it can be seen that for the minimal perceptible erythema the exposure dose required at 335 nm is approximately 100 times that at

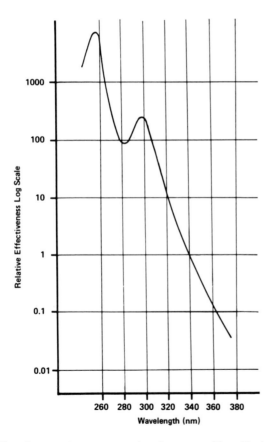

Fig. 4. The UV-erythema action spectrum plotted on a semi-logarithmic scale to include wavelengths in the UV-A.

300 nm. For 365 nm the exposure dose is some 1000 times that required at 300 nm. A number of studies[1, 2, 3] with wide band UV-A sources (320–400 nm), with a preponderance of wavelengths around 365 nm, have confirmed that the MED for the longer UVR is around 30 J cm^{-2}.

A comparison using the band UV-B from the Westinghouse FS40 sunlamp fluorescent tubes gave a value of 30 mJ cm^{-2}, confirming the dose ratio of 1000:1 for the two wavelength regions.[4] For erythema due to 335 nm radiation recent studies do not produce such well matched results: laser radiation at 337·1 nm requires 10 to 30 J cm^{-2} to elicit a minimal erythema,[5] and our own series with broad band 335 nm radiation (half maximum bandwidth: 30 nm) shows an average of around 10 J cm^{-2} for the MED. The fall in erythemal effectiveness with increasing wavelength is therefore probably more rapid than is shown for the idealized action spectrum in Figure 4.

The time course and dose response relationships for erythemas due to these longer wavelengths appear to vary within the UV-A range; the concept of a typical UV-A erythema is therefore doubtful. The 337·1 nm laser radiation induced erythema resembles that for UV-B in that it has a latent period of some hours and reaches its peak intensity about 24 h after exposure. When the irradiance is high, an immediate erythema due to a local heating effect may be observed.[5] With a broad band UV-A source in which the 365 nm region predominates, or with solar-simulating UV-A sources, the exposure dose required to elicit a delayed erythema is such that an immediate erythema is also produced.[6, 7, 8] In one report, this immediate erythema fades to be replaced by the delayed response at around 24 h.[9] Parrish and his colleagues state that a delayed erythema

1. Parrish, J. A., Ying, C. Y., Pathak, M. A. and Fitzpatrick, T. B. (1974). Erythemogenic properties of long-wave ultraviolet light. In 'Sunlight and Man' (Ed., Fitzpatrick, T. B.), p. 131. University of Tokyo Press, Tokyo.
2. Tannenbaum, L., Parrish, J. A., Pathak, M. A., Anderson, R. R. and Fitzpatrick, T. B. (1975). Tar phototoxicity and phototherapy for psoriasis. Arch. Derm. **111**, 467.
3. Willis, I. and Cylus, L. (1977). UV-A erythema in skin: Is it sunburn? J. invest. Derm. **68**, 128.
4. Parrish, J. A., Anderson, R. R., Urbach, F. and Pitts, D. (1978). 'UV-A. Biological Effects of Ultraviolet Radiation with Emphasis on Human Responses to Longwave Ultraviolet', p. 119. Plenum Press, New York.
5. Parrish, J. A., Anderson, R. R., Ying, C. Y. and Pathak, M. A. (1976). Cutaneous effects of pulsed nitrogen gas laser irradiation. J. invest. Derm. **67**, 603.
6. Hausser, I. (1938). Über spezifische Wirkungen des Langwelligen ultravioletten Lichts auf die Menschliche Haut. Strahlentherapie **62**, 315.
7. Bachem, A. (1955). Time factors of erythema and pigmentation produced by ultraviolet rays of different wavelength. J. invest. Derm. **25**, 215.
8. Buettner, K. J. K. (1968). The effects of natural sunlight on human skin. In 'The Biologic Effects of Ultraviolet Radiation (with emphasis on skin)' (Ed., Urbach, F.), p. 257. Pergamon Press, Oxford.
9. Pathak, M. A., Riley, F. C. and Fitzpatrick, T. B. (1962). Melanogenesis in human skin following exposure to long-wave ultraviolet and visible light. J. invest. Derm. **39**, 435.

may be produced by 365 nm radiation with no immediate erythemal response provided sufficiently low irradiances on fair skinned subjects are used.[1] However, according to Hauser,[2] a typical 385 nm erythema is produced at the end of the exposure which reaches a maximum intensity by about 5 h and then rapidly fades to be replaced by pigmentation. The detection of the immediate erythema may be confused by an immediate pigmentation which is also characteristically produced by these longer wavelengths.[3] The studies of Willis, Kligman and Epstein[4] were concerned mainly with the effect of this immediate pigmentation response in relation to the subsequent skin reactions to UV-B irradiation. They showed that UV-A exposures of three to six times that required for an immediate reaction of either erythema or pigmentation failed to produce an erythema which persisted for 24 h. A further study[5] showed that the UV-A dose required for an immediate erythema is some four times that required for immediate pigmentation, but the threshold erythema fades by 4–6 h. To obtain a reaction which persists for 24 h, the UV-A exposure is approximately four times the immediate erythema dose. Our own studies with solar simulating UV-A have produced results in agreement with the latter view; the threshold immediate erythema fades rapidly. It is suggested that this erythema might be a localized heating effect due to the absorption of non-specific energy.[6] However, the reaction is apparently specific for the longer wavelengths of the UV spectrum and the energy required is less than that calculated to be necessary for the production of a heat erythema alone.[7]

It is obvious from the above discussion that the investigations of the erythema action spectrum have failed in most of the criteria for "ideal" action spectroscopy. Perhaps the most noticeable point of difference between the study of erythema in man and the investigations of wavelength dependency in ideal systems is that there appear to be three

1. Parrish, J. A., Anderson, R. R., Urbach, F. and Pitts, D. (1976). 'UV-A, Biological Effects of Ultraviolet Radiation with Emphasis on Human Responses to Longwave Ultraviolet', p. 119. Plenum Press, New York.
2. Hausser, I. (1938). Über spezifische Wirkungen des langwelligen ultravioletten Lichts auf die menschliche Haut. *Strahlentherapie* **62**, 315.
3. Buettner, K. J. K. (1968). The effects of natural sunlight on human skin. *In* 'The Biologic Effects of Ultraviolet Radiation (with emphasis on skin)' (Ed., Urbach, F.), p. 237. Pergamon Press, Oxford.
4. Willis, I., Kligman, A. M. and Epstein, J. H. (1972). Effects of long ultraviolet rays on human skin: Photoprotective or photoaugmentative? *J. invest. Derm.* **59**, 416.
5. Kaidbey, K. H. and Kligman, A. M. (1978). The acute effects of long-wave ultraviolet radiation on human skin. *J. invest. Derm.* **72**, 253.
6. Bücker, H. (1960). Zur Abgrenzung des UV-Erythems durch das unspezifische strahlungserythem. *Strahlentherapie* **111**, 404.
7. Berger, D. S. (1969). Specification and design of solar ultraviolet simulators. *J. invest. Derm.* **53**, 192.

separate mechanisms for the production of vasodilatation at the various wavelength regions used in the study. Nevertheless, investigations of erythema action spectra have played a major role in establishing the characteristics of these different mechanisms. Moreover, the investigation of these effects has in itself initiated much fruitful research.

III. EPIDERMAL HYPERPLASIA AND SUNBURN

Thickening of the epidermis is a significant component of a mild sunburn reaction, and also of the reaction produced by moderate doses of either UV-B or UV-C. In the first 48 h after exposure there is some thickening due to inter- and intracellular oedema, but by 72 h there is an increased mitotic rate of the cells in the basal layer leading to hyperplasia. When the acute inflammatory stage has subsided, all layers of the epidermis appear thickened. In the absence of further stimulation, the epidermis returns to normal after about 2 months.

Epidermal homeostasis is a complex process involving a number of interacting mechanisms.[1,2,3] Epidermal chalone is thought to effect control of mitosis in the basal layer by a negative feed back inhibition,[4,5,6] and it is feasible that the chalone–adrenalin complex responsible for this inhibition is directly inactivated by UVR. The delay in the increased basal mitotic rate may be explained by the damaging UVR effects on the basal cells themselves. However, a release from mitotic inhibition may be better explained, as in the cases of wound responses and the hyperplasia following tape stripping by an interruption of the synthesis of chalone brought about by damage to the cells which produce it.[7,8] In skin exposed to UVR there is a significant, transient blocking of DNA synthesis and

1. Jarrett, A. (1973). Epidermal kinetics. In 'The Physiology and Pathophysiology of the Skin' (Ed., Jarrett, A.), Vol. 1, The Epidermis, p. 91. Academic Press, London, Orlando and New York.
2. Halprin, K. M. (1977). The control of epidermal cell proliferation: cyclic nucleotides and prostaglandins as 'second messengers'. In 'Psoriasis. Proceedings of the Second International Symposium' (Eds, Frabe, E. M. and Coc, A. J.), p. 122. Yorke Medical Books, New York.
3. Weinstein, G. D. (1979). Epidermal cell kinetics. In 'Dermatology in General Medicine'. 2nd Edition. (Eds, Fitzpatrick, T. B., Eisen, A. Z., Wolff, K., Freedberg, I. M. and Austen, K. F.), p. 85. McGraw-Hill, New York.
4. Iversen, O. H. and Evensen, A. (1962). Experimental skin carcinogenesis in mice. *Norweg. Monographs Med. Sci.* Norweg. Univ. Press, Oslo.
5. Bullough, W. S. (1972). The control of epidermal thickness. *Br. J. Derm.* **87**, 167.
6. Bullough, W. S. (1975). Mitotic control in adult mammalian tissues. *Biol. Rev.* **50**, 99.
7. Bullough, W. S. (1972). The control of epidermal thickness. *Br. J. Derm.* **87**, 187.
8. Pinkus, H. (1952). Examination of the epidermis by the strip method. *J. invest. Derm.* **19**, 431.

mitosis[1] with some indication of a disturbance in mitochondrial function,[2] but unfortunately there seems to have been no direct study of chalone activity in UV-irradiated skin.

Another aspect of the effect of UVR on epidermal cell turnover is illustrated by quantitative studies on the response of mouse ear epidermis to single exposure. Analysis of the results suggested that the increase in mitotic activity was caused by substances released from UV-damaged cells.[3] A later extension of this work demonstrated that growth stimulating substances could be extracted from UV-irradiated skin although no attempt was made to establish their identity.[4] More recently, it has been shown that UV-irradiation of the skin induced ornithine decarboxylase activity in the epidermis resulting in the synthesis of growth promoting polyamines such as spermine and spermidine.[5, 6]

The increased synthesis of prostaglandins following exposure of the skin to UVR may also have an effect on epidermal cell proliferation. However, the exact nature of this involvement is not clear. Greaves suggests that the formation of prostaglandin E_2 in the epidermis should result in a decreased epidermal cell turnover through increased levels of cellular cyclic adenosine monophosphate (cAMP).[7] This hypothesis is based on the association of decreased cAMP levels with increased proliferative states both *in vitro* and *in vivo*. However, this association is not clearly defined,[8] the increase in prostaglandin content of UV-irradiated skin is followed by an increase in DNA synthesis, and the intradermal injection of prostaglandin E_2 actually increases the number

1. Epstein, J. H., Fukuyama, K. and Fye, K. (1970). Effects of ultraviolet radiation on the mitotic cycle and DNA, RNA and protein synthesis in mammalian epidermis *in vivo*. *Photochem. Photobiol.* **12**, 57.

2. Johnson, B. E., Daniels, F., Jr and Magnus, I. A. (1968). Response of human skin to ultraviolet light. *In* 'Photophysiology', Vol. IV (Ed., Giese, A. C.), p. 139, Academic Press, London, Orlando and New York.

3. Soffen, G. A. and Blum, J. F. (1961). Quantitative measurements of changes in mouse skin following a single dose of ultraviolet light. *J. cell. comp. Physiol.* **58**, 81.

4. Blum, H. F. (1968). Hyperplasia induced by ultraviolet light: possible relationship to cancer induction. *In* 'The Biologic Effects of Ultraviolet Radiation (with emphasis on skin)' (Ed., Urbach, F.), p. 83. Pergamon Press, Oxford.

5. Lowe, N. J., Verma, A. K. and Boutwell, R. K. (1978). Ultraviolet light induces epidermal ornithine decarboxylase. *J. invest. Derm.* **71**, 417.

6. Verma, A. K., Lowe, N. J. and Boutwell, R. K. (1979). Induction of mouse epidermal ornithine decarboxylase activity and DNA synthesis by ultraviolet light. *Cancer Res.* **39**, 1035.

7. Greaves, M. W., Hensby, C. N., Black, A. K., Plummer, N. A., Fincham, N., Warin, A. P. and Camp, R. (1978). Inflammatory reactions induced by ultraviolet irradiation. *Bull. Cancer* **65**, 299.

8. Adachi, K. (1977). Epidermal cyclic AMP system and its possible role in proliferation and differentiation. *In* 'Biochemistry of Cutaneous Epidermal Differentiation' (Eds, Seiji, M. and Bernstein, I. A.), p. 288. University Park Press, Baltimore.

of DNA-synthesizing cells.[1] Moreover, although others have suggested that the increase in cAMP follows the UV-induced synthesis of prostaglandin which regulates cyclic nucleotide metabolism,[2] these increased cAMP levels in UV-irradiated pig skin occur later associated with the hyperplasia, rather than with the earlier inhibition of mitosis and DNA synthesis.[3] None the less, with repeated exposures to UVR, some reduction of the epidermal turnover rate occurs and the generalized hyperplasia is reduced to a greater extent than can be explained by an increase of protective mechanisms such as hyperpigmentation or hyper-keratosis.

Although melanin pigmentation has been proposed as the major protective component of the skin against UVR damage, the horny layer also plays a significant part. This is most clearly illustrated by the difficulty in eliciting a UV erythema in the skin of the palms of the hands or the soles of the feet. Calculations based on the relative thickness of the palmar and plantar horny layers have shown that a dose many thousand times the MED on trunk skin would be required. Even vitiliginous skin may be rendered less sensitive to UVR by repeated exposures,[4, 5] and Guillaume attributed this effect to the increased thickness of the horny layer.[6] This view was shared by Everett who demonstrated that epidermal hyperplasia and the resultant thickening of the horny layer was significantly greater in vitiliginous skin than in normally pigmented white skin following exposure to the same amount of radiation.[7]

In sun-tanned skin, the erythema threshold returns to normal at about the same time as the hyperplasia, well before the hyperpigmentation has faded.[8, 9 10] With mild UVR damage, in which only the outer layers of the

1. Eaglstein, W. H. and Weinstein, G. D. (1975). Prostaglandin and DNA synthesis in human skin: possible relationship to ultraviolet light effects. *J. invest. Derm.* **64**, 386.
2. Adachi, K., Yoshikawa, K., Halprin, K. M. and Levine, V. (1975). Prostaglandins and cyclic AMP in epidermis. *Br. J. Derm.* **92**, 381.
3. Halprin, K. M. (1976). Cyclic nucleotides and epidermal cell proliferation. *J. invest. Derm.* **66**, 339.
4. With, C. (1920). Studies of the effect of light on vitiligo. *Br. J. Derm.* **32**, 145.
5. Meyer, P. S. (1924). Gewöhnung vitilignöser Hautstellen an Ultraviolettes Licht und andere Reize. *Arch. Dermatol. u. Syphilis* **147**, 238.
6. Guillaume, A. C. (1926). Le pigment épidermique, la pénétration des rayons uv et la mécanisme de protection de l'organisme vis-à-vis de ces radiations. *Bull. mém. soc. méd. hôp. Paris* **50**, 1133.
7. Everett, M. A. (1961). Protection from sunlight in vitiligo. *Arch. Derm.* **84**, 997.
8. Perthes, G. (1924). Über Strahlenimmunität. *Munch. med. Wochschr.* **71**, 1301.
9. Schall, L. and Alius, H. J. (1928). Zur Biologie des Ultraviolettlichts. IV. Die Reaktion der menschlichen Haut auf widerholte Ultraviolettlichbestrahlung (Lichtschutz). *Strahlentherapie* **27**, 769.
10. Van der Leun, J. C. (1965). Delayed pigmentation and U.V. erythema. *In* 'Recent Progress in Photobiology'. Proceedings of the 4th International Photobiology Congress (Ed., Bowen, E. J.), p. 387. Blackwell Scientific Publications, Oxford.

viable epidermis are affected, the thickness of the protective stratum corneum is obviously an important factor. If the site for the primary photoreaction which is responsible for a threshold erythema response resides in the outermost living cells of the epidermis, then the horny layer must be the main physiological barrier to the radiation. Thus, the thickening of this layer following UV-induced hyperplasia is the major protective adaptation for these milder reactions. However, the mechanisms involved in this adaptation appear to be more complex than a simple thickening of the cell layers, since UV-induced changes in the protein content of the horny layer may on their own result in a decreased transmission of the radiation.[1] Also, Miescher showed that isolated horny layer did indeed become increasingly opaque to the sunburn wavelengths during exposure.[2]

IV. BIOCHEMICAL CHANGES IN UV-IRRADIATED SKIN

The morphologic characteristics of the various acute and chronic reactions of normal skin to sunlight are well established. However, the intermediate steps between the absorption of UVR in the skin and the development of these reactions have not been defined. In fact, neither the anatomical site nor the molecular nature of a primary target for the UV-induced changes in skin, has been determined. Some photochemical changes in complex molecules involve the production of free radicals and the detection of these reactive groupings in UV-irradiation skin may give some indication as to the nature of the target molecule involved. The majority of biomolecules may be affected by UVR but the wavelengths required may be in the short UV-C region and therefore the effects are not relevant to skin reactions to sunlight. However, in some cases, although the most effective wavelengths are in the UV-C, UV-B may also cause some effects. Deoxyribonucleic acid is probably the most likely candidate as the primary target for the biological effects of UVR and this will be discussed here in some detail. Thus, there is a great deal of information available from studies on micro-organisms and cells in culture, but also more attention has been recently paid to changes in living irradiated skin. Less is known about protein, carbohydrate and lipid, but there are good reasons for considering changes in these skin constituents as being of lesser importance. None the less, the processes

1. Hausmann, W. and Spiegel-Adolph (1927). Über Lichtschutz durch vorbestrahle Eiweisslosungen. *Klin. Wochschr.* **6**, 2182.
2. Miescher, G. (1980). Das Problem des Lichtschutzes und der Lichtgewöhnung. *Strahlentherapie* **35**, 403.

involved in sunburn and the chronic changes of premature ageing and carcinogenesis are complex and may well involve more than one kind of target molecule.

A. Free Radicals[1, 2]

Reactive free radicals are not necessarily involved in the photochemical events leading to the overall acute and chronic skin reactions to UVR. None the less, they have been detected in human skin exposed to moderate doses (30 to 60 mJ cm^{-2}) of 254 nm radiation.[3] Although low temperatures are required for their detection, the observation is probably relevant as a part of the overall reaction in living skin. Also with very high doses of wavelengths of up to 320 nm being virtually all UV-B irradiation, free radicals were detected in irradiated skin. Free radical signals were also detected in UV-irradiated negro specimens, but the yield was lower for the corresponding dose in white skin. Wavelengths beyond 320 nm failed to induce a free radical signal in "white" skin but were shown to enhance the natural, stable free radical, characteristic of melanin, in black skin.[4, 5]

B. Nucleic Acids

The possible role of nucleic acids in skin reactions to UVR was not examined in detail until after 1968, possibly because of technical difficulties.[6, 7] Some advance has been made since then[7] but interpretation of the findings of *in vitro* techniques in relation to the *in vivo* situation remains difficult. The relevance of the mass of data obtained with micro-organisms and cells in culture to the acute and chronic reactions of skin to sunlight is certainly not obvious.

1. Blois, M. S. (1961). 'Free Radicals in Biological Systems'. Academic Press, Orlando, New York and London.
2. Slater, T. F. (1972). 'Free Radical Mechanisms in Tissue Injury'. Pion Ltd, London.
3. Norins, A. L. (1962). Free radical formation in the skin following exposure to ultraviolet light. *J. invest. Derm.* **39**, 445–447.
4. Pathak, M. A. and Stratton, K. (1968). Free radicals in human skin before and after exposure to light. *Arch. Biochim. Biophys.* **123**, 468–476.
5. Pathak, M. A. and Stratton, K. (1969). Effects of ultraviolet and visible radiation and the production of free radicals in skin. *In* 'The Biologic Effects of Ultraviolet Radiation' (Ed., Urbach, F.), pp. 207–222. Pergamon Press, Oxford.
6. Johnson, B. E., Daniels, F., Jr and Magnus, I. A. (1968). Response of human skin to ultraviolet light. *In* 'Photophysiology Current Topics', Vol. IV (Ed., Giese, A. C.), pp. 139–202 Academic Press, Orlando, New York and London.
7. Johnson, B. E. (1978). Formation of thymine containing dimers in skin exposed to ultraviolet radiation. *Bull. Cancer* **65**, 283–298.

1. DNA as a Target for the Biologic Effects of UVR

The importance of DNA as a target for the biologic effects of UVR was first emphasized in 1928 when Gates showed the similarity between the absorption spectrum of the nucleic acid and the wavelength dependence for the killing of bacteria (Fig. 5).[1] The same relationship obtains for UVR-induced mutations.[2] The nucleus of animal cells was shown to be the major target for UVR effects by cytological engineering methods and the use of micro-beam UV-irradiation so that different cellular components could be irradiated separately.[3] The unique genetic and metabolic control exercised through nuclear DNA would suggest that while UV damage to other duplicating biomolecules such as RNA may have little effect on the cell as a whole, a similar amount of molecular damage to its DNA would be catastrophic.

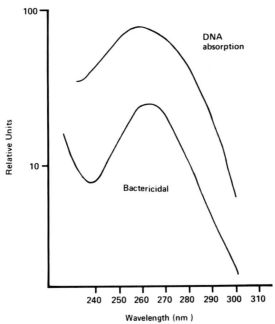

Fig. 5. The absorption spectrum of DNA and a typical action spectrum for the UV-induced killing of bacteria.

1. Gates, F. L. (1928). On nucleic derivatives and the lethal action of ultraviolet light. *Science* **68**, 479.
2. Zelle, N. R. and Hollaender, A. (1955). Effects of radiation on bacteria. *In* 'Radiation Biology' (Ed., Hollaender, A.), Vol. II, pp. 365–430. McGraw-Hill, New York.
3. Giese, A. C. (1964). Studies on ultraviolet radiation action upon animal cells. *In* 'Photophysiology', Vol. II (Ed., Giese, A. C.), pp. 203–246. Academic Press, Orlando, New York and London.

2. Pyrimidine Dimers as the Effective Photochemical Targets in DNA

Despite extensive investigations of DNA photochemistry[1,2] the results had little relevance to the biologic effects of UVR until 1960 when Beukers and Berrends[3] demonstrated the major photoproducts in UV-irradiated frozen aqueous solutions of thymine as being cyclobutyl dimers. These dimers, formed by photoaddition at the 5, 6 positions of the thymine molecules were later isolated from UV-irradiated bacteria, including *Haemophilus influenzae*[4,5,6] and from various eukaryote cell types in culture[7,8] (Fig. 6).

Most studies of the photochemical changes of DNA have used 3H-thymidine labelling techniques and radiochemical analysis. The isolated dimers have, therefore, necessarily contained thymine. However, cytosine containing dimers are also formed.[9] Because both thymine–thymine (TT) and thymine–cytosine (TC) dimers are included in the radiochemical assay results, these photochemical lesions in DNA are best termed pyrimidine dimers or thymine containing dimers.

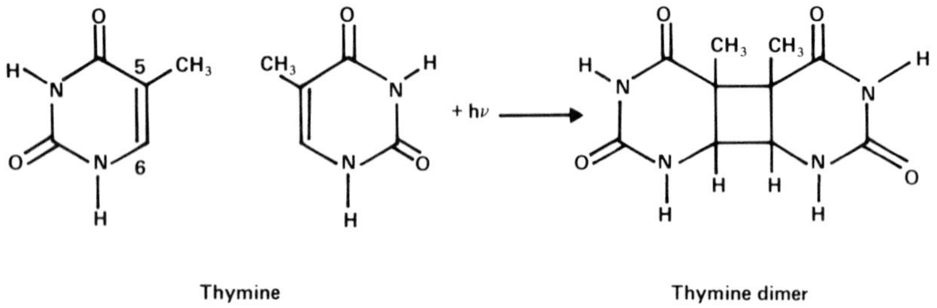

Thymine   Thymine dimer

Fig. 6. The UV-induced formation of cyclobutane type dimer of thymine at the 5,6 double bond.

1. McLaren, A. D. and Shugar, D. (1964). *In* 'Photochemistry of Proteins and Nucleic Acids'. Pergamon Press Inc., New York.
2. Smith, K. C. and Hanawalt, P. C. (1969). *In* 'Molecular Photobiology', Academic Press, London, Orlando and New York.
3. Beukers, R. and Berrends, W. (1960). Isolation and identification of the product of thymine. *Biochim. Biophys. Acta* **41**, 550–551.
4. Wacker, A., Dellweg, H. and Weinblum, D. (1960). Strahlenschemische Veranderung der Nucleinsauren *in vivo* und *in vitro*. I. *Mitteil. Naturwiss* **47**, 477.
5. Smith, K. C. (1964). Photochemistry of the nucleic acids. *In* 'Photophysiology', Vol. II (Ed., Giese, A. C.), pp. 329–388. Academic Press, Orlando, New York and London.
6. Setlow, R. B. and Setlow, J. K. (1962). Evidence that ultraviolet-induced thymine dimers in DNA cause biological damage. *Proc. natn. Acad. Sci. U.S.A.* **48**, 1250–1257.
7. Trosko, J. E., Chu, E. H. Y. and Carrier, W. L. (1965). The induction of thymine dimers in ultraviolet-irradiated mammalian cells. *Radiation Res.* **24**, 667–672.
8. Painter, R. B. (1970). The action of ultraviolet light on mammalian cells. *In* 'Photophysiology', Vol. V (Ed., Giese, A. C.), pp. 169–190. Academic Press, Orlando, New York and London.
9. Setlow, R. B. and Carrier, W. L. (1966). Pyrimidine dimers in ultraviolet-irradiated DNAs. *J. mol. Biol.* **17**, 237–254.

In native DNA, dimers may only be formed between neighbouring bases on the same strand. Figure 7 shows how TT dimers may appear in UV-irradiated DNA.

Pyrimidine dimers may interfere with the transcription process by which the metabolic activity of the cell is controlled and this effect may be lethal. Moreover, the presence of dimers in the replication template may result in blocks in the DNA synthesis sequence. If the dimers are by-passed, the daughter strand DNA will contain gaps which will result in the death of the new generation cells. Any repair at this stage is "error prone" and may give rise to lethal or non-lethal mutations in the new generation.

In an aqueous solution of thymine, dimers formed by exposure to 280 nm radiation revert to the monomer when exposed to shorter wavelength UVR around 240 nm. This aspect of photochemistry represents a wavelength dependent equilibrium reaction in which the

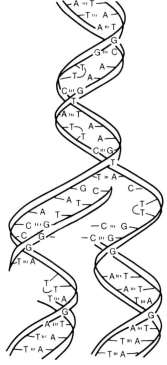

Fig. 7. The double helix of DNA during semi-conservative replication containing UV-induced thymine dimers. On the right hand replication fork, the dimer had blocked DNA synthesis while on the left, a gap has been left in the newly formed daughter strand.

steady-state conditions favour the monomer at shorter wavelengths.[1] This short wavelength reversal phenomenon appears to be specific for pyrimidine dimers. Therefore, the finding that the induced inactivation of the "infectivity" of transforming DNA by 280 nm radiation is also reversed by subsequent exposure to 240 nm radiation, is good evidence that these dimers are involved in this particular biologic effect of UVR.[2]

To reach equilibrium conditions a high proportion of adjacent pyrimidines must be in dimer form, and the dose requirement for such a state, even in prokaryote cell types (i.e. bacteria with relatively small genomes) is some 100 times the mean lethal dose (about $10 \, J \, m^{-2}$)[3] Therefore, it must be emphasized that short wavelength reversal cannot be used to demonstrate pyrimidine dimers in reactions of higher cellular systems. However, the greater the number of adjacent thymines present in a given DNA species, the greater is the UV-induced damage.[4] Also photoreactivation, a non-damaging form of dimer reversal extensively reviewed by Setlow[5] and Cook,[6] exists in most cell types. Such photoenzymatic repair[7] (PER) was described by Kelner[8] with respect to bacteria and by Dulbecco[9] with reference to bacteriophage. This type of repair is dependent on long wavelength UVR (320–390 nm). Even the longer UVR and visible radiation are also able to induce enzymatic splitting of the pyrimidine dimers.

The photoreactivating enzyme has been observed in varying amounts in all genera examined, but it could not be detected in plancental mammals. More recently, an apparent photoenzymic repair has been

1. Setlow, R. B. (1961). The action spectrum for the reversal of the dimerization of thymine induced by ultraviolet light. *Biochim. Biophys. Acta* **49**, 237–238.
2. Setlow, R. B. and Setlow, J. K. (1962). Evidence that ultraviolet-induced thymine dimers in DNA cause biological damage. *Proc. natn. Acad. Sci. U.S.A.* **48**, 1250–1257.
3. Jagger, J. (1976). Ultraviolet inactivation of biological systems. *In* 'Photochemistry and Photobiology of Nucleic Acids' (Ed., Wang, S. Y.), Vol. 2, pp. 147–186. Academic Press, Orlando, New York and London.
4. Setlow, J. K. (1964). Effects of UV on DNA: correlations among biological changes, physical changes and repair mechanisms. *Photochem. Photobiol.* **3**, 405–413.
5. Setlow, J. K. (1966). The molecular basis of biological effects of ultraviolet radiation and photoreactivation. *In* 'Current topics in Radiation Research', Vol. 2 (Eds, Ebert, M. and Howard, A.), pp. 195–248.
6. Cook, J. S. (1970). Photoreactivation in animal cells. *In* 'Photophysiology', Vol. V (Ed., Giese, A. C.), pp. 191–233. Academic Press, Orlando, New York and London.
7. Rubert, C. S. (1964). Photoreactivation of ultraviolet damage. *In* 'Photophysiology', Vol. II (Ed., Giese, A. C.), pp. 283–327. Academic Press, Orlando, New York and London.
8. Kelner, A. (1949). Effect of visible light on the recovery of Streptomyces griseus conidia from ultraviolet irradiation injury. *Proc. natn. Acad. Sci. U.S.A.* **35**, 73–79.
9. Dulbecco, R. (1949). Reactivation of ultraviolet inactivated bacteriophage by visible light. *Nature* **163**, 949–950.

identified in human cells,[1,2] but photoreactivation of UVR effects in mammalian systems does not seem to be a common event. In transforming DNA, short wavelength reversal and PER are complementary. In various cell types, UV-induced inhibition of DNA synthesis, mutagenesis and cell death were reversed by "PER" and therefore probably result from pyrimidine dimer formation.

A second repair mechanism was first recognized in 1963.[3] Following irradiation UVR-resistant strains of *E. coli* overcame blocks produced in their DNA synthesis when incubated in the dark, but UV-sensitive strains did not show this recovery. The processes involved in this dark recovery, defined as "excision repair" include the recognition of the lesion in the DNA, the enzymatic incision into the strand, and the removal of the lesion. The resulting gap in the DNA strand is filled in by the synthesis of the required nucleotide sequence of the partner strand. The finding that thymine containing dimers were present in acid soluble extracts of UV-irradiated cells at a time when the numbers of dimers in the DNA itself were apparently decreasing[4,5] have been amplified by studies which demonstrated the repair synthesis stage[6] and identified the enzymes involved.[7] The excision of pyrimidine dimers from UV-irradiated mammalian cells was first observed by Regan and his colleagues in human cells.[8] Earlier studies had mainly used rodent cell lines[9,10] which have little or no excision repair capacity.[11] "Unscheduled DNA synthesis" after UV-irradiation was demonstrated autoradiographically ("light

1. Sutherland, B. M. (1974). Photoreactivating enzyme from human leukocytes. *Nature* **248**, 109–112.

2. Sutherland, B. M. (1978). Photoreactivation in mammalian cells. *Int. Rev. Cytol.* Supplement **8**, 301–334.

3. Setlow, R. B., Swenson, P. A. and Carrier, W. L. (1963). Thymine dimers and inhibition of DNA synthesis by ultraviolet irradiation of cells. *Science* **142**, 1464–1466.

4. Setlow, R. B. and Carrier, W. L. (1964). The disappearance of thymine dimers from DNA: an error correcting mechanism. *Proc. natn. Acad. Sci. U.S.A.* **51**, 226–251.

5. Boyce, R. P. and Howard-Flanders, P. (1964). Release of ultraviolet light-induced thymine dimers from DNA in *E. coli* K-12. *Proc. natn. Acad. Sci. U.S.A.* **51**, 293–300.

6. Pettijohn, D. and Hanawalt, P. (1964). Evidence for repair-replication of ultraviolet damaged DNA in bacteria. *J. mol. Biol.* **9**, 395–410.

7. Grossman, L. (1974). Enzymes involved in the repair of DNA. *In* 'Advances in Radiation Biology', Vol. 4, pp. 77–129.

8. Regan, J. P., Trosko, J. E. and Carrier, W. L. (1968). Evidence for excision of ultraviolet-induced pyrimidine dimers from the DNA of human cells *in vitro. Biophys. J.* **8**, 319–325.

9. Trosko, J. E., Chu, E. H. Y. and Carrier, W. L. (1965). The induction of thymine dimers in ultraviolet-irradiated mammalian cells. *Radiat. Res.* **24**, 667–672.

10. Klimek, M. (1966). Thymine dimerisation in L-strain mammalian cells after irradiation with ultraviolet light and the search for repair mechanisms. *Photochem. Photobiol.* **5**, 603–607.

11. Meyn, R. E., Vizard, D. I., Hewitt, R. R. and Humphrey, R. M. (1974). The fate of pyrimidine dimers in the DNA of ultraviolet-irradiated Chinese hamster cells. *Photochem. Photobiol.* **20**, 221–226.

labelling") by the uptake of 3H-thymidine into the DNA of cells which were not in the S phase of normal replication.[1] This process is almost certainly a manifestation of repair replication, being the base insertion part of the excision repair process. Normal human skin fibroblasts can excise up to 70% of pyrimidine dimers, and they possess efficient excision repair with a high degree of unscheduled DNA synthesis after UV-irradiation. The importance of pyrimidine dimers as photochemical lesions in human cells following UV radiation is demonstrated by the decreased excision repair efficiency of fibroblasts and other cell lines from patients with xeroderma pigmentosum.[2, 3] The increased sensitivity of some variants of xeroderma pigmentosum cells to at least the lethal effects of UVR, whilst still exhibiting a normal level of excision repair, appears related to a deficiency in a third repair process known as post replication repair. Semi-conservative DNA synthesis can take place when the parental DNA contains thymine dimers but the newly formed, daughter strand will have gaps where the template was damaged (Fig. 8). Post replication repair (or daughter strand repair) is directed to the filling in of these gaps by processes which are not, as yet, exactly defined.[4, 5] This latter repair process may be very important for rodent cell lines which appear to be deficient in excision repair. The evidence for the primary role of pyrimidine dimers in the UV-induced damage to isolated DNA and also to transforming DNA appears incontrovertible. As the cellular organization becomes increasingly complex, the involvement of other DNA lesions must be considered. For example, in radiation-resistant organisms whose repair processes for pyrimidine dimers are very efficient, DNA-protein linking may be the main cause of damage.[6] None the less, the evidence obtained from the pyrimidine dimer repair studies at all levels of cellular organization suggests that these dimers do play a major role in UVR-induced inhibition of DNA synthesis, mutagenesis and cell death.

The repair of UV-induced damage to DNA has been actively investigated. As the complex molecular mechanisms involved are

1. Rasmussen, R. E. and Painter, R. B. (1966). Radiation-stimulated DNA synthesis in cultured mammalian cells. *J. Cell Biol.* **29**, 11.
2. Cleaver, J. E. (1970). DNA damage and repair in light-sensitive human skin diseases. *J. invest. Derm.* **54**, 181–195.
3. Cleaver, J. E. (1973). Xeroderma Pigmentosum, DNA repair and carcinogenesis. *In* 'Current Research in Oncology' (Eds, Anfinsen, G. B., Potter, N. and Schechter, A. N.), pp. 15–42. Academic Press, Orlando, New York and London.
4. Rupp, W. D. and Howard-Flanders, P. (1968). Discontinuities in the DNA synthesised in an excision defective strain of *Escherichia coli* following ultraviolet irradiation. *J. mol. Biol.* **31**, 291–304.
5. Lehmann, A. R. (1974). Post replication repair of DNA in mammalian cells. *Life Sci.* **15**, 2005–2016.
6. Smith, K. C. (1966). Physical and chemical changes induced in nucleic acids by ultraviolet light. *Radiat. Res.* Supplement **6**, 54–79.

unravelled, they appear similar to those due to chemical and ionizing radiation damage. The three major pathways for repair are illustrated in simple diagrammatic form in Fig. 8. These will be referred to later in the section on xeroderma pigmentosum and other related light sensitivity conditions (see page 2522).

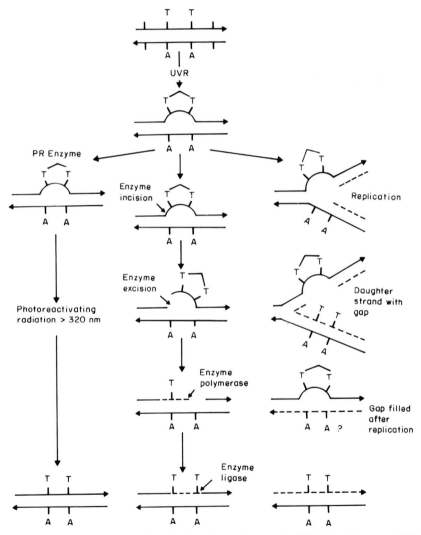

Fig. 8. Diagrammatic representation of the 3 major repair process for UV-induced damage to DNA. T = Thymine; A = Adenine; TT = Thymine dimer. On the left is Photoreactivation. In the centre is Excision repair. On the right is the so-called Post Replication repair.

There are a number of excellent reviews of the subject[1,2,3] which include discussions of more recent findings concerning single base excision compared with nucleotide excision mechanisms. The latter is an emergency repair process involved in trans-dimer DNA synthesis.

3. DNA as a Target for the Effects of UVR on Skin

Just as the similarity of the bacteriocidal action spectrum to the absorption spectrum of DNA was taken as evidence that DNA may be the primary target site, so the short wavelength peak of the erythema action spectrum[4] was thought to indicate that DNA is a target for UV-erythema. However, on these grounds the erythema action spectrum could well have protein or even sterol as its primary target, the complex shape of the curve being attributed to the filtering effects of the stratum corneum. The loss of basophilia and Schiff base staining of epidermal nuclei after UV-irradiation[5] does not appear until some 8–24 h after exposure, and may be due to nuclear oedema resulting from secondary rather than primary damage to DNA. There is little quantitative change in the DNA of mouse skin exposed to massive doses of UVR *in vitro* although certain phospholipids were decreased.[6]

Epstein and his colleagues,[7] using hairless mice, first showed that DNA changes occurred early in UVR effects on the skin. Within 1 h of an exposure to 4.5×10^3 J m^{-2} of polychromatic radiation below 320 nm, both the epidermal mitotic rate and DNA synthesis were significantly decreased. This UVR dose appears to be some eight times the threshold for producing vascular reactions in hairless mouse skin but is still probably an order of magnitude less than that required for enzyme inactivation. A block in the DNA template may well explain the inhibition of DNA synthesis, as this occurs in irradiated micro-organisms

1. Hanawalt, P. C. and Setlow, R. B. (1975). (Eds). Molecular mechanisms for repair of DNA Parts A and B. Plenum Press, New York.
2. Friedberg, E. C., Cook, K. H., Duncan, J. and Mortelmans, K. (1977). DNA repair enzymes in mammalian cells. *In* 'Photochemical and Photobiological Reviews' (Ed., Smith, K. C.), Vol. 2, pp. 263–322.
3. Hanawalt, P. C., Cooper, P. K., Ganesan, A. K. and Smith, C. A. (1979). DNA repair in bacteria and mammalian cells. *Ann. Rev. Biochem.* **48**, 783–836.
4. Johnson, B. E., Daniels, F., Jr and Magnus I. A. (1968). Response of human skin to ultraviolet light. *In* 'Photophysiology Current Topics', Vol. IV (Ed., Giese, A. C.), pp. 139–202. Academic Press, Orlando, New York and London.
5. Hamperl, H., Henschke, V. and Schulze, R. (1939). Vergleich der Hautreaktionen beim Bestrahlungserythem und bei der direkten Pigmentierung. *Virchows Arch. Path. Anat.* **304**, 19–33.
6. Tickner, A. (1963). Changes in phospholipids of mouse skin after ultraviolet irradiation *in vitro*. *Biochem. J.* **88**, 80–84.
7. Epstein, J. H., Fukuyama, K. and Epstein, W. L. (1968). UVL induced stimulation of DNA synthesis in hairless mouse epidermis. *J. invest. Derm.* **51**, 455.

and cells in culture. There is also inhibition of DNA synthesis in human epidermis after *in vivo* irradiation,[1] in hairless mouse,[2] rabbit[3] and guinea-pig[4] skin. In whole, haired albino mouse skin the maximum inhibition of DNA synthesis is apparent 2 h after exposure regardless of the dose or wavelength used. With fluorescent sunlamps (Westinghouse FS 20, 285–335 nm; peak 310 nm) the threshold dose for producing a vascular reaction, approximately 1×10^3 J m^{-2}, results in 20% inhibition of DNA synthesis. An exposure dose of $1 \cdot 3 \times 10^4$ J m^{-2} results in 80% inhibition of DNA synthesis and produces a marked vascular reaction with stasis followed by necrosis.

Autoradiographic studies of Epstein and his colleagues[5] using 3H-thymidine and UV-irradiated hairless mouse skin was the first demonstration of "light-labelling" of skin irradiated *in vivo*. This very sparse labelling was present in all layers of the epidermis within 5 min of exposure, maximal at 20 min and markedly reduced after 2 h. This may represent the repair replication phase of a deficient repair process as occurs in cultured rodent cells. If this is so, it is good evidence that DNA is directly damaged in living skin exposed to UVR. Also, because pyrimidine dimers are the major photochemical lesions in irradiated DNA and undergo this style of repair, this has been taken as evidence for the presence of pyrimidine dimers in UV-irradiated skin.[2] A typical pattern of "sparse" labelling also occurs in normal human skin exposed to UVR *in vivo* (Fig. 9), but not in irradiated skin from xeroderma pigmentosum patients which has an excision repair deficiency.[1, 6] This again is indirect evidence that UVR damages DNA in living skin and that the damage may be pyrimidine dimers.

Damage to the DNA of both epidermal and dermal cells in living human and mouse skin exposed to UVR has also been demonstrated

1. Epstein, W. L., Fukuyama, K. and Epstein, J. H. (1969). Early effects of ultraviolet light on DNA synthesis in human skin *in vivo*. *Arch. Derm.* **100**, 84–89.
2. Jung, E. G., Johnert, E., Erbs, G., Knobloch, G. C. and Muller, S. (1971). Wavelength dependence of UV induced alterations of epidermal cells in hairless albino mice. *Arch. Derm. Forsch.* **241**, 284–291.
3. Cripps, D. J., Ramsay, C. A., Carter, J. and Boutwell, R. K. (1972). Effect of monochromatic UV radiation on DNA synthesis with *in vivo* and *in vitro* autoradiography. *J. invest. Derm.* **58**, 312–314.
4. Kramer, D. M., Bathak, M. A., Kornhauser, A. and Wiskermann, A. (1974). Effect of ultraviolet irradiation on biosynthesis of DNA in guinea pig skin *in vivo*. *J. invest. Derm.* **62**, 388–393.
5. Epstein, J. H., Fukuyama, K. and Epstein, W. L. (1968). UVL induced stimulation of DNA synthesis in hairless mouse epidermis. *J. invest. Derm.* **51**, 445.
6. Epstein, J. H., Fukuyama, K., Reed, W. B. and Epstein, W. L. (1970). Defect in DNA synthesis in skin of patients with xeroderma pigmentosum demonstrated *in vivo*. *Science* **168**, 1477–1478.

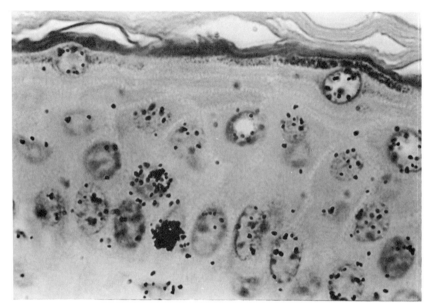

Fig. 9. Excision repair in epidermis exposed to UVR *in vivo* as indicated by sparse labelling throughout all cell layers with tritiated thymidine. Heavy labelling over one nucleus of the basal layer is indicative of normal semi-conservative DNA replication. (Courtesy of John H. Epstein, M.D.)

using fluorescent antibodies to UV-irradiated native DNA.[1,2] Studies using radioimmune assay techniques with amphibian cells in which UV-induced pyrimidine dimers are reversed by photoreactivation, have shown that antibodies mounted against UV-irradiated DNA have a high specificity for these dimers.[3] However, the sensitivity of the fluorescence method appears to be low; the threshold dose for positive fluorescence after 254 nm radiation in hairless mouse skin is at least $2100 \, \text{J m}^{-2}$, some five times that for the classical radiochemical method which itself is also very insensitive when used under *in vivo* conditions.[2] Moreover, small amounts of pyrimidine dimers are detectable in mammalian cells exposed to natural sunlight.[4] However, using "solar simulator UVR", no nuclear

1. Tan, E. M. and Stoughton, R. B. (1969). Ultraviolet light induced damage to deoxyribonucleic acid in human skin. *J. invest. Derm.* **52**, 537–541.
2. Jarzabek-Chorzelska, M., Zarebska, Z., Wolska, H. and Rzesa, G. (1976). Immunological phenomena induced by UV rays. *Acta dermatogener.* **56**, 15–18.
3. Cornelis, J. J., Rommelaere, J., Urbain, J. and Errera, M. (1977). A sensitive method for measuring pyrimidine dimers in situ. *Photochem. Photobiol.* **26**, 241–246.
4. Trosko, J. E., Krause, D. and Isoun, M. (1970). Sunlight-induced pyrimidine dimers in human cells *in vitro*. *Nature* **228**, 358–359.

fluorescence could be detected, even with 40 times the exposure dose required to elicit a minimal, visible skin reaction.

4. Identification of Thymine-Containing Dimers in UV-Irradiated Skin

Pathak and his colleagues[1] were the first to isolate thymine-containing dimers from UV-irradiated skin by radiochemical analysis. Bowden and his colleagues[2] also successfully isolated pyrimidine dimers from irradiated living mouse skin. The extraction of DNA was accomplished by a similar method to that of the Pathak group, but the dimer separation was achieved by two-dimensional paper chromatography.[3] The complex procedure for labelling the basal cell DNA that was used in these studies illustrates the technical problem of employing radiochemical techniques. Because the dimer yield is expressed as a percentage of the total DNA radioactivity in the dimer peak, and because this may be as little as 0·04%, a high efficiency of labelling is essential. Cooke and Johnson[4] obtained areas of synchronous growth with high DNA synthesis rates by plucking the flanks of albino mice to stimulate the hair growth cycle.

Ley and his colleagues[5] demonstrated the induction of pyrimidine dimers in mouse skin epidermis by the assay of endonuclease-sensitive sites in DNA. The method appears to be as sensitive as the radiochemical method, and 89% of endonuclease-sensitive sites were identified as pyrimidine dimers by the use of a yeast photoreactivating enzyme. The identification, isolation and quantitation of pyrimidine dimers in living human skin exposed to UVR or sunlight requires a more sensitive methodology, and this may now be available in the form of monoclonal antibody labelling techniques. See ref. 6 for more recent information.

5. Pyrimidine Dimer Yields in UV-Irradiated Skin

The difficulties in studies involving living skin were illustrated by our

1. Pathak, M. A., Kramer, D. M. and Gungerich, V. (1972). Formation of thymine dimers in mammalian skin by ultraviolet radiation *in vivo*. *Photochem. Photobiol.* **15**, 177–185.
2. Bowden, G. T., Trosko, J. E., Shapas, B. G. and Boutwell, R. K. (1975). Excision of pyrimidine dimers from epidermal DNA and nonsemiconservative epidermal DNA synthesis following ultraviolet irradiation of mouse skin. *Cancer Res.* **35**, 3599–3607.
3. Carrier, W. L. and Setlow, R. B. (1971). The excision of pyrimidine dimers (the detection of dimers in small amounts). *In* 'Methods in Enzymology' (Eds, Grossman, L. and Moldave, K.), Vol. XXI, pp. 230–237. Academic Press, New York.
4. Cooke, A. and Johnson, B. E. (1978). Dose response, action spectrum and rate of excision of ultraviolet radiation-induced thymine dimers in mouse skin DNA. *Biochim. biophys. Acta* **517**, 24–30.
5. Ley, R. D., Sedita, A., Grube, D. D. and Fry, R. J. M. (1977). Induction and persistence of pyrimidine dimers in the epidermal DNA of two strains of hairless mice. *Cancer Res.* **37**, 3243–3248.
6. Sutherland, B. M., Harber, L. C. and Kochevar, I. (1980). Pyrimidine dimer formation and repair in human skin. *Cancer Res.* **40**, 3181–3185.

work. Using monochromatic 260 nm radiation $(260 \pm 7.8 \, nm)$,[1] we obtained dimer yields of 0·07% with 2000 J m^{-2} and 0·16% with 5200 J m^{-2}: these low figures are explained by the fact that whole skin was assayed for dimers and much of the DNA was at a depth not reached by the incident UVR. The technique is therefore weighted against a high dimer yield. Similar results were obtained with 290 ± 7.8 nm radiation for which there was a greater overall dimer yield (Table 5). This shows two effects, one directly related to the formation of dimers at a single level within the skin, and the other which is dependent on the formation of dimers at deeper levels as the exposure dose is increased. The dimer yields with "sunlamp" fluorescent tube exposure (Westinghouse FS-20, emission 280–400 nm, peak 315 nm) were also low: a total UVR dose of between 12 and 13 000 J m^{-2} produced only 0·08% dimers.

The dimer yield obtained from guinea-pig skin by Pathak's group appears rather high for the dose of UVR given (Table 6). This was

Table 6

Pyrimidine dimers in skin irradiated *in vivo*

Wavelenth (nm)	Exposure dose (J m^{-2})	Dimer radioactivity as % of total in DNA
254	640	1·2, 0·46
285–350	600	0·4, 0·6, 0·6
320–400	194000	0
Pathak, Kramer and Gungerich (1972)		
254	420	0·076
	840	0·130
	1680	0·196
	5040	0·566
	8000	0·560
Bowden, Trosko, Shapas and Boutwell (1975)		
260	2000	0·070
	5200	0·160
290	500	0·016
	1000	0·045
	1500	0·105
	2000	0·144
	3000	0·177
	4000	0·137
	8000	0·240
Cooke and Johnson (1978)		

1. Cooke, A. and Johnson, B. E. (1978). Dose response, action spectrum and rate of excision of ultraviolet radiation-induced thymine dimers in mouse skin DNA. *Biochim. biophys. Acta* **517**, 24–30.

irrespective of whether the UVR was from a low pressure mercury arc (99% 254 nm), or from a medium pressure source 285–350 nm): the most effective radiation being in the 297–313 nm region. With the latter source, an increase in exposure dose gave rise to an increase in dimer yield, but the dose response relationship is extremely complex. Bowden and his colleagues[1] used 254 nm radiation exclusively and were unable to obtain as high a dimer yield. The dose response curve is almost linear over an order of magnitude before a plateau is reached at what appears to be a low yield value.

Ley and his colleagues[2] using "sunlamp" radiation reported a yield of 0.9×10^{-10} endonuclease sensitive sites per dalton of DNA per J m^{-2}. For an exposure of 10 000 J m^{-2}, this is equivalent to approximately 0.2% radioactivity in the dimer region which compares favourably with our results.

In vitro studies have shown that dimer yields with 254 or 260 nm radiation increase linearly with increasing dose over a range from 50 to 1000 J m^{-2}. Yields for an exposure dose of 100 J m^{-2} from the results of various studies with cells in monolayer culture are shown in Table 7. The basal layer of guinea-pig or mouse skin might be considered as a monolayer of cells, shielded against radiation by the superficial epidermal cell layers. An approximation of the exposure dose at the basal layer level could be obtained by calculation based on the known transmittance of mouse epidermis or, alternatively, human stratum corneum. For 254 nm radiation, these values are 5% and 8% respectively and they have been used to calculate the dimer yield produced by 100 J m^{-2} at the basal cell layer from the data obtained by Pathak's group and also by Bowden and his colleagues. The calculations show that the results obtained by Bowden fit well with the data obtained *in vitro*, but those of Pathak's group show a yield which is greater by a factor of at least four.

6. Wavelength Dependence for Pyrimidine Dimer Formation

An action spectrum for thymine dimer formation in aqueous thymine solutions shows a peak around 260 nm with a rapid fall off at longer wavelengths so that the relative effectiveness of 290 nm radiation is 10% of the maximum, and that of 300 nm radiation only about 2.5%.[3] The

1. Bowden, G. T., Trosko, J. E., Shapas, B. G. and Boutwell, R. K. (1975). Excision of pyrimidine dimers from epidermal DNA and nonsemi-conservative epidermal DNA synthesis following ultraviolet irradiation of mouse skin. *Cancer Res.* **35**, 3599–3607.
2. Ley, R. D., Sedita, A., Grube, D. D. and Fry, R. J. M. (1977). Induction and persistence of pyrimidine dimers in the epidermal DNA of two strains of hairless mice. *Cancer Res.* **37**, 3243–3248.
3. Deering, R. A. and Setlow, R. B. (1963). Effects of ultraviolet light on thymidine dinocleotide and polynucleotide. *Biochim biophys. Acta* **68**, 526–534.

Table 7

Pyrimidine dimers formed by 100 J m^{-2} 254 or 260 nm radiation in a variety of cells and in skin. Expressed as % of total DNA radioactivity

Cells	Hamster	Trosko et al. (1965)[1]	0·47
		*Meyn et al. (1974)[2]	0·41
	Mouse	Klimek (1966)[3]	0·14
		Horikawa et al. (1968)[4]	0·24
		Ben-Ishai and Peleg (1974)[5]	0·42
			0·49
		London et al. (1976)[6]	0·46
	Human	Cleaver (1970)[7]	0·48
Skin			
	Guinea-pig	Pathak et al. (1972)[8]	1·6 (a)
			2·4 (b)
	Mouse	*Bowden et al. (1975)[9]	0·19 (a)
			0·32 (b)

* Extrapolation from given data based on linearity from 50–1000 J m^{-2}.
(a) Adjusted for 8% transmittance of 260 nm through human stratum corneum.
(b) Adjusted for 5% transmittance of 260 nm through mouse epidermis.

1. Trosko, J. E., Chu, E. H. Y. and Carrier, W. L. (1965). The induction of thymine dimers in ultraviolet-irradiated mammalian cells. *Radiat. Res.* **24**, 667, 672.
2. Meyn, R. E., Vizard, D. I., Hewitt, R. R. and Humphrey, R. M. (1974). The fate of pyrimidine dimers in the DNA of ultraviolet-irradiated Chinese hamster cells. *Photochem. Photobiol.* **20**, 221–226.
3. Klimek, M. (1966). Thymine dimerisation in L-strain mammalian cells after irradiation with ultraviolet light and the search for repair mechanisms. *Photochem. Photobiol.* **5**, 603–607.
4. Horikawa, M., Mikaido, O. and Sugahara, T. (1968). Dark reactivation of damage induced by ultraviolet light in mammalion cells *in vitro*. *Nature* **218**, 489–491.
5. Ben-Ishai, R. and Peleg, L. (1975). Excision repair in primary cultures of mouse embryo cells and its decline in progressive passages and established cell lines. *Basic Life Sci.* **58**, 607–610.
6. London, D. A., Carter, D. M. and Condit, E. S. (1976). Effect of pigment on photomediated production of thymine dimers in cultured melanoma cells. *J. invest. Derm.* **67**, 261–264.
7. Cleaver, J. E. (1970). DNA damage and repair in light-sensitive human skin diseases. *J. invest. Derm.* **54**, 181–195.
8. Pathak, M. A., Kramer, D. M. and Gungerich, V. (1972). Formation of thymine dimers in mammalian skin by ultraviolet radiation *in vivo*. *Photochem. Photobiol.* **15**, 177–185.
9. Bowden, G. T., Trosko, J. E., Shapas, B. G. and Boutwell, R. K. (1975). Excision of pyrimidine dimers from epidermal DNA and nonsemiconservative epidermal DNA synthesis following ultraviolet irradiation of mouse skin. *Cancer Res.* **35**, 3599–3607.

wavelength dependence for thymine containing dimer induction in micro-organisms shows a shift in maximum effectiveness to 270 nm.[1]

A study of unscheduled DNA synthesis in normal human fibroblasts revealed a complex wavelength dependency with little difference between 260 and 280 nm radiation. The effectiveness of 300 nm was consistently less, while no unscheduled DNA synthesis was induced with 320 nm radiation.[2] In hairless mouse epidermis irradiated *in vivo*, the peak of effectiveness for producing "sparse labelling" was around 280–290 nm. The 300–320 nm region was some 10 times less effective, and, surprisingly, so was the 250–260 nm region.[3] Fluorescent antibody technique showed that UVR from 254 to 300 nm was effective in inducing photochemical lesions in the DNA of hairless mouse epidermis, irradiated *in vivo*.[4] Approximately four times more radiant energy was required at 310 nm, but with this wavelength some indication of DNA damage in the dermis was also observed. Although the "labelling" technique may not be specific for pyrimidine dimers, the fluorescence method probably is, and it is a pity that a more detailed action spectrum study was not undertaken.

Tyrrell[5] induced pyrimidine dimers in *E. coli* with 365 nm radiation. However, as the exposure dose required to obtain 0.1% radioactivity in the dimer region was in the order of 2×10^7 J m^{-2}, this would appear to have little practical meaning in the present context. Work with guinea-pig skin *in vivo* employed different sources of radiation in the skin, 254 nm, 285–350 nm and 320–400 nm. Beyond 320 nm dimers were not produced with intensities of approximately 2×10^5 J m^{-2} of radiation. Equivalent exposure doses of 254 nm and 285–350 nm produced approximately the same dimer yield, but transmittance differences of these two wavelengths through the superficial epidermis result in different levels of irradiance of the basal cells. Human stratum corneum transmits 8% of 260 nm, 10% of 290 nm, 20% of 300 nm, and 35% of 310 nm radiations. An intensity of

1. Setlow, J. K. and Boling, M. E. (1965). The resistance of *Micrococcus radiodurans* to ultraviolet radiation. II. Action spectra for killing, delay in DNA synthesis and thymine dimerization. *Biochim. biophys. acta* **108**, 259–265.
2. Ichihashi, M. and Ramsay, C. A. (1976). The action spectrum and dose response studies of unscheduled DNA synthesis in normal human fibroblasts. *Photochem. Photobiol.* **23**, 103–106.
3. Jung, E. G., Bohnert, E., Erbs, G., Knobloch, G. V. and Muller, S. (1971). Wavelength dependence of UV induced alterations of epidermal cells in hairless albino mice. *Arch. Derm. Forsch.* **241**, 241–291.
4. Tan, E. M., Freeman, R. G. and Stoughton, R. B. (1970). Action spectrum of ultraviolet light-induced damage to nuclear DNA *in vivo*. *J. invest. Derm.* **55**, 439–443.
5. Tyrrell, R. M. (1973). Induction of pyrimidine dimers in bacterial DNA by 365 nm radiation. *Photochem. Photobiol.* **17**, 69–73.
6. Trosko, J. E. and Kasschau, M. R. (1967). Study of pyrimidine dimers in mammalian cells surviving low doses of ultraviolet radiation. *Photochem. Photobiol.* **6**, 215–219.

$640 \, J \, m^{-2}$ of 254 nm radiation at the skin surface would therefore deliver approximately $50 \, J \, m^{-2}$ of energy at the basal layer while an incident dose of $600 \, J \, m^{-2}$ of the longer wavelengths would be in the region of $120 \, J \, m^{-2}$ at the bottom of the epidermis. Therefore, the changes in basal cell irradiation due to differences in wavelength transmission in living skin would give a result which approaches the results obtained *in vitro*.

Cooke and Johnson[1] studied the wavelength dependence for thymine-containing dimer formation in mouse skin *in vivo* using a single dose level of $2 \times 10^3 \, J \, m^{-2}$ at 260, 280, 290, 300 and 310 nm. With this system, 290 nm was the most effective wavelength, while the yields obtained with 280 and 300 nm appear approximately equal. The shortest radiation is slightly less effective but the yield with 310 nm is only 10% of that with 290 nm. The low yield with 310 nm radiation is similar to that obtained with the "sunlamp" fluorescent tube which, although only 10% of that obtained at 290 nm, has a greater relevance for skin exposed to natural sunlight (Fig. 10).

This action spectrum is also dependent upon the variable penetration into the skin of the different wavelengths. The dimer yield could be adjusted by taking into account the known transmittance of whole mouse epidermis. When this is done, it becomes apparent that an action spectrum is obtained which closely resembles that for cells in monolayer culture (Table 8). This is of value in that it illustrates how an action spectrum having little relationship to the absorption spectrum for thymine is produced when the photochemical reaction occurs within a complex medium such as skin.

7. The Persistence of Dimers in UV-Irradiated Skin

The original investigations of excision repair in mammalian cells used rodent cell lines where no dimer excision was detected.[2, 3] However, thymine containing dimers were found in high yield in post replication DNA.[4] In contrast, normal human cells revealed efficient dimer

1. Cooke, A. and Johnson, B. E. (1978). Dose response, action spectrum and rate of excision of ultraviolet radiation-induced thymine dimers in mouse skin DNA. *Biochim. biophys. Acta* **517**, 24–30.
2. Trosko, J. E. and Kasschau, M. R. (1967). Study of pyrimidine dimers in mammalian cells surviving low doses of ultraviolet radiation. *Photochem. Photobiol.* **6**, 215–219.
3. Klimek, H. (1966). Thymine dimerisation in L-strain mammalian cells after irradiation with ultraviolet light and the search for repair mechanisms. *Photochem. Photobiol.* **5**, 603–607.
4. Meyn, R. E., Vizard, D. I., Hewitt, R. R. and Humphrey, R. M. (1974). The fate of pyrimidine dimers in the DNA of ultraviolet-irradiated Chinese hamster cells. *Photochem. Photobiol.* **20**, 221–226.

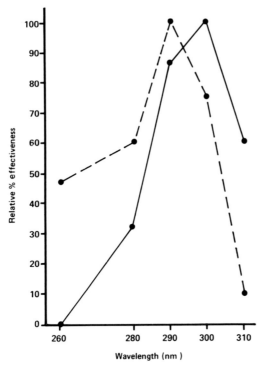

Fig. 10. Action spectra for UV-induced thymine dimer formation (– – – –) and for inhibition of DNA synthesis (———) in mouse skin.

Table 8

Transmittance of mouse epidermis wholeskin dimer yield and adjusted dimer yield at different wavelengths of UVR

Wavelength (nm)	Transmittance (%)	Dimer yield	Adjusted dimer yield
260	5	0·068	1·36
280	7	0·087	1·24
290	16	0·144	0·90
300	40	0·108	0·27
310	48	0·015	0·03

excision[1, 2] and low levels of excision were later detected in rodent cells exposed to low doses of UVR.[3, 4]

Autoradiographic studies have shown a high degree of "sparse labelling" in a specific mouse cell line.[5] Mouse embryo cells in early culture exhibit efficient excision of dimers which is lost in older cultures.[6] The significance of this observation in relation to adult mouse skin is difficult to assess, as Bowden and his colleagues demonstrated repair replication in irradiated living mouse skin. They suggest that the basal layer cells exist in a quasi-embryonic state so that they retain their excision function, and therefore the results do not conflict with the data obtained from the cultural studies. Unfortunately, there is no correlation between the data presented for repair replication and that for loss of dimers; moreover, the small number of animals used in the dimer study introduces problems in assessing the significance of the decreased dimer yield.

Ley and his group were unable to detect a decrease in endonuclease sensitive sites in UV-irradiated mouse skin over a 24-h period and suggest that the results obtained by Bowden and his co-workers depend upon the loss of a population of cells containing a high dimer concentration rather than being due to an excision of dimers. Cooke and Johnson were unable to detect any decrease in dimer yield 24 h after exposure of 8×10^3 J m^{-2} of 290 nm radiation, but with a lower dose, 2×10^3 J m^{-2}, the dimer yield showed a continuing decrease over a 72-h period. These results related to dimers present in whole skin, and thus there is a strong possibility that they represent a loss of dimer-containing superficial cells whilst unaffected 3H-thymidine labelled cells persist in the deeper region. If dimer excision does occur here, it is less efficient than in normal human cells *in vitro*. Dimer excision in normal human skin *in vivo* is probably similar to that demonstrated *in vitro*, so that, although this form of repair may play an important part in the reactions of human skin to UVR, some other repair process is involved in mouse skin.

1. Regan, J. P., Trosko, J. E. and Carrier, W. L. (1968). Evidence of excision of ultraviolet induced pyrimidine dimers from the DNA of human cells *in vitro*. *Biophys J.* **8**, 319–325.
2. Painter, R. B. and Cleaver, J. E. (1969). Repair replication, unscheduled DNA synthesis and the repair of mammalian DNA. *Radiat. Res.* **37**, 451–466.
3. Lehmann, A. R. (1972). Post replication repair of DNA in ultraviolet irradiated mammalian cells. *Eur. J. Biochem.* **31**, 433–445.
4. Setlow, R. B., Regan, J. D. and Carrier, W. L. (1972). Different levels of excision repair in mammalian cell lines. Abstr. 16th Annual Biophysical Society Meeting, Toronto, p. 19a.
5. Zajdella, F., Yoshikura, H. and Szafarz, D. (1977). DNA repair in cultured mouse cells induced by UV irradiation or polycyclic aromatic hydrocarbons; influence of caffeine. Colloques internationaux du C.N.R.S. Canceroganese Chimique, No. 256, 389–405.
6. Peleg, L., Haz, E. and Ben-Ishai, R. (1976). Changing capacity for DNA excision repair in mouse embryonic cells *in vitro*. *Exp. Cell Res.* **104**, 301–307.

There is now unequivocal evidence that thymine-containing dimers are formed in mammalian skin exposed to UVR *in vivo*. Any reaction such as cell death, inhibition of DNA synthesis, or the induction of mutation, might be ascribed to pyrimidine dimer formation in other UV-irradiated biological systems and, therefore, can also be reasonably related to such reactions in skin. At the present time, however, there is no good evidence for a cause–effect relationship. There is some direct evidence that UV-induced DNA-protein linking occurs in skin,[1] and indirect evidence that this is of importance in the inhibition of cell proliferation in the skin after exposure to UV.[2, 3]

8. RNA in Skin Photobiology

The major UV-induced changes in RNA are the formation of uracil dimers and the hydration of cytosine; protein binding may also occur[4] The majority of studies have been with viruses in which RNA is the genetic determinant and UV-irradiation results in inactivation.[5] In higher organisms, photochemical lesions of transfer, messenger or ribosomal RNA would be expected to interfere with the nucleotide coding for protein synthesis.

There is an immediate inhibition of RNA synthesis in UV-irradiated skin[6] which, with moderate exposure doses, is restricted to the suprabasal layers of the epidermis.[7] Such inhibition may well be due to photobiological changes in the nuclear DNA. However, because it occurs so rapidly, there is also probably an inhibition of protein synthesis due to direct damage to ribosomal RNA.[8]

1. Pathak, M. A. and Zimmermann, E. (1974). Biochemical changes in epidermal nucleic acids following UV irradiation. In 'Progress in Photobiology', Proc. of VI International Congress on Photobiology. (Ed., Schenck, G. O.). Deutsche Gesellschaft für Lichtforschung e.V., Frankfurt.
2. Cooke, A. and Johnson, B. E. (1976). Deoxyribonucleic acid in skin reactions to ultraviolet radiation. *J. invest. Derm.* **66**, 262, Abs.
3. Shetlar, M. D. (1980). Cross-linking of proteins to nucleic acids by ultraviolet light. In 'Photochemical and Photobiological Reviews' (Ed., Smith, K. C.), pp. 105–197. Plenum Press, New York.
4. Smith, K. C. and Hanawalt, P. C. (1969). 'Molecular Photobiology', Academic Press, London, Orlando and New York.
5. Wang, S. Y. (Ed.) (1976). 'Photochemistry and Photobiology of Nucleic Acids'. Academic Press, London, Orlando and New York.
6. Baden, H. P. and Pearlman, C. (1964). The effect of ultraviolet light on protein and nucleic acid synthesis in the epidermis. *J. invest. Derm.* **48**, 71–75.
7. Fukuyama, K., Epstein, W. L. and Epstein, J. H. (1967). Effect of ultraviolet light on RNA and protein synthesis in differentiated epidermal cells. *Nature* **216**, 1031–1032.
8. Epstein, J. H., Fukuyama, K. and Fye, K. (1970). Effects of ultraviolet radiation on the mitotic cycle and DNA, RNA, and protein synthesis in mammalian epidermis *in vivo*. *Photochem. Photobiol.* **12**, 57–65.

C. Changes in Irradiated Proteins

Protein absorption spectra, showing a peak around 280 nm (Fig. 11) due mainly to the aromatic amino acids, tryptophan and tyrosine, are similar to the action spectra of UV-induced damage to micro-organisms and other cells in culture.[1,2] This stimulated studies of protein photochemistry. However, the successful correlation of photochemical lesions in DNA with the various biologic effects of UVR has been more widely accepted.[3,4]

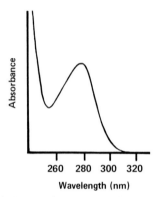

Fig. 11. The absorption of a typical protein (serum albumin) showing peak around 280 nm due to the aromatic amino-acid constituents.

Dose levels required to affect proteins in living cells are high and, therefore, marked effects of UVR on skin proteins exposed *in vivo* are unlikely to be demonstrated. Photochemical reactions in proteins, induced by small doses of radiation, are likely to be restricted to relatively minor structural changes. Thus, photolysis of amino acids such as tryptophan and the rupture of hydrogen and disulphide bonds, due to damage to the aromatic residues, are the major changes observed. Some enzymes are progressively inactivated as their tryptophan content is

1. McLaren, A. D. and Shugar, D. (1964). 'Photochemistry of Proteins and Nucleic Acids'. Pergamon Press, Oxford.
2. Giese, A. C. (1964). Studies on ultraviolet radiation action upon animal cells. *In* 'Photophysiology', Vol. II (Ed., Giese, A. C.), pp. 203–246. Academic Press, London, Orlando and New York.
3. Smith, K. C. and Hanawalt, P. C. (1969). 'Molecular Photobiology', Academic Press, London, Orlando and New York.
4. Painter, R. B. (1970). The action of ultraviolet light on mammalian cells. *In* 'Photophysiology' (Ed., Giese, A. C.), Vol. V. Academic Press, London, Orlando and New York.

destroyed, while in other enzymes, such as trypsin, the integrity of the disulphide bonds is essential for their activity. If such photochemical protein reactions occur in UV-irradiated skin the enzyme inactivation could result in breakdown of normal cell metabolism.

The changes in sulphur-containing groups in UV-irradiated skin are complex. There is an initial decrease in disulphide, but its relation to changes in enzyme activity is not clear.[1]

Polarographic studies appeared to show that psoriatic scales and dermal protein might be changed but normal epidermal protein appeared stable to UVR.[2] With high exposure doses, UV-irradiation may reduce the activity of skin enzymes such as succinic dehydrogenase, ATPase, acid phosphatase, beta glucuronidase, DNase and tyrosinase.[3, 4]

Also, glycolysis[5, 6] transaminase activity, glucose oxidation[7] and a number of respiratory dehydrogenases[8] are reduced in UV-irradiated skin, but there has been little attempt to determine the exposure doses required.

Studies of UV-induced enzyme inactivation *in vitro* appear to have little relevance to the reactions of living skin to sunlight as the exposure dose levels were high and 254 nm radiation was mainly used. Enzyme activity in isolated mitochondria is susceptible to this treatment,[9, 10] and similar changes have been detected in skin exposed to 20 times the minimally reactive dose, but lactic acid dehydrogenase, a free cytoplas-

1. Kusuhara, M. and Knox, J. M. (1962). Changes in the sulfhydryl and disulfide groups in animal skin following a single exposure to ultraviolet light. *J. invest. Derm.* **39**, 287–294.

2. Ogura, R., Knox, J. M. and Kusuhara, M. (1963). A polarographic study on the effects of ultraviolet light on scales, epidermis, dermis and serum. *J. invest. Derm.* **40**, 37–41.

3. Seiji, M. and Itakura, H. (1966). Enzyme inactivation by ultraviolet irradiation and protective effect of melanin *in vitro. J. invest. Derm.* **47**, 507–509.

4. Ogura, R., Kinoshita, A., Shimada, T., Murakami, M. and Knox, J. (1977). Effect of anti-inflammatory agents on the release of acid phosphatase in the epidermis following ultraviolet light exposure. *The Kurume Medical Journal* **24**, 121–129.

5. Wolgemuth, J. and Ikebata, T. (1927). Über die Milchsaurebildung in der Haut und ihre Beeinglusung durch verschiedene Strahlenarten. *Biochem. Z.* **186**, 43.

6. Rothman, S. (1954). *In* 'Physiology and Biochemistry of the Skin'. The Univ. of Chicago Press, Chicago, Illinois.

7. Coffey, W., Finkelstein, P. and Laden, K. (1963). The effect of UV irradiation on enzyme systems in the epidermis. *J. Soc. cosmet. Chem.* **14**, 55–63.

8. Im, M. J. C. (1969). Effect of ultraviolet light on some dehydrogenase activities in the epidermis of the rhesus monkey (Macaca multatta). *J. invest. Derm.* **52**, 329.

9. Barber, A. A. and Ottolenghi, A. (1957). Effect of ethylenediamine tetra-acetate on lipid peroxide formation and succinoxidase inactivation by ultraviolet light. *Proc. Soc. exp. Biol. Med.* **96**, 471–000.

10. Beyer, R. E. (1959). The effect of ultraviolet light on mitochondria. I. Inactivation and protection of oxidative phosphorylation during far-ultraviolet irradiation. *Arch. Biochem. Biophys.* **79**, 269–275.

mic enzyme, was unaffected.[1, 2] Under similar conditions, acid phosphatase activity was also reduced[3, 4] but, as discussed later (see page 2464), disruption of the mitochondrial and lysosomal membranes could produce similar effects. Also the decrease of amino acid incorporation into proteins and of nucleotides into RNA and DNA following UV-irradiation[5, 6] is better explained in terms of template damage rather than inactivation of the enzymes. Repair enzymes for damaged DNA are clearly not affected.[7] We have demonstrated that the exposure required to marginally inactivate enzymes for DNA synthesis is twice that required to produce an 80% inhibition of 3H-thymidine incorporation;[8] such a dose causes complete necrosis of mouse skin.

Also the decrease in collagen in chronically UVR exposed skin[9] appears to be a secondary rather than a direct effect on protein.[10] Depending on the nature of the collagen isolated, and the experimental conditions, *in vivo* irradiation can lead to increased cross link formation or their degradation.[11, 12, 13, 14] Increased cross linking also occurs in mammalian skin exposed to high doses of UVR.[15, 16] However, the doses used are well beyond likely exposure levels, and no such effect was observed by even a $50 \times$ MED exposure.[10]

1. Daniels, F., Jr and Johnson, B. E. (1974). Normal, Physiologic and Pathologic Effects of Solar Radiation on the Skin. *In* 'Sunlight and Man' (Ed., Fitzpatrick, T. B.), pp. 117–130. University of Tokyo Press, Tokyo.
2. Johnson, B. E. (1968). Ultraviolet Radiation and lysosomes in skin. *Nature* **219**, 1258–1259.
3. Fand, I. (1972). The protective effect of a sunscreen upon the lysosomes of ultraviolet-irradiated skin. *Dermatologica* **144**, 237–247.
4. Grossie, V. B., Jr and Black, H. S. (1977). The effect of ultraviolet light (UVL) on the lysosomes of hairless mouse epidermis. *Experientia* **33**, 425–426.
5. Baden, H. P. and Pearlman, C. (1964). The effect of ultraviolet light on protein and nucleic acid synthesis in the epidermis. *J. invest. Derm.* **48**, 71–75.
6. Epstein, J. H., Fukuyama, K. and Fye, K. (1970). Effects of ultraviolet radiation on the mitotic cycle and DNA, RNA and protein synthesis in mammalian epidermis *in vivo*. *Photochem. Photobiol.* **12**, 57–65.
7. Epstein, W. L., Fukuyama, K. and Epstein, J. H. (1969). Early effects of ultraviolet light on DNA synthesis in human skin *in vivo*. *Arch Derm.* **100**, 84–89.
8. Cooke, A. (1976). Doctoral Thesis in the University of Dundee, Scotland.
9. Sams, W. M., Jr and Smith, J. G., Jr (1965). Alterations in human dermal fibrous connective tissue with age and chronic sun damage. *In* Advances in Biology of the Skin', Vol. VI, 'Ageing' (Ed., Montagna, W.), pp. 199–210. Pergamon Press, Oxford.
10. Lovell, W. W. (1973). Ultraviolet irradiation of dermal collagen *in vivo*. I. Single doses of radiation. *Trans. St. John's Hosp. Derm. Soc.* **59**, 166–174.
11. Fujimori, E. (1966). Ultraviolet light irradiated collagen macromolecules. *Biochem.* **5**, 1034.
12. Davidson, R. J. and Cooper, D. R. (1967). The effect of ultraviolet irradiation on acid-soluble collagen. *Biochem. J.* **105**, 965.
13. Consden, R. and Kirrane, J. A. (1967). Action of ultraviolet light on soluble collagens. *Nature* **215**, 165.
14. Raab, W. (1969). Effects of ultraviolet light on human dermal collagen *in vitro*. *Arch. Klin. Exp. Derm.* **234**, 36.
15. Bottoms, E. and Shuster, S. (1963). Effect of ultraviolet light on skin collagen. *Nature* **199**, 192.
16. Bottoms, E., Cater, C. W. and Shuster, S. (1966). Effect of ultraviolet irradiation on skin collagen. *Nature* **211**, 97.

D. Effects of Irradiation on Carbohydrate[1,2]

Carbohydrate photochemistry in relation to photobiology is mainly concerned with the possible role in damage to deoxyribose in DNA. Although chain breakage may result from experimental photosensitization of deoxyribose, this is not a major photobiological event. Carbohydrate generally does not absorb wavelengths longer than 230 nm so that direct effects of UVR on skin carbohydrate would seem unlikely. Hyaluronic acid is depolymerized by UVR *in vitro*[3,4] and such an affect in the dermis would have important consequences in terms of water binding and its viscosity. However, dermal depolymerization *in vitro* requires high doses and this may not be detected until 24 h later. Any such change in skin *in vivo* is probably secondary, and this also applies to changes in glycosaminoglycans in chronically exposed skin.[5,6] Similarly, increased epidermal glycogen, resulting from an acute UV-exposure appears to be the result of the non-specific injury response, rather than a direct effect of UVR.[7,8] A decrease of the small amount of glycogen normally in the epidermis during the first 4 h following exposure is thought to be related to an increased cytoplasmic alpha-glucosidase activity, possibly following lysosome membrane damage.[9]

E. Urocanic Acid

Urocanic acid is an imidazole compound (4-imidazole acrylic acid, Fig. 12), first observed in relation to skin as a constituent of human sweat,[10] although this was probably an artefact.[11] It was shown to be a major UV-

1. McLaren, A. D. and Shugar, D. (1964). 'Photochemistry of Proteins and nucleic acids'. Pergamon Press, Oxford.
2. Smith, K. C. (1977). Ultraviolet Radiation Effects on Molecules and Cells. *In* 'The Science of Photobiology' (Ed., Smith, K. C.), pp. 113–142. Plenum Press, New York.
3. Balazs, E. A., Laurent, T. C., Howe, A. F. and Varga, L. (1959). Irradiation of mucopolysaccharides with ultraviolet light and electrons. *Radiat. Res.* **11**, 149.
4. Hvidberg, E., Kvorning, S. A., Schmidt, A. and Schon, J. (1959). Effect of ultraviolet irradiation on hyaluronic acid *in vitro. Acta Pharmacol. Toxicol.* **15**, 356.
5. Smith, J. C., Davidson, E. A. and Taylor, R. W. (1965). Human cutaneous acid mucopolysaccharides: the effects of age and chronic sun damage. *In* 'Ageing: Advances in Biology of Skin', Vol. VI (Ed., Montagna, W.), pp. 211–218. Pergamon Press, Oxford.
6. Summerly, R. and Jefferson, B. M. (1969). Sulphated acid mucopolysaccharides in actinic elastosis. *Br. J. Derm.* **81**, 51–55.
7. Daniels, F., Jr, Brophy, D. and Lobitz, W. C., Jr (1961). Histochemical responses of human skin following ultraviolet irradiation. *J. invest. Derm.* **37**, 351–356.
8. Ohkawara, A. and Halprin, K. M. (1967). Ultraviolet light and glycogen formation in the human epidermis. *Arch. Derm.* **95**, 416–420.
9. Ohkawara, A., Halprin, K. M. and Levine, V. (1972). Glycogen metabolism following ultraviolet irradiation. *J. invest. Derm.* **59**, 264–268.
10. Zenisek, A. and Kral, J. A. (1953). Occurrence of urocanic acid in human sweat. *Biochim. biophys. Acta* **12**, 479–480.
11. Brusilow, S. W. and Ikai, K. (1968). Urocanic acid in sweat: an artifact of elution from the epidermis. *Science* **160**, 1257.

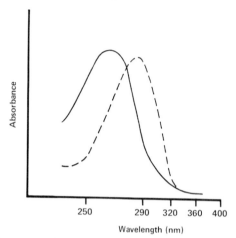

Fig. 12. The absorption spectra of Urocanic acid in different vehicles. ———— Aqueous. - - - - -
Ethanol. From: Parrish, J. A., Pathak, M. A. and Fitzpatrick, T. B. (1972). Topical protection
against germicidal radiation. *Arch. Surg.* **104**, 276.

absorbing component of human stratum corneum[1] and guinea-pig
epidermis.[2] At neutral pH, it exhibits an absorption spectrum peaking
around 270–280 nm extending into the region of sunburn UVR. Because
it is a deamination product of histidine urocanic acid is a normal
constituent of human epidermis.[3, 4] It persists in this situation because
urocanase, the enzyme responsible for its further degradation, is not
present in the skin.[5]

In unexposed skin, urocanic acid is present as the trans isomer. In
addition a photochemical change is observed *in vivo* as well as *in vitro*,
which involves a trans to cis isomerization; the absorbed energy being
dissipated by a dark reaction in the reverse direction.[5, 6, 7]

1. Spier, H. W. and Pascher, G. (1959). Die wasserloslichen Bestandteile der peripheren
   Hornschicht (Hautoberflache). Quantitative Analysen V. Das Substrat der UV-Absorption
   des Wasserloslichen. Urocaninsauregehalt der Hornschicht. *Arch. Klin. Exp. Derm.* **209**,
   181–193.
2. Tabachnick, J. (1957). Urocanic acid, the major acid soluble, ultraviolet absorbing compound in
   guinea pig epidermis. *Arch. Biochim. Biophys.* **70**, 295–297.
3. Everett, M. A., Anglin, J. H. and Bever, A. T. (1961). Ultraviolet induced biochemical
   alterations in skin. I. Urocanic acid. *Arch. Derm.* **84**, 717–719.
4. Baden, H. P. and Pathak, M. A. (1965). Urocanic acid in keratinizing tissue. *Biochim. biophys. Acta*
   104, 200–201.
5. Baden, H. P. and Pathak, M. A. (1967). The metabolism and function of urocanic acid in skin. *J.
   invest. Derm.* **48**, 11–17.
6. Anglin, J. H., Bever, A. T., Everett, M. A. and Lamb, J. H. (1961). Ultraviolet light-induced
   alterations in urocanic acid *in vivo*. *Biochim. biophys. Acta* **53**, 408–409.
7. Baden, H. P., Pathak, M. A. and Butler, D. (1966). Trans to cis isomerization of urocanic acid.
   Nature **210**, 732–733.

The cis isomer content of human epidermis is increased during the summer months.[1] Although the total urocanic acid content of epidermis may be decreased by exposure to UVR,[2] this requires a high dose and both isomer forms are equally reduced.[3] A single exposure to sunlight sufficient to produce erythema, results in a delayed increase in total urocanic acid,[4, 5] which may be due to an induced increase in histidase activity.[6]

Since the findings that urocanic acid in the trans isomer form might act as an endogenous sunscreen against UV-B effects,[3, 5] opinions have become divided, and it has been clearly stated that urocanic acid has no significant physiologic protection effect against UV-B, at least in the concentrations found in normal skin.[7]

Relatively high exposures of UVR result in the formation of a photodimer when urocanic acid is irradiated *in vitro*. This dimer has been isolated from guinea-pig skin exposed to approximately 8 MEDs of wavelengths between 280 and 320 nm.[8] Although this alternative photochemical change has been dismissed as irrelevant to amounts of radiation causing moderate skin damage,[5] it may yet prove to have an important role in reactions to prolonged exposure to UVR.

F. Lipid Involvement

While it is difficult to envisage metabolic lipids being involved in UV-induced damage to biological systems, structural lipid may certainly be one of the primary targets for such damage because of its importance in the maintenance of membrane integrity. Metabolic activities occur within discrete compartments comprising the complex membrane–vacuolar system of the cell. It has been suggested that barrier breakdown with enzyme release results from damage to the membrane

1. Pascher, G. (1962). Cis und Trans-Urocaninsaure als Bestandteile der Stratum corneum. *Arch. Klin. Exp. Derm.* **214**, 234–238.
2. Anglin, J. H., Bever, A. T., Everett, M. A. and Lamb, J. H. (1961). Ultraviolet light-induced alterations in urocanic acid *in vivo*. *Biochim. biophys. Acta* **53**, 408–409.
3. Baden, H. P. and Pathak, M. A. (1967). The metabolism and function of urocanic acid in skin. *J. invest. Derm.* **48**, 11–17.
4. Hais, I. M. and Strych, A. (1969). Increase of urocanic acid content in human epidermis following insolation. *Collection Czech. Chem. Commun.* **34**, 649–655.
5. Hais, I. M., Strych, A., Spacek, J., Zenisek, A. and Kral, J. A. (1970). The increase of epidermal imidazoleacrylic acid following insolation. *J. invest. Derm.* **55**, 39–46.
6. Anglin, J. H., Jones, D. H., Bever, A. T. and Everett, M. A. (1966). The effect of ultraviolet light and thiol compounds on guinea pig skin histidase. *J. invest. Derm.* **46**, 34–39.
7. Parrish, J. A., White, H. A. D. and Pathak, M. A. (1979). Photomedicine. *In* 'Dermatology in General Medicine' (Ed., Fitzpatrick, T. B.), 2nd edition, Eisen, A. Z., Wolff, K., Freedberg, I. M. and Austen, K. F., pp. 942–994. McGraw-Hill Book Co., New York.
8. Anglin, J. H. and Everett, M. A. (1964). Photodimerization of urocanic acid *in vitro* and *in vivo*. *Biochim. biophys. Acta* **68**, 492–501.

system, leading to a cessation of ordered cellular function and finally cell death.[1]

The exact molecular structure of cellular membranes remains to be elucidated, but it is clear that phospholipids, by virtue of hydrophilic groups at one end of the molecule, and insoluble fatty acids at the other, play a major role in the maintenance of membrane integrity. Cholesterol within critical limits appears to act as an additional stabilizing factor in membranes.

Light-induced changes to cholesterol have been known since the beginning of this century and there is a considerable literature relating to its photochemistry.[2] The importance of 7-dehydrocholesterol as a precursor for vitamin D in the skin has tended to divert attention from the possible involvement of cholesterol itself in UV-induced changes in biological systems.

Apart from sterols, lipids appear to exhibit little UV-absorbance above about 250 nm. However, an oxygen dependent lipid peroxidation may be induced by free radicals produced from isolated polyunsaturated fatty acids due to longer wavelength UV-irradiation.[3]

Biologic membranes may be disrupted by the addition of UV-irradiated polyunsaturated fatty acid,[4] and a similar disruption may follow the UV-induced lipid peroxidation of biomembranes.[5] The presence of polyunsaturated fatty acids, therefore, gives rise to a locus of potential instability within membranes. The formation of such lipid peroxide foci in the unsaturated fatty acids of membrane phospholipid may lead to large areas of potential instability. Such autoxidation can be counteracted by naturally occurring antioxidants such as alpha tocopherol and SH groups as well as by free-radical scavengers. However, alpha tocopherol is itself destroyed by UVR of wavelength 250–320 nm.[6] It would therefore appear that biomembranes are susceptible to UV

1. Bacq, Z. M. and Alexander, P. (1961). 'Fundamentals of Radiobiology', 2nd Edition, pp. 263–269. Pergamon Press, Oxford.
2. Mier, P. D. and Cotton, D. W. K. (1976). 'The molecular biology of skin'. Blackwell Scientific Publications, Oxford.
3. Wilbur, K. M., Bernheim, F. and Shapiro, D. W. (1949). The thiobarbituric acid reagent as a test for the oxidation of unsaturated fatty acids by various agents. *Arch. Biochem. Biophys.* **24**, 305.
4. Ottolenghi, A., Bernheim, F. and Wilbur, K. M. (1955). The inhibition of certain mitochondrial enzymes by fatty acids oxidized by ultraviolet light or ascorbic acid. *Arch. Biochem. Biophys.* **56**, 157–164.
5. Desai, I. D., Swant, P. L. and Tappel, A. L. (1964). Peroxidative and radiation damage to isolated lysosomes. *Biochim. biophys. Acta* **86**, 277–285.
6. |Kay, R. E. and Bean, R. D. (1970). Effects of radiation on artificial lipid membranes. *In* 'Advances in Biological and Medical Physics', Vol. 13 (Eds, Lawrence, J. H. and Gofman, J. W.), pp. 235–253. Academic Press, London, Orlando and New York.

damage by virtue of changes in their contained phospholipid, and cholesterol. However, studies of UV-induced haemolysis have shown that protein, rather than lipid, might be the membrane component that is specifically damaged.[1, 2] Nevertheless, in cell membranes generally, protein crosslinking and polyunsaturated fatty acid oxidation follow separate pathways in damaged membranes, and it is not clear whether one is more important than the other in the overall cellular effects of UVR.[3] What remains certain is that biomembranes can be damaged by UV-B radiation.

A decrease in freely extractable cholesterol in living human skin exposed to UVR or sunlight[4] can be shown to result from direct photochemical damage rather than to changes in metabolic function.[5] Lipid peroxides are formed in skin irradiated *in vivo* and the major site of reactivity appears to be the viable epidermis rather than surface lipids [6, 7, 8] (see below). The biologic consequences of lipid membrane damage in UV-irradiated skin, whether caused by cholesterol oxidation, or polyunsaturated fatty acid peroxidation in the phospholipid moiety,[9] may be mediated through two major pathways. The first results from an increase in membrane permeability, or rupture.[10, 11] The second depends on the release of fatty acid precursors resulting in the synthesis of prostaglandins and related compounds.[12]

Mitochrondrial oxidative respiration is somewhat impaired by ex-

1. Cook, J. S. (1956). Some characteristics of haemolysis by ultraviolet light. *J. Cell comp. Physiol.* **47**, 55–84.

2. Keohane, K. W. and Metcalf, W. K. (1959). *Physics Med. Biol.* **4**, 140–147.

3. Kochevar, I. E. (1980). Cell membrane damage due to ultraviolet radiation. *Abs. J. invest. Derm.* **74**, 256.

4. Rauschkolb, E. W., Farrell, G. and Knox, J. M. (1967). Effects of ultraviolet light on skin cholesterol. *J. invest. Derm.* **49**, 632–635.

5. Lo, W. B. and Black, H. S. (1972). Formation of cholesterol-derived photoproducts in human skin. *J. invest. Derm.* **58**, 278–281.

6. Dubouloz, P. and Dumas, J. (1954). Sur la formation de peroxides lipidiques dans la peau sous l'action des radiations. *In* 'Proceedings of the First International Photobiology Congress', pp. 247–248. Veenman and Zonen, Wageningen, The Netherlands.

7. Meffert, H. v. and Reich, P. (1969). Beeinflussung der Lipoperoxide der menschlichen Hautoberflache durch ultraviolette Strahlung *in vitro* und *in vivo*. *Derm. Mschr.* **155**, 948–954.

8. Meffert, H. v. and Reichmann, G. (1972). Lipidperoxydation an der menschlichen Hautoberflache durch erythemwirksame UV-Strahlung. *Acta biol. med. germ.* **28**, 667–673.

9. Tickner, A. (1963). Changes in the phospholipids of mouse skin after irradiation *in vitro*. *Biochem. J.* **88**, 80–88.

10. Johnson, B. E. and Daniels, F., Jr (1969). Lysosomes and the reactions of skin to ultraviolet radiation. *J. invest. Derm.* **53**, 85–94.

11. Daniels, F., Jr and Johnson, B. E. (1974). Effects of Solar Radiation on the Skin. *In* 'Sunlight and Man' (Ed., Fitzpatrick, T. B.), pp. 117–130. Univ. of Tokyo Press, Tokyo.

12. Black, A. K., Fincham, N., Greaves, M. W. and Hensby, C. N. (1980). Time course changes in levels of arachidonic acid and prostaglandins D, E, F, in human skin following ultraviolet B irradiation. *Br. J. clin. Pharmac.* **10**, 453–457.

posure to UVR *in vitro*,[1,2] probably due to membrane disturbance, and this occurs in UV-irradiated skin.[3] Unless there is massive membrane disruption, microsomes and endoplasmic reticulum do not appear to be greatly affected by UVR, although there may be a temporary inhibition of macromolecule synthesis. Minor damage to lysosome membranes, however, may have far reaching secondary effects which extend beyond the immediate photochemical event. The hydrolytic nature of the enzymes contained within lysosomes could result in digestion of vital cell constituents. At present, autolysis due to lysosome enzyme action is thought to result from cell death rather than to cause it, and lysosomes are considered as pleomorphic and multifunctional organelles.[4,5] None the less, there is evidence for their involvement in a number of pathological conditions, including radiation damage.

Hydrolytic enzymes including proteases are released from isolated rat liver lysosomes by treatment with vitamin A and a similar effect is obtained with UVR.[6] Both these actions are inhibited by hydrocortisone. The UV-induced enzyme release from lysosomes may be correlated with the UV exposure dose, free radical formation and with lipid per-oxidation.[7,8] Moreover, for a given dose, lipid peroxide effects on membranes are greater in lysosomes than in mitochondria.[7] These studies suggest that UV-induced changes in cells may in part be due to lysosome membrane damage. Microsomes are more susceptible to peroxide formation than lysosomes,[9] and it would appear that lipid peroxidation may produce a potential membrane defect which does not necessarily of itself lead to increased permeability or breakdown. The lysosome membrane seems to be a special case because the initial peroxidation may

1. Montgomery, P. O'B. and Reynolds, R. C. (1964). Cellular responses to ultraviolet radiation. *Lab. Invest.* **13**, 1243–1251.
2. Beyer, R. E. (1959). The effect of ultraviolet light on mitochondria I. Inactivation and protection of oxidative phosphorylation during far ultraviolet irradiation. *Arch. Biochem. Biophys.* **79**, 269–275.
3. Johnson, B. E. (1965). Doctoral Thesis, University of London.
4. Dingle, J. T. and Fell, H. B. (Eds) (1969–1975). 'Lysosomes in Biology and Pathology' (4 Vols). American Elsevier, New York.
5. Lazarus, G. S., Hatcher, V. B. and Levine, N. (1975). Lysosomes and the skin. *J. invest. Derm.* **65**, 259–271.
6. Weissman, G. and Dingle, J. T. (1961). Release of lysosomal protease by UV irradiation and inhibition by hydrocortisone. *Exp. Cell Res.* **25**, 207–210.
7. Desai, I. D., Sawant, P. L. and Tappel, A. L. (1964). Peroxidative and radiation damage to isolated lysosomes. *Biochim. biophys. Acta* **86**, 277–285.
8. Tappel, A. L., Sawant, P. L. and Shibko, S. (1963). Lysosomes: Distribution in animals, hydrolytic capacity and other properties. *In* 'Ciba Foundation Symposium on Lysosomes' (Eds, De Reuck, A. V. S. and Cameron, J.), pp. 78–108. Churchill, London.
9. Wills, E. D. and Wilkinson, A. E. (1967). The effect of irradiation on lipid peroxide formation in subcellular fractions. *Radiat. Res.* **31**, 732–741.

result in a membrane which is susceptible to enzymatic digestion[1] by its contained enzymes such as cathepsin and phospholipase.

Lysosomal acid phosphatase was rapidly decreased in mouse skin irradiated *in vivo*, indicating an enzyme leakage through damaged membranes because lactic dehydrogenase was unaffected.[2, 3] UV damage to foetal rat skin could be inhibited by hydrocortisone.[4] This action of hydrocortisone is probably due to its stabilizing effect on cell membranes. A histochemical study of lysosomal acid phosphatase in UV-irradiated human skin provided evidence of a gradually increasing permeability of the lysosomal membranes within keratinocytes with the enzyme being detected in abnormal nuclear and inter-cellular locations 6 h after irradiation.[5] Confirmation of these findings has been provided at biochemical, histochemical and ultrastructural levels,[6, 7, 8, 9] but the evidence that lysosomal membrane damage is the primary cause of UV effects on the skin remains inconclusive. There is evidence that other cellular components are damaged preferentially after UV-irradiation of the skin.[10] Moreover, the release of hydrolytic enzymes from the epidermis after *in vivo* irradiation cannot be detected in skin perfusates,[11] nor are enzymes detected in early suction blister fluid from irradiated skin.[12] However, this may only indicate that the released lysosomal enzymes remaining within the damaged cells are bound to extracellular target sites.

1. Watkins, K. K. (1970). High oxygen effect for the release of enzymes from isolated mammalian lysosomes after treatment with ionizing radiation. *In* 'Advances in Biological and Medical Physics', Vol. 13 (Eds, Lawrence, J. H. and Gofman, J. W.), pp. 289–305. Academic Press, London, Orlando and New York.
2. Johnson, B. E. (1968). Ultraviolet radiation and lysosomes in skin. *Nature* **219**, 1258.
3. Johnson, B. E. (1965). Doctoral Thesis, University of London.
4. Weismann, G. and Fell, H. B. (1962). The effect of hydrocortisone on the response of foetal rat skin in culture to ultraviolet irradiation. *J. exp. Med.* **116**, 365.
5. Johnson, B. E. and Daniels, F., Jr (1969). Lysosomes and the reactions of skin to ultraviolet radiation. *J. invest. Derm.* **53**, 85.
6. Fand, I. (1972). The protecting effect of a sunscreen upon the lysosomes of ultraviolet irradiated skin. *Dermatologica* **144**, 237.
7. Grossie, V. B. and Black, H. S. (1977). The effect of ultraviolet light (UVL) on the lysosomes of hairless mouse epidermis. *Experientia* **33**, 425.
8. Ogura, R., Kinoshita, A., Shimada, T., Murakami, M. and Knox, J. M. (1977). Effect of anti-inflammatory agents on the release of acid phosphatase in the epidermis following ultraviolet light exposure. *The kurume Med. J.* **24**, 121.
9. Wilgram, G. F., Kidd, R. L., Krawczk, W. S. and Cole, P. L. (1970). Sunburn effects on keratin osomes. *Arch. Derm.* **101**, 505.
10. Honigsmann, H., Wolff, K. and Konrad, K. (1974). Epidermal lysosomes and ultraviolet light. *J. invest. Derm.* **63**, 337.
11. Greaves, M. W. and Sondergaard, J. (1970). Pharmacologic agents released in ultraviolet inflammation studied by continuous skin perfusion. *J. invest. Derm.* **54**, 365.
12. Volden, G. (1978). Acid hydrolases in blister fluid. 4. Influence of ultraviolet radiation. *Br. J. Derm.* **99**, 53.

V. HISTOLOGICAL AND HISTOCHEMICAL CHANGES

A. Histological Changes

Microdissection combined with microanalysis techniques has made it possible to perform biochemical determinations related to specific skin zones such as the dermis, epidermis, the appendages and the horny layer. However, for the accurate localization of enzyme activity or a specific biomolecule within the skin histochemical and cytochemical methods are essential. The changes in experimentally sunburned skin were established by the studies of Keller,[1] Miescher,[2] and Uhlmann.[3] At the time of the appearance of erythema, or shortly after, intracellular oedema was observed in the epidermis, and with exposures over 10 times the MED leucocyte migration also occurred. By 24 h following exposure, there was degeneration of the keratinocytes, and after the acute stage of inflammation had subsided the epidermis became thickened.

Miescher[4] correlated the histologic picture of irradiated white skin with its clinical appearance and, therefore, indirectly with the exposure dose. Slight erythema was associated with some cell damage of the uppermost cell layers of the epidermis, but with more intense erythema, the damage extended downwards to the basal layer. More recent studies have confirmed the earlier reported UV-B damage to keratinocytes with intra-epidermal vesiculation and liquefaction degeneration of the basal cells 24–48 h after exposure.[5, 6] Complete epidermal necrosis occurred in blistering reactions with damage to the dermis shown by lack of staining of fibroblasts and endothelial cells.

Over a period of 10 days the major stages of a severe sunburn reaction are: (1) At 24 h, many damaged keratinocytes. (2) At 2 days, epidermal disorganization and arborization of melanocytes. (3) At 3 days, epidermal regeneration and desquamation. (4) At 4 days, regeneration of keratinocytes and melanocyte hypertrophy. (5) At 6 days, re-establishment of the horny layer with continued melanocyte hyper-

1. Keller, P. (1924). Über die Wirkung des ultravioletten Lichtes auf die Haut unter besonderer Berücksichigung der Dosierung. III. Histologie der Lichtungzundung. *Strahlentherapie* **16**, 537.
2. Miescher, G. (1930). Das Problem des Lichtschutzes und der Lichtgewöhnung. *Strahlentherapie* **35**, 403.
3. Uhlmann, E. (1931). Über histologische Untersuchungen der mit Vitalux-Lampe bestrahlten Haut. *Strahlentherapie* **40**, 765.
4. Miescher, G. (1932). Untersuchungen über die Bedeutung des Pigments für den UV-Lichtschutz der Haut. *Strahlentherapie* **45**, 201.
5. Willis, I. and Cylus, L. (1977). UV-A erythema in skin: is it sunburn? *J. invest. Derm.* **66**, 128.
6. Rosario, R., Mark, G. J., Parrish, J. A. and Mihm, M. C. (1979). Histological changes produced in skin by equally erythemagenic doses of UV-A, UV-B, UV-C, and UV-A with psoralens. *Br. J. Derm.* **101**, 209.

trophy. (6) At 10 days, epidermal thickening and diminished melanocyte activity.[1]

With smaller doses, there are usually only scattered damaged keratinocytes (Fig. 13) or a number of dyskeratotic cells within the epidermis 24 h after exposure. At 72 h, increased numbers of mitotic figures appear in the basal layer and the damaged cells now form a compressed band just beneath the stratum corneum (Fig. 14).

The epidermis is significantly thickened 6 days after exposure with a parakeratotic horny layer beneath the original normal keratin layer.[2]

Ultrastructural studies of predominantly UV-B irradiated human and guinea-pig skin have revealed numerous cytoplasmic vacuoles in basal and higher epidermal cells.[3] Also nuclear vacuolation and filament aggregation[4] occur shortly after exposure. At 12 h, irregular dense bodies were present in the basal layer and later similar bodies develop in the prickle cells. There was a decrease in the number of keratinosomes, which may be evidence of damage to lysosomes.[5] The granular layer was unchanged until 12 h after exposure, at which time an increase in the number and thickness of the tonofibrils was observed. By 72 h, the basal cell vacuoles had disappeared,[3] but there was a generalized increase in the thickness of the granular layer associated with the development of cytoplasmic inclusions and vacuolization.[6] After 1 week, the granular layer had reverted to normal. The first changes in the region of the horny layer developed at 72 h: at this time, a thick, parakeratotic zone was observed beneath the original normal horny layer. Not only did this zone contain nuclei, but the horny layer was replaced here by large, spheroidal, ill-defined cells. Melanosomes were present and groups of dense particles were dispersed within the keratin.[7] The 72-h specimens

1. Clark, W. M., Jr and Pathak, M. A. (1966). Cited by Johnson, B. E., Daniels, F., Jr and Magnus, I. A. (1968). In 'Response of Human Skin to Ultraviolet Light', in 'Photophysiology', Vol. IV (Ed., Giese, A. C.), p. 139. Academic Press, London, Orlando and New York.
2. Daniels, F., Jr, Brophy, D. and Lobitz, W. C. (1961). Histochemical responses of human skin following ultraviolet irradiation. *J. invest. Derm.* **37**, 351.
3. Nix, T. E., Jr, Nordquist, R. E., Scott, J. R. and Everett, M. A. (1965). Ultrastructural changes induced by ultraviolet light in human epidermis: basal and spinous layers. *J. invest. Derm.* **45**, 52.
4. Wier, K., Fukuyama, K. and Epstein, W. L. (1971). Nuclear changes during light-induced depression of ribonucleic acid and protein synthesis in human epidermis. *Lab. Invest.* **25**, 451.
5. Wilgram, G. F., Kidd, R. L., Krawczyk, W. S. and Cole, P. L. (1970). Sunburn effect of keratinosomes. *Arch. Derm.* **101**, 505.
6. Nix, T. E., Jr, Nordquist, R. E. and Everett, M. A. (1965). Ultrastructural changes induced by ultraviolet light in human epidermis: granular and transitional cell layers. *J. Ultrastruct. Res.* **12**, 547.
7. Nix, T. E., Jr, Nordquist, R. E., Scott, J. R. and Everett, M. A. (1964). Ultrastructural changes in stratum corneum induced by ultraviolet light. *J. invest. Derm.* **43**, 301.

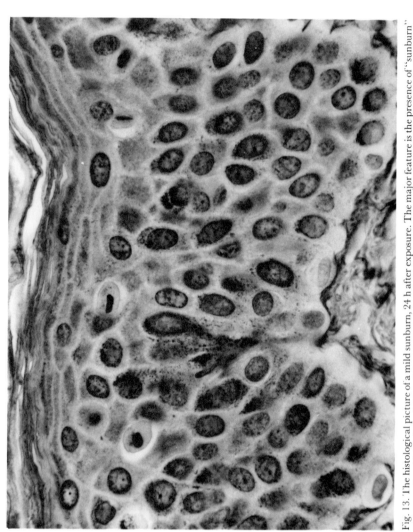

Fig. 13. The histological picture of a mild sunburn, 24 h after exposure. The major feature is the presence of "sunburn" or apoptotic cells in the prickle cell layer. (Courtesy of Farrington Daniels, Jr, M.D.)

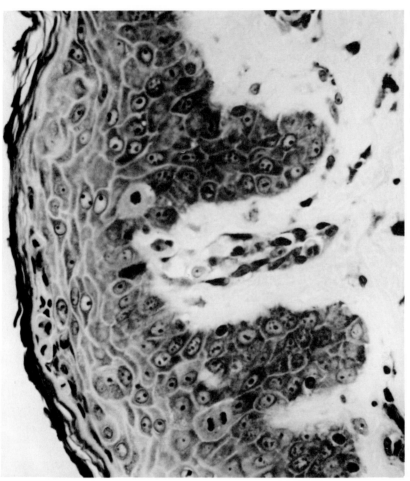

Fig. 14. The histological picture of a mild sunburn at 72 h after exposure. Damaged cells form a band beneath the original stratum corneum, mitotic figures are clearly seen in the basal layer and both increased nucleolar size and increased cytoplasmic staining in the suprabasal layers are indicative of the increased protein synthesis accompanying hyperplasia. (Courtesy of Farrington Daniels, Jr, M.D.)

showed an increase in size of the keratinocyte nuclei[1] which was correlated with increased epidermal thickness and may be an indication of increased protein synthesis. This could be confirmed by light microscopy (Fig. 14). There was an increase in cytoplasmic metachromasia of the basal cell layer as early as 7 h after exposure, and by 48 h this was present throughout the epidermis. The metachromasia is consistent with an increase in cellular RNA, and this was confirmed by more specific staining methods.[2] It indicates a relatively rapid recovery in RNA and protein synthesis following their initial blockage which could be demonstrated by autoradiographic methods.[3]

Autoradiographic studies of DNA synthesis in UV-irradiated skin also demonstrated its early inhibition in the epidermis,[4] indicating that DNA may be a primary target for the action of UVR. A decrease in Feulgen staining of the nuclei of UV-irradiated epidermal cells has been cited as evidence that DNA is the specific target for UV-R in skin.[5] However, this effect was only observed 24 h after exposure.[6] Like the decrease in the activities of mitochondrial enzymes, lactic acid dehydrogenase, alkaline phosphatase, and non-specific esterases in UV-irradiated mouse skin and the reported increase in oxidase and peroxidase activities,[7] this probably represents a secondary change.

In the absence of cellular damage there was no change in succinic acid dehydrogenase, alkaline phosphatase, sulphydryl or disulphide reactions following irradiation of human skin, but deposits of glycogen were detected in the basal layer 12 h after an erythema-producing exposure.[8] The irregular dense bodies observed with the electron microscope were

1. Nix, T. E., Jr (1967). Ultraviolet-induced changes in epidermis. *In* 'Ultrastructure of Normal and Abnormal Skin' (Ed., Zelickson, A. S.), p. 304. Henry Kimpton, London.

2. Johnson, B. E., Daniels, F., Jr and Magnus, I. A. (1968). Response of human skin to ultraviolet light. *In* 'Photophysiology', Vol. IV (Ed., Giese, A. C.), p. 139. Academic Press, London, Orlando and New York.

3. Fukuyama, K., Epstein, W. L. and Epstein, J. H. (1967). The effect of ultraviolet light on RNA and protein synthesis in differentiated epidermal cells. *Nature* **216**, 1031.

4. Epstein, W. L., Fukuyama, K. and Epstein, J. H. (1969). Early effects of ultraviolet light on DNA synthesis in human skin *in vivo*. *Arch. Derm.* **100**, 84.

5. Hamperl, H., Henschke, U. and Schulze, R. (1930). Über den Primärvorgang bei der Erythemerzügung durch ultraviolette Strahlung. *Naturwiss.* **27**, 486.

6. Ewert, G., Bottchep, K. and Wiskemann, A. (1974). DNA staining in human epidermal cells irradiated by 254 and 300 nm. *In* 'Progress in Photobiology'. Proc. VI Int. Congr. Photobiol. (Ed., Schenck, G. O.). Deutsche Gesellschaft für Lichtforschung, e.V., Frankfurt.

7. Hanke, W. (1961). Die Bedeutung von latenzeiten für u.v. strahlenbedingte Veräderungen am lebenden Gewebe. *In* 'Progress in Photobiology'. Proc. III Int. Congr. Photobiol. (Eds, Christensen, B. C. and Buchmann, B.), p. 336. Elsevier, Amsterdam.

8. Danils, F., Jr, Brophy, D. and Lobitz, W. C. (1961). Histochemical responses of human skin following ultraviolet irradiation. *J. invest. Derm.* **37**, 351.

considered to be glycogen,[1] and its appearance in the basal layer after 12 h and still later in the prickle cells probably represents a non-specific wounding response.[2] With high doses of UV-B or UV-C, mast cell degranulation[3] and damage to fibroblast DNA[4, 5] may occur. However, the major changes with moderate doses are restricted to the epidermis, the most obvious of which is the appearance of the so-called "sunburn cells". These are individually damaged cells within the epidermis and appear between 6 h and 48 h following exposure.[6, 7, 8, 9] Their number increases with increasing dose up to a maximum, but when minimal UV-erythema is produced some are inevitably present 24 h after the exposure.[10, 11] Moreover, sunburn cells appear after exposures which fail to elicit a vascular reaction. There is a superficial resemblance between the distribution of these cells and Langerhans cells (see Fig. 13) and preliminary studies produced some evidence that Langerhans cells were damaged in UV-irradicated skin.[12, 13] However, evidence for cytolysis of the Langerhans cell as a specffic epidermal effect of UVR was not forthcoming[14] and the keratinocyte derivation of the majority of sunburn

1. Nix, T. F., Jr (1967). Ultraviolet-induced changes in epidermis. In 'Ultrastructure of Normal and Abnormal Skin' (Ed., Zelickson, A. S.), p. 304. Henry Kimpton, London.
2. Lobitz, W. C. and Holyoke, J. B. (1954). The histochemical response of the human epidermis to controlled injury glycogne. J. invest. Derm. **22**, 189.
3. Valtonen, E. J., Janne, J. and Siimes, M. (1964). The effect of the erythemal reaction caused by ultraviolet irradiation on mast cell degranulation in the skin. Acta Dermato-Venereol. **44**, 269.
4. Epstein, W. L., Fukuyama, K. and Epstein, J. H. (1969). Early effects of ultraviolet light on DNA synthesis in human skin in vivo. Arch. Derm. **100**, 84.
5. Tan, E. M., Freeman, R. G. and Stoughton, R. B. (1970). Action spectrum for ultraviolet light induced damage to nuclear DNA in vivo. J. invest. Derm. **55**, 439.
6. Rost, G. A. and Keller, P. (1929). In 'Handbuch der Haut- und Geschlecht-skrankheiten', Vol. 5, Part 2, p. 1. Springer, Berlin.
7. Daniels, F., Jr, Brophy, D. and Lobitz, W. C. (1961). Histochemical responses of human skin following ultraviolet irradiation. J. invest. Derm. .**37**, 351.
8. Johnson, B. E. and Daniels, F., Jr (1969). Lysosomes and the reactions of skin to ultraviolet radiation. J. invest. Derm. **53**, 85.
9. Wilgram, G. F., Kidd, R. L., Krawczyk, W. S. and Cole, P. L. (1970). Sunburn effect on keratinosomes. A report with special note on ultraviolet-induced dyskeratosis. Arch. Derm. **101**, 505.
10. Johnson, B. E., Mandell, G. and Daniels, F., Jr (1972). Melanin and cellular reactions to ultraviolet radiation. Nature New Biol. **235**, 147.
11. Woodcock, A. and Magnus, I. A. (1976). The sunburn cell in mouse skin: preliminary quantitative studies on its production. Br. J. Derm. **95**, 459.
12. Fan, J., Schoenfeld, R. J. and Hunter, R. (1959). A study of the epidermal clear cells with special reference to their relationship to the cells of Langerhans. J. invest. Derm. **32**, 445.
13. Zelickson, A. S. and Rottaz, J. (1970). The effects of sunlight on human epidermis. Arch. Derm. **101**, 312.
14. Wolff, K. and Winkelmann, R. K. (1967). The influence of ultraviolet light on the Langerhans cell population and its hydrolytic enzymes in guinea pigs. J. invest. Derm. **48**, 531.

cells has been confirmed by light and electron microscope studies.[1, 2, 3, 4]

Nevertheless, the more recent findings that the characteristic surface membrane markers of Langerhans cells are particularly susceptible to UVR may have some relevance for skin reactions involving the immune system.[5, 6]

Sunburn cells appear to be individual abnormal keratinized cells. The findings of abnormal sites of lysosomal enzymes in the epidermis of UV-irradiated skin has been taken as evidence for the lysosome membrane being the primary UVR target in the keratinocytes.[3, 7, 8, 9] Their release may also be related to the development of the sunburn cells. However, it is not proven that lysosomes are damaged in sunburn cells,[10] and the fact that these cells exhibit a decreased DNA repair capacity[11] as well as being produced by 8-MOP photosensitization[12] suggests that they result from damage to their DNA. Daniels[13] noted that they were not "typically dyskeratotic" and they might be considered as "apoptotic cells". These

1. Daniels, F., Jr (1967). Ultraviolet radiation and dermatology. *In* 'Therapeutic Electricity and Ultraviolet Radiation', 2nd Ed. (Ed., Licht, S.), p. 379. Elizabeth Licht, New Haven, Connecticut.

2. Nix, T. E., Jr, Nordquist, R. E., Scott, R. J. and Everett, M. A. (1969). Ultrastructural changes induced by ultraviolet light in human epidermis: basal and spinous layers. *J. invest. Derm.* **45**, 52.

3. Wilgram, G. F., Kidd, R. L., Krawczyk, W. S. and Cole, P. L. (1970). Sunburn effect on keratinosomes. A report with special note on ultraviolet-induced dyskeratosis. *Arch. Derm.* **101**, 505.

4. Olson, R. L., Gaylor, J. and Everett, M. A. (1974). Ultraviolet-induced individual cell keratinization. *J. cut. Pathol.* **1**, 130.

5. Toews, G. B., Bergstresser, P. R., Streilein, J. W. and Sullivan, S. (1980). Epidermal Langerhans cell density determines whether contact hypersensitivity or unresponsiveness follows skin painting with DNFB. *J. Immunol.* **124**, 445.

6. Aberer, W., Schuler, G., Stingl, G., Hönigsmann, H. and Wolff, K. (1981). Ultraviolet light depletes surface markers of Langerhans cells. *J. invest. Derm.* **76**, 202.

7. Olson, R. L. and Everett, M. A. (1969). Alterations in epidermal lysosomes following ultraviolet light exposure. *In* 'The Biologic Effects of Ultraviolet Radiation with Emphasis on the Skin' (Ed., Urbach, F.), p. 473. Pergamon Press, Oxford.

8. Johnson, B. E. and Daniels, F., Jr (1969). Lysosomes and the reactions of skin to ultraviolet radiation. *J. invest. Derm.* **53**, 85.

9. Fand, I. (1972). The protective effect of a sunscreen upon the lysosomes of ultraviolet-irradiated skin. *Dermatologica* **144**, 237.

10. Hönigsmann, H., Wolff, K. and Konrad, K. (1974). Epidermal lysosomes and ultraviolet light. *J. invest. Derm.* **63**, 337.

11. Brenner, W. and Gschnait, F. (1979). Pathogenesis of epidermal UV injury. Reduced DNA repair in sunburn cells. *Arch. derm. Res.* **261**, 113.

12. Young, A. R. and Magnus, L. A. (1981). An action spectrum for 8-MOP induced sunburn cells in mammalian epidermis. *Br. J. Derm.* **104**, 541.

13. Daniels, F., Jr (1963). Ultraviolet carcinogenesis in man. *Nat. Cancer Inst. Monogr.* **10**, 407.

are produced by individual cell shrinkage and necrosis as a basic biological phenomenon of cell deletion involved in the control of cell populations.[1]

B. UV-A Radiation and Skin

The development of sunburn cells in human epidermis exposed to moderate doses of radiation from an unfiltered mercury arc was described in 1939.[2] The authors also examined the histopathology of skin exposed to UV-A in sufficient amounts to induce immediate pigmentation but were unable to detect any sign of damage to either the epidermis or dermis. Miescher[3] extended these studies using exposures of UV-A (principally 365 nm) in erythema-producing doses. There was little evidence of epidermal change but significant damage to the vascular endothelium was observed. High dose UV-A damage to the endothelium produced cellular swelling, nuclear damage as evidenced by the presence of nuclear dust and the extravasation of red blood cells. There was also a marked cellular infiltrate, but no damage to the epidermis, and these findings have been confirmed later by a number of light microscopy studies,[4, 5, 6, 7] and by electron microscopy.[8] When solar simulating radiation is used, there is evidence of epidermal damage similar to that obtained with equally erythemogenic doses of UV-B, although there may be some augmenting influence of wavelengths around 320 nm. However, the dermal changes observed are restricted to the development of a mild inflammatory infiltrate.[9] It would appear that the UV-A dose level required to produce damage to the vascular endothelium is greater than is usually encountered in natural sunlight under normal conditions.

1. Kerr, J. F. R., Wyllie, A. H. and Currie, A. R. (1972). Apoptosis: a basic biological phenomenon with wide ranging implications in tissue kinetics. *Br. J. Cancer* **26**, 239.
2. Hamperl, H., Henschke, U. and Schulze, R. (1939). Vergleich der Hautreaktionen beim Bestrahlungserythem und bei des direkten Pigmentierung. *Arch. Path. Anat.* **304**, 19.
3. Miescher, G. (1957). Zur Histologie der lichbedingten Reaktionen. *Dermatologica* **115**, 345.
4. Stern, W. K. (1972). Anatomic localization of the response to ultraviolet radiation in human skin. *Dermatologica* **145**, 361.
5. Willis, J. and Cylus, L. (1977). UV-A erythema; is it sunburn? *J. invest. Derm.* **68**, 128.
6. Parrish, J. A., Anderson, R. R., Urbach, F. and Pitts, D. (1978). 'UV-A Biological Effects of Ultraviolet Radiation with Emphasis on Human Responses to Longwave Ultraviolet'. Plenum Press, New York.
7. Rosario, R., Mark, G. J., Parrish, J. A. and Mihm, M. C. (1979). Histological changes produced in skin by equally erythemogenic doses of UV-A., UV-B., UV-C and UV-A with psoralens. *Br. J. Derm.* **101**, 299.
8. Kumakiri, N., Hashimoto, K. and Willis, I. (1977). Biologic changes due to longwave ultraviolet irradiation on human skin: Ultrastructural study. *J. invest. Derm.* **60**, 392.
9. Willis, I., Kligman, A. and Epstein, J. H. (1973). Effects of long ultraviolet rays on human skin: photoprotective or photoaugmentative. *J. invest. Derm.* **59**, 416.

However, if such damage were achieved with solar simulating radiation this would be accompanied by very damaging dose levels of UV-B radiation to the epidermis.

VI. PHARMACOLOGIC ASPECTS OF UV-INDUCED INFLAMMATION

Early investigations of UV-induced vasodilatation showed that when the blood was excluded from an irradiation site during the exposure, the reaction obtained was more severe than usual. This was taken to indicate that under normal conditions of exposure, the blood protects against UV-damage to the blood vessel walls.[1,2] The first measurements of UV-transmittance through the epidermis resulted in the discarding of this idea because the wavelengths causing vasodilatation were completely absorbed within the epidermis. However, more recent measurements, indicate that about 10% of wavelengths around 300 nm are transmitted through the epidermis, and this has revived interest in a dermal effect of UVR. Despite this it is difficult to reconcile the effect on blood vessel walls as being the primary mechanism for delayed vasodilatation. A more likely result of this damage would be vasoconstriction and bleeding into the dermis as the cells first swell and then disintegrate. A direct effect of UVR on isolated blood vessels has been described[3] but the immediate contraction observed seems to have little relevance to the delayed onset of the persistent erythema seen in irradiated skin. With very high exposure doses, vascular stasis occurs which is more consistent with the expected effect of UVR on blood vessels.[4]

Other factors which are cited as evidence for an indirect effect of UVR in erythema production were the long latent period of the reaction and the histological findings in which the cellular damage appeared to be restricted to the prickle cell layer of the epidermis.[5] Over a period of time, various hypotheses have been developed to explain this indirect effect in terms of a diffusible mediator of vasodilatation. This mediator could be

1. Finsen, N. R. (1899). Über die Bedeutung der chemischen Strahlen des Lichts für Medicin und Biologie. Vogel, Leipsig.
2. Wucherfennig, V. (1931). Biologie und praktische Verwendbarkeit der Erythemschwelle des UV. *Strahlentherapie* **40**, 201.
3. Sams, W. M., Jr and Winkelmann, R. K. (1969). The effect of ultraviolet light on isolated blood vessels. *J. invest. Derm.* **53**, 79.
4. Grice, K., Ryan, T. J. and Magnus, I. A. (1970). Fibrinolytic activity in lesions produced by monochromator ultraviolet irradiation in various photodermatoses. *Br. J. Derm.* **83**, 637.
5. Blum, H. F. (1945). Physiological effects of sunlight on man. *Physiol. Rev.* **25**, 483.

formed directly in the epidermis by the action of UVR, by the photochemical alteration of histidine into histamine,[1] or as a result of UV-induced damage to the epidermis. The latent period for the development of erythema would depend on the time taken for the formation of the mediator and its diffusion from the epidermis to the affected blood vessels. The complex aspects of diffusion processes in the skin in relation to UV-erythema are fully discussed by van der Leun.[2]

Lewis has likened the sunburn response to that obtained with histamine, and suggested that the "H" substance was the mediator involved.[3] However, neither histamine depletion[3, 4] nor the administration of antihistamines[5, 6, 7, 8] had an effect on the delayed phase of the sunburn reaction in either man or experimental animals. The immediate reaction, obtained in some animals with high doses of UV-B and UV-C, can be inhibited by antihistamines,[9, 10] but it is doubtful that this has any counterpart in the UV-induced reactions of human skin. Apart from this high dose reaction, possibly due to a direct effect of UVR on dermal mast cells,[11] histamine does not appear to have a role in the responses of skin to UVR.

In the rat, the early phase of UV-induced reactions appears to be mediated by serotonin (5-HT),[9] and this may also be involved in the delayed phase seen in this species.[12] The results of *in vitro* studies suggest that 5-HT may be derived from a UV-induced photochemical alteration

1. Ellinger, F. (1951). Die Histaminhypothese der biologischen Strahlenwirkungen. *Schweiz. Med. Woschr.* **81**, 61.
2. Van der Leun, J. C. (1966). 'Ultraviolet erythema. A study of diffusion processes in human skin'. Thesis. University of Utrecht.
3. Lewis, T. (1927). 'The blood vessels of the human skin and their responses'. Shaw, London.
4. Partington, M. W. (1954). The vascular response of the skin to ultraviolet light. *Clin. Sci.* **13**, 405.
5. Valtonen, E. J. (1965). Studies of the mechanism of ultra-violet erythema formation. *Acta dermvenereol.* **45**, 199.
6. Klouwen, H. H. and Mighorst, J. C. A. (1957). Untersuchungen über das Entstehen des Ultraviolett-Erythems. 1. Wird das Erythem durch Histamin verursacht? *Strahlentherapie* **104**, 618.
7. Partington, M. W. (1954). The vascular response of the skin to ultraviolet light. *Clin. Sci.* **13**, 425.
8. Lloyd, J. and Johnson, B. E. (1965). Triprolidine and the response of skin to ultraviolet radiation. *Br. J. Derm.* **77**, 244.
9. Logan, G. and Wilhelm, D. L. (1966). Vascular permeability changes in inflammation. 1. The role of endogenous permeability factors in ultraviolet injury. *Br. J. exp. Pathol.* **47**, 300.
10. Sim, M. P. (1964). The response of mouse skin to ultraviolet irradiation and its modification by drugs. *Excerpta Medica Internatl. Congress Series* **82**, 207.
11. Valtonen, V. J. (1968). Studies of the mechanism of ultraviolet erythema formation. V. Changes in the fine structure of the skin during the process of ultraviolet erythema caused by waveband UV-C. *Acta derm-venereol.* **48**, 203.
12. Claesson, S., Juhlin, L. and Wettermark, G. (1969). The action of ultraviolet light on skin with and without horny layer: the effect of 48-/80 and methotrimeprazine. *Acta derm-venereol.* **39**, 3.

of skin tryptophan,[1] but there is no evidence that such a reaction is involved in the sunburn response of human skin.

Epstein and Winkelmann[2] reported the presence of kinin activity in perfusates from UV-irradiated skin, but this was transient being present at 20 min, but not 3 h after exposure. Moreover, Greaves and Sondergaard were unable to detect any difference in the kinin levels of perfusates from irradiated and control skin.[3] It appears that kinins are not directly involved in either the production or the persistence of delayed sunburn erythema. However, the unidentified vasodilator substances referred to in the early sunburn literature as being present in the skin and circulating blood of UV-irradiated animals[4] may have been kinins. However, it seems more likely that they were prostaglandins or prostaglandin-related compounds.[5] Greaves and Sondergaard likened the major vaso-active agent in their dermal perfusates from UV-irradiated human skin to prostaglandin and Mathur and Gandhi identified prostaglandins in the UV-irradiated skin of man and albino rats.[6] There is a reasonable correlation between the anti-rheumatic properties of non-steroidal anti-inflammatory agents and their ability to suppress UV-erythema in guinea-pigs.[7] Indomethacin in particular, appears to act through the inhibition of prostaglandin synthetase[8] and when administered orally, topically or intradermally it suppresses to varying degrees the erythemas due to UV-C and UV-B in man and experimental animals.[9-16] However, it has no effect on the reactions

1. Doepfmer, W. and Cerietti, A. (1958). Über die Entstehung von Serotonin und 5-Hydroxytryptophan nach UV-Bestralung. *Experentia* **14**, 376.
2. Epstein, J. H. and Winkelmann, R. K. (1967). Ultraviolet light-induced kinin formation in human skin. *Arch. Derm.* **95**, 532.
3. Greaves, M. W. and Sondergaard, J. (1970). Pharmacological agents released in ultraviolet inflammation studied by continuous skin perfusion. *J. invest. Derm.* **54**, 365.
4. Blum, H. F. (1945). The physiological effects of sunlight on man. *Physiol. Rev.* **25**, 483.
5. Sondergaard, J. (1974). Prostaglandins in normal and pathological skin. *J. cut. Pathol.* **1**, 275.
6. Mathur, G. P. and Gandhi, V. M. (1972). Prostaglandin in human and albino rat skin. *J. invest. Derm.* **58**, 291.
7. Winder, C. V., Max, J., Burr, V., Been, M. and Rosiere, C. E. (1958). A study of pharmacological influences on ultraviolet erythema in guinea pigs. *Arch. int. Pharmacodyn.* **116**, 261.
8. Greaves, M. W. and McDonald–Gibson, W. (1973). Effect of non-steroid anti-inflammatory drugs on prostaglandin biosynthesis by skin. *Br. J. Derm.* **88**, 47.
9. Gupta, N. and Levy, L. (1973). Delayed manifestation of ultraviolet reaction in the guinea pig caused by anti-inflammatory drugs. *Br. J. Pharmac.* **47**, 240.
10. Snyder, D. S. and Eaglestein, W. H. (1974). Topical indomethacin and sunburn. *Br. J. Derm.* **90**, 91.
11. Snyder, D. S. and Eaglstein, W. H. (1974). Intradermal anti-prostaglandin agents and sunburn. *J. invest. Derm.* **62**, 47.
12. Snyder, D. S. (1975). Cutaneous effects of topical indomethacin, an inhibitor of prostaglandin synthesis, on UV-damaged skin. *J. invest. Derm.* **64**, 322.

induced by UV-A alone or those following 8-methoxypsoralen photo-sensitization.[1, 2] The concentrations of arachidonic acid and pro-staglandins E_2 and F_2 in suction blister fluid from irradiated skin show similar changes in both UV-C and UV-B erythemas. There is a slow increase which reaches maximum levels around 18–24 h after either UV-C or UV-B exposure. However, with the UV-C the erythema fades after 48 h, and the arachidonic acid and prostaglandin levels also fall at this time. A similar fall occurs in prostaglandins with UV-B, but the maximum intensity of erythema is maintained. With the moderately high doses given, this time course follows that of the UV-C erythema, but with UV-B the intensity of the erythema remains.

It is difficult to explain this persistent vasodilatation as a response to prostaglandins which are not present in sufficient amounts to produce a "bolus" effect, and are no longer detectable in the skin.[3, 4, 5] In this series of experiments by Greaves and his colleagues, it was shown that oral indomethacin completely blocked the UV-induced synthesis of pro-staglandins in the skin. Arachidonic acid concentrations, however, still increased, and reached levels greater than those in control UV-irradiated skin without indomethacin. The vascular reactions to UV-B were only slightly affected, and even the UV-C erythema was not totally sup-pressed. Obviously the role of prostaglandins E_2 and F_2^x in the sunburn reaction is not as clear cut as was first envisaged,[6] and it may be that they

1. Morison, W. L., Paul, B. S. and Parrish, J. A. (1977). The effect of indomethacin on long-wave ultraviolet-induced delayed erythema. *J. invest. Derm.* **68**, 120.
2. Gschnait, F. and Pehamberger, H. (1977). Indomethacin does not affect PUVA induced erythema. *Arch. derm. Res.* **259**, 109.
3. Black, A. K., Greaves, M. W., Hensby, C. N. and Plummer, M. A. (1978). Increased prostaglandins E and F in human skin at 6 and 24 h after ultraviolet B irradiation (290–320 nm²). *Br. J. clin. Pharmac.* **5**, 431.
4. Camp, R. D., Greaves, M. W., Hensby, C. N., Plummer, M. A. and Warin, A. P. (1978). Short wavelength ultraviolet irradiation of human skin: effect of indomethacin on prostaglandin and arachidonic acid activity. *Br. J. clin. Pharmac.* **6**, 145.
5. Black, A. K., Greaves, M. W., Hensby, C. N., Plummer, M. A. and Warin, A. P. (1978). Effects of indomethacin on arachidonic acid, prostaglandin E and F in horny skin 24 h after UVB and UVC irradiation. *Br. J. clin. Pharmac.* **6**, 261.
6 Greaves, M. W., Hensby, C. N., Black, A. K., Plummer, M. A., Fincham, N., Warin, A. P. and Camp, R. (1978). Inflammatory reactions induced by ultraviolet irradiation. *Bull. Cancer* **65**, 299.

13. Eaglestein, W. H. and Marsico, A. R. (1975). Dichotomy in response to indomethacin in UV-C and UV-B induced ultraviolet light inflammation. *J. invest. Derm.* **65**, 238.
14. Greenberg, R. A., Eaglstein, W. H., Turnier, H. and Hoyden, P. V. (1974). Orally given indomethacin and blood flow response to UVL. *Arch. Derm.* **111**, 328.
15. Kaidbey, K. H. and Kurban, A. K. (1976). The influence of corticosteroids and topical indomethacin on sunburn erythema. *J. invest. Derm.* **66**, 153.
16. Law, E. and Lewis, A. J. (1977). The effect of systemically and topically applied drugs on ultraviolet-induced erythema in the rat. *Br. J. Pharmac.* **59**, 591.

modulate the actions of other inflammatory agents rather than directly acting as vasodilators.[1] The delayed phase of the UV-B erythema may involve other members of the complex fatty acid/prostaglandin group of compounds. The finely balanced blood vessel endothelium–platelet relationship mediated through thromboxanes and prostacyclins may be involved in the persistent inflammatory response,[2] and changes here might also be related to the reported loss of fibrinolytic activity which accompanies this reaction.[3]

Although the cellular infiltrate associated with UV-erythema is less than that obtained with many inflammatory stimuli, there may still be a role for leukocytes, particularly in the later stages of the reaction to UV-B. This hypothesis was discarded as a result of one inconclusive study,[4] but it has been revived by the recent finding that the UV-B response in guinea-pigs made leukopenic with cyclophosphamide is significantly reduced both in intensity and duration compared with that in saline treated controls.[5]

Inhibition of UV-erythema may also be obtained with steroids,[6, 7, 8] but the effect is less pronounced than that of indomethacin.[9] The mechanism involved is not known. However, as well as inducing vasoconstriction and stabilizing lysosome membranes, steroids may inhibit the synthesis of prostaglandins.[10] Unlike the cyclo-oxygenase inhibiting effect of indomethacin, the steroids act by preventing the release of fatty acids from structural phospholipid, probably by the induction of a phospholipase inhibitor, and thereby limit the availability of prostaglandin precursors.[11] Even so, it is not clear how this effect could relate to inhibition of erythema.

1. Magnus, I. A. (1976). 'Dermatological Photobiology. Clinical and Experimental Aspects', p. 125. Blackwell Scientific Publications, Oxford.

2. Greaves, M. W., Hensby, C. N., Black, A. K., Plumner, M. A., Fincham, N., Warin, A. P. and Camp, R. (1978). Inflammatory reactions induced by ultraviolet irradiation. *Bull. Cancer* **65**, 299.

3. Grice, K., Ryan, T. J. and Magnus, I. A. (1970). Fibrinolytic activity in lesions produced by monochromator ultraviolet irradiation in various photodermatoses. *Br. J. Derm.* **83**, 637.

4. Logan, G. and Wilhelm, D. L. (1966). The inflammatory reaction in ultraviolet injury. *Br. J. exp. Path.* **47**, 286.

5. Eaglstein, W. H., Sakai, M. and Mizuno, N. (1979). Ultraviolet radiation induced inflammation and leukocytes. *J. invest. Derm.* **72**, 59.

6. Jarvinen, K. A. J. (1951). Effect of cortisone on reaction of skin to ultraviolet light. *Br. med. J.* **ii**, 1377.

7. Ljunggren, B. and Moller, H. (1973). Influence of corticosteroid on ultraviolet light erythema and pigmentation in man. *Arch. Dermatol. Forsch.* **248**, 1.

8. Law, E. and Lewis, A. J. (1977). The effect of systemically and topically applied drugs on ultraviolet-induced erythema in the rat. *Br. J. Pharmac.* **59**, 591.

9. Kaidbey, K. H. and Kurban, A. K. (1976). The influence of corticosteroids and topical indomethacin on sunburn erythema. *J. invest. Derm.* **66**, 153.

10. Greaves, M. W. and McDonald Gibson, W. (1972). Inhibition of prostaglandin biosynthesis by corticosteroids. *Br. med. J.* **ii**, 83.

11. Flower, R. J. and Blackwell, G. J. (1979). Anti-inflammatory steroids induce biosynthesis of a phospholipase A_2 inhibitor which prevents prostaglandin generation. *Nature* **278**, 456.

A major feature of the effects of either steroid or non-steroidal compounds on the skin reaction to UVR is that they appear to be directed solely against the vascular element of the reaction. Actual damage to the epidermis is apparently unaffected by these drugs.[1, 2]

Sunburn is one of the most common forms of inflammatory reaction in the skin and UV-erythema in animals has been used as an experimental model for studying the efficacy of anti-inflammatory agents.[3] However, the pharmacology of the reaction remains poorly understood. It is obviously complex, and it is doubtful whether a single mediator could account for all the various phases of the vascular reactions obtained.

VII. CHRONIC EFFECTS OF SOLAR RADIATION

The long-term effects of repeated solar exposure are changes in the skin which in some respects resemble premature ageing. These clinical alterations occur much earlier in those who work outside most of their lives and are more marked in Caucasians, particularly those of Celtic origin who have chosen to live in parts of the world where the amount of sunshine is greater than that of their country of origin. The macroscopic skin changes consist of dryness, wrinkling, yellow discolouration, loss of elasticity, and dilated superficial blood vessels particularly those of the face. Ecchymoses, known as senile purpura, develop on exposed sites such as the backs of the hands, together with pigmentary abnormalities leading to localized patches of hyper- and hypopigmentation. The skin of the back of the neck may become thickened and this is most common in those whose life work has been in agriculture or the fishing industries, the so-called "farmers" and "sailors" skin. Localized areas of abnormal epidermal activity develop which may lead to the formation of solar keratoses, and these may eventually progress to frank squamous cell carcinomata. The development of basal cell carcinomas on light exposed areas would seem to be related to long-term solar exposure, and such radiation may also play a part in the development of malignant melanomas.

1. Kaidbey, K. H. and Kurban, A. K. (1976). The influence of corticosteroids and topical indomethacin on sunburn erythema. *J. invest. Derm.* **66**, 153.
2. Law, E. and Lewis, A. J. (1977). The effect of systemically and topically applied drugs on ultraviolet-induced erythema in the rat. *Br. J. Pharmac.* **59**, 591.
3. Swingle, K. F. (1974). Evaluation of anti-inflammatory activity. *In* 'Anti-inflammatory Agents', Vol. 2 (Eds, Scherrer, R. A. and Whitehouse, M. W.), p. 34. Academic Press, London, Orlando and New York.

A. Changes in Skin due to Natural Ageing

Changes in the histology, biochemistry and biophysical properties of human and animal skin occur during the normal lifetime whether or not the skin is exposed to solar radiation. These have been discussed in an earlier volume by Jarrett.[1]

In unexposed skin the major changes due to ageing are thinning of the epidermis with a reduced number of cell layers together with flattening of the dermo-epidermal junction. In the atrophic epidermis the keratinocytes exhibit great variations in their size, shape and staining properties. However, in general the thickness and number of cell layers in the stratum corneum are not significantly altered.[2]

Ageing changes in the melanocyte system of the epidermis appear to be restricted to a decrease in the number of active cells compensated for by an increase in cell size of those remaining. The functional contacts in the normal epidermal melanin unit required for the distribution of the pigment throughout the keratinocyte system may be disorganized in the aged skin, resulting in its characteristic patchy pigmentation.[3]

Ageing changes in the dermal connective tissue are shown histologically by a thickening of the fibres in fixed tissue. There is a marked difference between thick, coarse fibres and the fine, delicate fibres seen in foetal skin. Rasmussen and his colleagues[4] studied the biophysical properties of human dermis from individuals over the wide range of 32 weeks of gestation to 88 years of age. They demonstrated changes which corresponded to an increase in the stability of collagen. This increased stability could be explained in terms of an increased polymerization of the basic trophocollagen molecule (see p. 919, Vol. 3). The total collagen of adult dermis is greater than that of younger skin and this appears to be due to an increase in the insoluble fraction.[5] With increasing age there is a continued increase in the insoluble collagen[6] together with an

1. Jarrett, A. (1974). 'The Physiology and Pathophysiology of the Skin' (Ed., Jarrett, A.), Vol. 3. Academic Press, London, Orlando and New York.
2. Montagna, W. (1965). Morphology of the aging skin: the cutaneous appendages. In 'Advances in Biology of Skin', Vol. 6 (Ed., Montagna, W.), p. 1. Pergamon Press, Oxford.
3. Fitzpatrick, T. B., Szabo, G. and Mitchell, Ruth E. (1965). Age changes in the human melanocyte system. In 'Advances in Biology of Skin', Vol. 6 (Ed., Montagna, W.), p. 35. Pergamon Press, Oxford.
4. Rasmussen, D. M., Wakim, K. G. and Winkelmann, R. K. (1965). Effect of aging on human dermis: studies of thermal shrinkage and tension. In 'Advances in Biology of Skin', Vol. 6 (Ed., Montagna, W.), p. 151. Pergamon Press, Oxford.
5. Sams, W. M., Jr and Smith, G., Jr (1965). Alterations in human dermal fibrous connective tissue with age and chronic sun damage. In 'Advances in Biology of Skin', Vol. 6 (Ed., Montagna, W.), p. 199. Pergamon Press, Oxford.
6. Elden, H. R. (1965). Biophysical aspects of aging in connective tissue. In 'Advances in Biology of Skin', Vol. 6 (Ed., Montagna, W.), p. 229. Pergamon Press, Oxford.

exponential decrease in the soluble fraction.[1] With this increase in insoluble, highly polymerized collagen, there is a concomitant increase in its tensile strength (see also Chapter 26, Vol. 3).

In unexposed skin ageing brings about a relatively slight increase in the dermal elastic tissue compared with exposed skin. The lysine content which is the precursor of desmosine and isodesmosine, and thus related to the cross linking of the units of elastic is decreased. This would indicate that a greater degree of cross linkage has taken place involving the free lysine radicals.

The ageing dermis also shows a steady fall in the hexosamine/hydroxyproline ratio: this probably represents a reduction in the mucopolysaccharide, compared with its collagen content. Such an alteration is probably due to an absolute increase in the insoluble collagen moiety, but it could also represent a decrease in acid mucopoly-saccharide. This change is steadily progressive from infancy through childhood into adolescence (Table 9).

Table 9

Chronic effects of solar radiation—acid mucopolysacharides (AMPS) of human skin: variation with age[1] (expressed as micromoles Uronic acid per g dry weight)

	Infant	Child	Adolescent	Adult	Solar elastosis
Hyaluronic acid	5·0	3·8	0·6	0·9	3·2
Chondroitin sulphate	4·2	1·0	1·0	1·3	1·6
Total AMPS	9·5	4·9	1·8	2·4	5·2

1. Smith, J. G., Jr, Davidson, E. A. and Taylor, R. W. (1965). Human cutaneous acid muco-polysaccharides: The effects of age and chronic sun damage. In 'Advances in Biology of Skin', Vol. 6 (Ed., Montagna, W.), p. 211. Pergamon Press, Oxford.

The major acid mucopolysaccharide components are hyaluronic acid and chondroitin sulphate B, and a similar decrease in sialic acid is thought to relate to a reduction in glycoprotein[2, 3] (see also p. 929, Vol. 3).

1. Verzar, F. (1964). Aging of the collagen fiber. 'International Review of Connective Tissue Research', Vol. 2 (Ed., Mall, D. A.), p. 243. Academic Press, London, Orlando and New York.
2. Smith, J. G., Jr, Davidson, E. A. and Taylor, R. W. (1965). Human cutaneous acid mucopolysaccharides: The effects of age and chronic sun damage. In 'Advances in Biology of Skin', Vol. 6 (Ed., Montagna, W.), p. 211. Pergamon Press, Oxford.
3. Cerimele, D. and Serri, F. (1972). Clinical and histological alteration of human skin from sunlight. In 'Research Progress in Organic, Biological and Medicinal Chemistry', Vol. III, pt II (Eds, Crallo, U. and Santmaria, L.), p. 623. North Holland, Amsterdam.

B. Ageing Changes in Exposed Skin

It is against this complex background of biochemical and biophysical changes in unexposed skin that the effects of chronic solar exposure have to be reviewed. In general it would appear that the changes in chronically exposed skin are an acceleration, and exaggeration of the normal ageing process. Atrophy, with pronounced flattening of the rete ridges, and marked variations in the size, distribution, and function of melanocytes has been observed.[1, 2, 3] The keratinization process tends to become disorganized[3] and there is some loss of cohesion between keratinocytes. The stratum corneum may be thicker than in unexposed ageing skin,[4] and there is alteration of the dermo-epidermal interface which after fixation appears reduplicated and thickened.

Haematoxylin and eosin staining of chronically exposed skin merely shows a vague dermal basophilia,[5, 6] Biochemical analysis shows a reduction of collagen as assessed by the amount of hydroxyproline per g weight of tissue, and it has been suggested that this is due to a reduction in the "insoluble" collagen fraction without a compensatory increase of the "soluble fraction".[7] On the other hand, experimental studies on animal skin *in vitro* using very high exposure doses (about 1 kJ cm^{-2}) showed an increase in the ratio of insoluble to soluble collagen,[8] and measured changes in the mechanical properties of the skin indicated that the UV radiation had increased the degree of cross-linking.[9] Similar changes have been recorded after UV-irradiation of isolated collagen,[10] but the relationship between the experimental results with such intense radiation to that of chronically exposed skin is difficult to evaluate.

1. Freeman, R. G., Cockerell, E. G., Armstrong, J. and Knox, J. M. (1962). Sunlight as a factor influencing the thickness of epidermis. *J. invest. Derm.* **39**, 295.
2. Everett, M. A., Nordquist, J. and Olsen, R. L. (1970). Ultrastructure of human epidermis following chronic sun exposure. *Br. J. Derm.* **84**, 248.
3. Mitchell, R. E. (1969). Chronic solar dermatitis—an electron microscopic study of the epidermis. *Aust. J. Derm.* **10**, 75.
4. Mackie, B. S. and McGovern, V. J. (1958). The mechanism of solar carcinogenesis. *Archs Derm.* **78**, 218.
5. Lever, W. F. and Schaumberg-Lever, G. (1975). 'Histopathology of the Skin', 5th ed., p. 249. J. B. Lippincott, Philadelphia.
6. Lund, A. Z. and Sommerville, R. L. (1957). Basophilic degeneration of the cutis. *Am. J. clin. Path.* **27**, 183.
7. Sams, W. M., Jr and Smith, J. G., Jr (1965). Alterations in human dermal fibrous connective tissue with age and chronic sun damage. *In* 'Advances in Biology of Skin', Vol. 6, 'Aging' (Ed., Montagna, W.), p. 199. Pergamon Press, Oxford.
8. Bottoms, E. and Shuster, S. (1965). Effect of ultraviolet light on skin collagen. *Nature* **199**, 192.
9. Bottoms, E., Cater, C. W. and Shuster, S. (1966). Effect of ultraviolet irradiation on skin collagen. *Nature* **211**, 97.
10. Fujimori, E. (1966). Ultraviolet light-induced change in collagen macromolecules. *Biochemistry* **5**, 1034.

The exposure of hairless mice to carcinogenic UV-irradiation ($0.9–1.8$ J cm^{-2} of UV-B per day) produced a 20% decrease in total collagen in 6 weeks, and this was associated with a decrease in such mechanical properties as tensile strength, ultimate strain and elasticity.[1] Total skin thickness was increased, but no increase in dermal elastic tissue was detected. In contrast to these findings, a much greater dose of UV-A (21.6 J cm^{-2}) had no effect.

A similar decrease in total collagen with UV-B was reported by Lovell[2] using a single high exposure of 50 J cm^{-2} on mouse skin *in vitro*, and it would therefore appear that some of the effects of chronic solar radiation can be simulated by UV-B irradiation but not with UV-A.

C. Mucopolysaccharides

It is of interest that in chronically exposed skin there is an increase in its mucopolysaccharide content,[3, 4] and this would appear to be due to an increase in the hyaluronic acid fraction together with an increase in the sialic acid content;[5, 6] however chondroitin sulphate levels were not significantly changed. Other techniques revealed a marked increase in argyrophilic fibres, but because these were almost completely extracted by 0.5 M acetic acid they were probably correctly considered to be collagen rather than reticulin.

Thus, it would seem that the overall picture presented by the effects of chronically irradiated skin differs from that seen in the normal ageing process of unexposed skin. The collagen content of the dermis is decreased rather than increased and there is evidence for the production of new young collagen. This, together with an increase in the hyaluronic acid content of the skin, is suggestive that solar irradiation has an effect on fibroblasts within the dermis rather more than a direct effect on the collagen itself.[2]

1. Alpermann, M. and Vogel, H. G. (1978). Effect of repeated ultraviolet irradiation on skin of hairless mice. *Arch. derm. Res.* **262**, 15.
2. Lovell, W. W. (1973). Ultraviolet irradiation of dermal collagen *in vivo*. I. Single doses of radiation. *Trans. St. John's Hosp. Derm. Soc.* **59**, 166.
3. Steiner, K. (1957). Mucoid substances and cutaneous connective tissue in dermatoses. II. Mucoid alterations in degenerative and congenital dermatoses. *J. invest. Derm.* **28**, 403.
4. Sams, W. M., Jr and Smith, J. G., Jr (1961). The histochemistry of chronically sun-damaged skin. *J. invest. Derm.* **37**, 447.
5. Smith, J. G., Jr, Davidson, E. A. and Taylor, R. W. (1965). Human cutaneous acid mucopolysaccharides: the effect of age and chronic sun damage. *In* 'Advances in Biology of Skin', Vol. 6 (Ed., Montagna, E.), p. 211. Pergamon Press, Oxford.
6. Cerimele, D. and Serri, F. (1972). Clinical and histological alterations of human skin from sunlight. *In* 'Research Progress in Organic, Biological and Medicinal Chemistry' (Eds, Gallo, U. and Santa-Maria, L.), p. 623. North-Holland, Amsterdam.

D. Elastic Tissue

Chronic solar radiation causes a marked increase in the orcein staining properties of dermal fibres. These fibres appear thickened and curled or they may be present in amorphous masses of orceinophilic material.[1,2] This is mainly located in the upper third of the dermis, but in severely solar damaged skin it can be seen throughout the whole dermis. Characteristically, the papillary dermis just beneath the epidermis is unaffected, and there is a clear zone between the epidermis and the densely staining orceinophilic material (see Vol. 3, Chapter 28, Fig. 11).

The derivation of orceinophilic material is not clear. Because collagen is normally the major dermal fibrous component and because there is a quantitative decrease in normal collagen content, it is possible that the elastotic masses are degraded collagen (see p. 849, Vol. 3). Electron microscopy,[3,4] differential staining,[1,5] and the effects of proteolytic enzymes[3,6] have all been used to investigate the relationship between degraded collagen and elastotic material. Banfield and Brindley considered that it is altered elastic tissue;[7] also the amino acid pattern of elastotic skin more closely resembles that of elastin than collagen.[8] Niebauer and Stockinger[9] suggest that a protein in collagen is identical with elastin, and this remains even when collagen is degraded. Electron microscope studies of mild solar degenerative changes in the dermis have revealed alterations in the elastic fibres which appear to be the initial stages of a degenerative process which could lead to the more severe manifestations of solar elastosis.[7,10] These initial changes are thought to consist of a thickening and an increased electron density of the fibre

1. Gillman, T., Penn, J., Bronks, D. and Roux, M. (1955). Abnormal elastic fibers. *Archs Path.* **59**, 733.
2. Smith, J. G., Jr and Finlayson, G. R. (1965). Dermal connective tissue altering with age and chronic sun damage. *J. Soc. cosmet. Chem.* **16**, 527.
3. Tunbridge, R. E., Tattersal, R. N., Hall, D. A., Astbury, W. T. and Reed, R. (1952). The fibrous structure of normal and abnormal human skin. *Clin. Sci.* **11**, 315.
4. Braun-Falco, O. (1969). Die Morphogenese der senil-aktinischen Elastose Eine elektronenmikroskopische Untersuchung. *Arch. klin. exp. Dermatol.* **235**, 138.
5. Burton, D., Hall, D. A., Keech, M. K., Reed, R., Saxl, E., Tunbridge, R. E. and Wood, M. J. (1955). Apparent transformation of collagen fibrils into 'elastin'. *Nature* **176**, 966.
6. Loewi, G., Glyn, L. C. and Dorling, J. (1960). Studies on the nature of collagen degeneration. *J. Path. Bact.* **80**, 1.
7. Banfield, W. G. and Brindley, D. C. (1963). Preliminary observations in Senile Elastosis using the electron microscope. *J. invest. Derm.* **41**, 9.
8. Smith, J. G., Jr, Davidson, E. A. and Hill, R. L. (1963). Composition of normal and pathological cutaneous elastin. *Nature* **197**, 1108.
9. Niebauer, G. and Stockinger, L. (1965). Über die senile Elastosis; Histochemische und electronen mikroskopische untersuchungen. *Arch. klin. exp. Dermatol.* **221**, 122.
10. Danielsen, L. and Kobayasi, T. (1972). Degeneration of dermal elastic in relation to age and light exposure. *Acta derm-venereol.* **52**, 1.

matrix. This is then followed by disruption of the fibres producing the typical masses of amorphous material. Long ago Unna suggested that the degradation of both elastin and collagen was involved in the development of elastosis,[1] and the light and electron microscope studies of Mitchell[2] support this view. An alternative explanation is that the elastotic masses are, in fact, the induced abnormal products of UV-damaged fibroblasts.[3, 4] However, although some of the changes in chronically sun-damaged skin may be due to altered fibroblast function, the evidence for an abnormal synthesis of elastotic material is not convincing.

Animal experiments designed to investigate UV-carcinogenesis have failed to reveal elastotic changes even after the development of squamous cell carcinomata. However, this may represent a species or, at least, a variety difference because Sams, Smith and Burk[5] clearly demonstrated elastotic degeneration in Dublin ICR strain mice within 3 months of daily UV-B exposure; and Nakamura and Johnson[6] demonstrated the development of abnormal elastic tissue in rat skin which had been irradiated for a period of some 27 weeks causing the disappearance of the normal elastic fibres. Using monochromatic radiation, 300 nm induced elastotic changes in mice, but high doses of 320 or 360 nm radiation were ineffective.[7] Kligman[8] has clearly illustrated the predominance of elastosis as the major change in chronically exposed skin. Elastic tissue changes were graded as simple hyperplasia through hypertrophy to massive degeneration on a 0–4 scale. The skin of the face from lightly pigmented subjects through age periods of 8 decades was studied. By the second decade 80% showed 1 + to 2 + changes: by middle age more than 50% had 3 + changes and over 70 all showed grade 4 elastosis. Although pigmented skin types showed less tendency to develop solar elastosis, none the less even the deeply pigmented skin of elderly negroes showed a grade

1. Unna, P. G. (1894). 'Die Histopathologie der Hautkrankheiten'. Hirschwald, Berlin.
2. Mitchell, R. E. (1967). Chronic solar dermatosis: A light and electron microscopic study of the dermis. *J. invest. Derm.* **48**, 203.
3. Ebner, H. (1969). Über die Entstehung des elastotischen Materials. Eine elektronenmikroskopische Studie. *Z. Haut Geschlechtskr.* **44**, 889.
4. Helwig, E. B. (1972). Diseases of elastic tissue. *In* 'Dermal Pathology' (Eds, Graham, J. H., Johnson, W. C. and Helwig, E. B.), p. 741. Harper and Row, New York.
5. Sams, W. M., Jr, Smith, J. G. and Burk, P. G. (1964). The experimental production of elastosis with ultraviolet light. *J. invest. Derm.* **43**, 467.
6. Nakamura, K. and Johnson, W. C. (1968). Ultraviolet light induced connective tissue changes in rat skin: A histopathologic and histochemical study. *J. invest. Derm.* **51**, 253.
7. Magnus, I. A. (1976). 'Dermatological Photobiology', p. 134. Blackwell Scientific Publications, Oxford.
8. Kligman, A. M. (1969). Early destructive effect of sunlight on human skin. *J. Am. Med. Ass.* **210**, 2377.

3 change in the face. The degree of elastosis in unexposed skin was markedly less than in exposed skin.[1]

An overall hypothesis for the changes in chronic solar damage would appear to include the following changes. The collagen already present in the skin is degraded. This may be due to a non-specific release of hydrolytic enzymes or by more specific UV-induced collagenolytic process. Fibroblast function reverts to a younger form with increased production of hyaluronic acid. There is an eventual decrease in fibroblast number and function with resulting alterations of the dermal connective tissue. The continuing UVR damage to the epidermis results in disordered keratinization and melanogenesis leading to keratotic abnormalities of the epidermis and observable changes in pigmentation. Also this repeated damage to the basal cell keratinocyte results in an abnormal thickened, basement membrane. There would appear to be little reason for concluding that the epidermal changes are secondary to those of the dermis, although Mackie and McGovern[2] argue convincingly for such a course of events.

E. The Reversal of Chronic Solar Changes

The possibility that benign chronic damage in skin exposed to sunlight might be reversible when further exposure is prevented is of obvious cosmetic importance. Moreover, if the serious skin changes related to long-term exposure require a changed stromal environment for their full expression, the possibility of such a reversal becomes of great interest. Gerstein and Freeman[3] investigated this by transplanting full thickness grafts from severely sun-damaged skin from the back of the neck to unexposed areas on the upper arm in 14 cases. Nine and a half months later, 11 of the grafts showed evidence of a return towards normal, both in the epidermis and the dermis. The elastotic masses appeared to regress most rapidly at the centre of the graft (Table 10). Papa and his colleagues[4] were unable to demonstrate a similar regression but it is not clear from their paper whether their results were in complete contradiction to those of Gerstein and Freeman. If chronically exposed skin is populated by fibroblasts which synthesize preferentially a young dermal

1. Kligman, A. M. (1974). Solar elastosis in relation to pigmentation. *In* 'Sunlight and Man' (Ed., Fitzpatrick, T. B.), p. 157. University of Tokyo Press, Tokyo.
2. Mackie, B. S. and McGovern, V. J. (1958). The mechanism of solar carcinogenesis. *Archs Derm.* **78**, 218.
3. Gerstein, W. and Freeman, R. G. (1963). Transplantation of actinically damaged skin. *J. invest. Derm.* **41**, 445.
4. Papa, C. M., Carter, D. M. and Kligman, A. M. (1970). The effect of autotransplantation on the progression or reversibility of aging in human skin. *J. invest. Derm.* **54**, 200.

Table 10

The effect of transplanting solar damaged skin to non-exposed areas[1]

Degree of improvement	No change	Slight improvement	Moderate improvement	Complete resolution
No. of subjects	3	5	5	1

1. Gerstein, W. and Freeman, R. G. (1963). Transplantation of actinically damaged skin. *J. invest. Derm.* **41**, 445.

connective tissue, then regression of the induced changes might be expected when the skin is removed from further insult. More complete studies of this aspect of the problem are clearly required.

VIII. PIGMENTATION

There are numerous good reviews dealing with pigment cell biology with special reference to melanin in the skin[1,2,3,4] and the subject is comprehensively discussed by Riley[5] (see Vol. 3).

The colour of human skin depends in the main on its content of three pigments—haemoglobin, carotene and melanin. The pink to red of lightly pigmented Caucasian skin is due to oxyhaemoglobin, while the reduced form gives rise to the blue tinge seen in superficial veins. The yellow coloration observed in the thick horny layer of the palms of the hands and soles of the feet, but rarely elsewhere, is due to accumulated carotenes. However, it is melanin which is primarily responsible for the varying skin shades of yellow, brown and black seen in the different races of man. This natural melanin content of the skin which varies from one individual to another is genetically controlled, and is termed "constitutive melanin pigmentation". Where a change in the colour of the skin

1. Riley, V. and Fortner, J. G. (Eds) (1963). 'The Pigment Cell: Molecular, Biological and Clinical Aspects'. New York Acad. Sci., New York.
2. Montagna, W. and Hu, F. (Eds) (1967). 'The Pigmentary System'. 'Adv. Biol. Skin', Vol. VIII. Pergamon Press, Oxford.
3. Riley. V. (1972). Pigmentation: its Genesis and Biologic Control. Appleton-Century-Crofts, Boston.
4. Jimbow, K., Quevedo, W. J., Jr, Fitzpatrick, T. B. and Szabo, G. (1976). Some aspects of melanin biology 1950–1975. *J.I.D.* **67**, 72.
5. Riley, P. A. (1974). The dendritic cell population of the epidermis. Part II of 'The Physiology and Pathophysiology of the Skin', Vol. 3. 'The Dermis and the Dendrocytes' (Ed., Jarrett, A.), p. 1104. Academic Press, London, Orlando and New York.

is induced by the action on the melanocyte system of hormones or chemical and physical agents, it is called "facultative melanin pigmentation".[1]

The dermatological photobiology of melanin is concerned with the changes in "constitutive" melanin pigmentation following exposure to UVR and that due to photosensitization (facultative pigmentation). This "facultative" melanin together with the varying degrees of "constitutive" pigmentation combine to protect against the effects of UVR.

The development of suntan in normally lightly pigmented skin following UV-stimulation is due to the redistribution of preformed melanosomes in the epidermis and the increased production of melanized melanosomes in the melanocytes and their subsequent transfer to the keratinocytes. The increased pigmentation of the hyperplastic epidermis affords increased protection against further UVR exposure. Increased activity of the melanocytes may be brought about by UV-C, UV-B or UV-A, but there are different mechanisms involved in the total response. With UV-B and UV-C, the previously described changes in keratinocyte behaviour occur concomitantly with the increase in melanin production, but with UV-A, there is little change in the keratinocytes. Although the tan obtained with UV-A may appear as intense as that with UV-B, the protection afforded is less, and it is therefore thought that changes other than just melanin production are involved in the protection afforded by a natural suntan. The importance of the horny layer in this respect has already been discussed and the effects of melanin on the transmission of UVR through the epidermis have been considered (see page 2403).

The genetically controlled variation in the form, distribution, and numbers of melanosomes responsible for racial variation in skin colour is also responsible for the racial variations in skin responses to UVR. In Negroid and Australoid epidermis, melanosomes are plentiful, large, and packaged singly in the lysosome system of the keratinocytes. In lightly pigmented Caucasoids, few fully melanized melanosomes are normally present. These are small and packaged as aggregates within keratinocyte lysosomes in which the protein moiety of the melanosomes is susceptible to proteolytic attack. In the more deeply pigmented Caucasoid and in tanned skin, the melanosomes are usually more varied in size, but the major difference is in the numbers produced and the greater persistence of the fully melanized melanosomes within the keratinocytes.

1. Quevedo, W. C., Jr, Fitzpatrick, T. B., Pathak, M. A. and Jimbow, K. (1974). Light and skin colour. In 'Sunlight and Man' (Ed., Fitzpatrick, T. B.), p. 165. University of Tokyo Press, Tokyo.

The mechanisms by which tyrosinase is stimulated are not understood, but they may include a non-specific wounding type of response in the lower epidermis combined with a UV-induced removal of an inhibitor to tyrosinase activity.

The immediate pigmentation reaction elicited in already pigmented skin by wavelengths between 360–420 nm is also a combined effect of the oxidation of "bleached melanin" already present within the keratinocytes and also a redistribution of preformed melanosomes within the melanocyte dendrites, and even possibly some transfer to neighbouring keratinocytes.

The pigmentary response obtained in photosensitization reactions is discussed in detail in the sections on Photochemotherapy and Drug and Chemical Induced Reactions (see pages 2571, 2579 and 2683).

The mechanisms by which melanin protects the skin against UVR and photosensitized damage are also not clearly defined. Some part of this protection may be through the neutral density filter effect of the melanosomes within the keratinocytes, but the complex molecular structure of the melanin polymer suggests a more complex protective mechanism. This may be related to its action as a semi-conductor material, diverting electron energy away from susceptible biological materials, or by acting as an electron trap in which such energy is dissipated harmlessly as heat.

IX. ULTRAVIOLET CARCINOGENESIS

The carcinogenic effects of ultraviolet radiation and natural sunlight have been well reviewed by Blum,[1] Epstein,[2] Urbach, Epstein and Forbes,[3] and Black,[4] and a good summary is presented by Magnus.[5]

In skin exposed to high intensity sunlight over long periods, the accelerated ageing changes are accompanied by the development of benign focal abnormalities of keratinization in the shape of solar

1. Blum, H. F. (1959). 'Carcinogenesis by Ultraviolet Light'. Princeton University Press, Princeton, New Jersey.
2. Epstein, J. H. (1971). Ultraviolet carcinogenesis. In 'Photophysiology', Vol. 5 (Ed., Giese, A. C.), p. 235. Academic Press, London, Orlando and New York.
3. Urbach, F., Epstein, J. H. and Forbes, P. D. (1974). Ultraviolet carcinogenesis: experimental, global and genetic aspects. In 'Sunlight and Man' (Ed., Fitzpatrick, T. B.), p. 259. University of Tokyo Press, Tokyo.
4. Black, H. S. and Chan, J. T. (1977). Experimental ultraviolet light-carcinogenesis. *Photochem. Photobiol.* **26**, 183.
5. Magnus, I. A. (1976). 'Dermatological Photobiology: Clinical and Experimental Aspects'. Blackwell Scientific Publications, Oxford.

keratoses, which may be succeeded by basal or squamous cell carcinomas. Evidence that solar UVR is responsible for skin carcinogenesis in humans is entirely epidemiologic, but nevertheless it is convincing. The majority of skin cancers, where no other carcinogenic influence is apparent, is produced in sun-exposed skin of lightly pigmented persons; such carcinogenesis is rare in Negroids. In matched populations, the incidence of skin cancer is higher in areas of more intense sunlight, and the tumours develop in the sites most exposed to the sun. This epidemiologic evidence is supported by data from numerous studies in which skin cancers were produced in experimental animals with controlled exposures to artificial UVR.

The carcinogenic action of sunlight appears to be derived from the mutagenic effects of UVR combined with the growth promoting action of wavelengths between 290 and 310 nm. Some suppression of the immune response through the induction of suppressor T lymphocytes may be a required step for this process and this effect of UV-B has been unequivocally demonstrated in experimental animals.[1] Some association between exposure to intense sunlight and the incidence of malignant melanoma is also postulated but the mechanisms involved here do not appear to be the same as for other skin cancers.

1. Kripke, M. L. (1980). Immunology of UV-induced skin cancer. Yearly Review. *Photochem. Photobiol.* **32**, 837.

Abnormal Reactions Associated with Skin Disorders

81

B. E. JOHNSON

Department of Dermatology, University of Dundee, Ninewells Hospital, Dundee, Scotland

I. THE PHOTODERMATOSES

A. Introduction

Polymorphic light eruption is the commonest of the idiopathic reactions of the skin to light in the British Isles.[1] This is probably still true whether actinic prurigo is considered as a separate entity or not. It is also commonly seen in other parts of Europe, in Scandinavia,[2] and in North

---

1. Frain-Bell, W. (1979). Dowling Oration. What is that thing called light? *Clin. exp. Derm.* **4**, 1.
2. Jansen, C. T. (1975). Monimuotienen valiohottuna. Kirjapaino Polytpos, Turku.

PHYSIOL. PATHOPHYSIOL. OF SKIN Vol. 8
ISBN 0 12 380608 9

America.[1] It is relatively rare in the Middle and Far East despite greater intensities of solar radiation. Although photosensitivity is present in both polymorphic light eruption and in actinic prurigo, it is the major feature of the former. Actinic prurigo is often a perennial eruption affecting both covered and exposed skin and in some instances the photosensitivity component may be less obvious.

Hydroa vacciniforme is characterized by blistering of the exposed skin: this may be large and often followed by scarring.[2, 3] Vesicles may also be a feature of the skin reaction to light in some children in association with actinic prurigo,[4] and these too may lead to pitted scarring. Solar urticaria is also included in the group of idiopathic photodermatoses. In photosensitivity dermatitis there is a persistent reaction to light in association with contact allergic sensitivity[4] or an initial photoallergy.[5] The reaction is eczematous but in the most severely affected subjects it may be associated with a pseudolymphomatous reaction, in which case the term "actinic reticuloid" is applied.[6, 7] The relative incidence of these so-called idiopathic photodermatoses is shown in Table 1.

B. Polymorphic Light Eruption

Polymorphic light eruption most commonly affects females, usually for

Table 1

The relative incidence of so-called idiopathic photodermatoses[4]

Type of disorder	No. of patients
Polymorphic light eruption/Actinic prurigo	336
Solar urticaria	21
Hydroa vacciniforme	5
Photosensitivity dermatitis and actinic reticuloid	136

1. Epstein, J. H. (1980). Continuing medical education. Polymorphous light eruption. *J. Am. Acad. Derm.* **3**, 32.
2. McRae, J. D., Jr and Perry, H. A. (1970). Hydroa Vacciniforme. *Archs Derm.* **87**, 124.
3. Bickers, D. R., Demar, L. K., DeLeo, V., Poh-Fitzpatrick, M. B., Aronberg, J. M. and Harber, L. C. (1978). Hydroa Vacciniforme. *Archs Derm.* **114**, 1193.
4. Frain-Bell, W. (1979). Dowling Oration. What is that thing called light? *Clin. exp. Derm.* **4**, 1.
5. Wilkinson, D. S. (1962). Further experience with halogenated salicylanilides. *Br. J. Derm.* **74**, 295.
6. Ive, F. A., Magnus, I. A., Warin, R. P. and Wilson Jones, E. (1969). 'Actinic Reticuloid': chronic dermatosis associated with severe photosensitivity and histological resemblance to lymphoma. *Br. J. Derm.* **81**, 469.
7. Frain-Bell, W., Lakshmipathi, T., Rogers, J. and Willock, J. (1974). The syndrome of chronic photosensitivity dermatitis and actinic reticuloid. *Br. J. Derm.* **91**, 617.

the first time in late adolescent or early adult life although it can start in childhood, and may persist for years. It is essentially an itchy erythematous papular eruption in which there is often a diffuse oedematous erythema with or without an urticicarial element. Although usually confined to exposed skin, the eruption can involve covered areas, but this is thought to be a result of the penetration of thin fabrics by the responsible wavelengths of the solar spectrum. The reason why certain exposed sites such as the skin of the face do not show the eruption remains obscure. It is usually only present during the sunshine months, but it can recur following exposure to winter sunshine. An element of "desensitization" or "hardening" is not uncommon as the reaction to sunlight tends to lessen as the summer progresses. This feature may be relevant to the relatively low incidence in countries nearer the equator, and also to the use of phototherapy for the treatment of polymorphic light eruption.

Close relatives of polymorphic light eruption subjects may have a similar photodermatosis although there is the possibility that the high incidence recorded in some reports is due to the inclusion of other types of the photodermatoses. Thus, the variation in reported familial incidence as listed in Table 2 probably indicates different clinical and photobiological criteria used by different investigators in the diagnosis of polymorphic light eruption.

Table 2

Familial incidence in polymorphic light eruption

	No. of subjects	Familial incidence (%)
Epstein[1]	84	14
Birt and Davis[2]	128	75
Jansen[3]	91	56
Frain-Bell[4]	310	21

The relationship between polymorphic light eruption and the atopic state is not clear. There is evidence that asthma, hay fever, eczema, are more frequently found in individuals with polymorphic light eruption or in their close relatives, than in the general population.

1. Epstein. J. H. (1966). Polymorphic Light Eruption. *Ann. Allergy* **24**, 397.
2. Birt, A. R. and Davis, R. A. (1975). Hereditary Polymorphic Light Eruption of American Indians. *Int. J. Derm.* **14**, 105.
3. Jansen, C. T. (1978). Heredity of Polymorphic Light Eruption. *Archs Derm.* **114**, 188.
4. Frain-Bell, W. (1979). Dowling Oration. What is that thing called light? *Clin. exp. Derm.* **4**, 1.

The additional element of urticaria noted in some subjects with polymorphic light eruption as an immediate response to light suggests the possible involvement of defined immunological and pharmacological mechanisms. Significantly elevated IgE and other immunoglobins in patients with polymorphic light eruption compared with a control population has been reported.[1] Evidence for cell mediated allergic reactions, as demonstrated by the *in vitro* correlates, has been demonstrated by some[2] but not by others.[3,4] In addition, UV-induced damage to DNA appears to undergo normal repair.[5]

Polymorphic light eruption and cutaneous lupus erythematosus have certain histological features in common. This has led to the suggestion that these conditions are in some way related. In both there may be evidence of UV-B photosensitivity, and the ability to reproduce either eruption by artificial irradiation of the skin has been reported.[6] However, antinuclear factors, haematological abnormalities and the presence of dermo–epidermal zone immunofluorescence have not been conclusively demonstrated in polymorphic light eruption. The typical clinical and histopathological features of PLE are shown in Fig. 1.

The photobiological features of polymorphic light eruption are of interest but the variable findings reported over the years have been such that the diagnosis still mainly depends on clinical features. The use of conventional phototesting for the determination of an action spectrum for erythema only occasionally provides evidence of photosensitivity.[6,7,8,9] In fact, an apparently normal action spectrum, despite undoubted clinical photosensitivity, is a common finding. However, some polymorphic light eruption subjects can be shown to have abnormal action spectrum for erythema usually confined to the UV-B wavelengths, but occasionally extending into the UV-A and even the visible range above

1. Jansen, C. T. (1977). Elevated serum immunoglobulin levels in PLEs. *Acta derm-venereol.* **57**, 331.
2. Horkay, I. and Meszaos, C. S. (1971). A study on lymphocyte transformation in light dermatoses. *Acta derm-venereol. (Stockholm)* **51**, 268.
3. Raffle, E. J., MacLeod, T. M. and Hutchinson, F. (1973). *In vitro* lymphocyte studies in chronic polymorphic light eruption. *Br. J. Derm.* **89**, 143.
4. Jansen, C. T. and Helander, I. (1976). Cell mediated immunity in chronic PLEs. *Acta derm-venereol. (Stockholm)* **56**, 121.
5. Jung, E. G. and Bohnert, E. (1974). Chronisch polymorphe Lichtdermatose; Untersuchungen an Lymphozyten *in vitro. Dermatologica* **148**, 209.
6. Epstein, J. H. (1980). Continuing medical education—polymorphic light eruption. *J. Am. Acad. Derm.* **3**, 329.
7. Frain-Bell, W. (1979). Dowling Oration. What is that thing called light? *Clin. exp. Derm.* **4**, 1.
8. Magnus, I. A. (1976). 'Dermatological Photobiology. Clinical and Experimental Aspects'. Blackwell Scientific Publications, Oxford.
9. Magnus, I. A. (1964). Studies with a monochromator in the common idiopathic photodermatoses. *Br. J. Derm.* **76**, 389.

400 nm. A similar wavelength activation of the abnormal papular reaction is also present.

A persistent erythema may follow immediate urtication on phototesting subjects with solar urticaria, and this may be the explanation, in some instances, for the unexpected breadth of the action spectrum in polymorphic light eruption. In some subjects with polymorphic light eruption the minimal dose for erythema is the same as that required to produce the delayed papular response, but multiples of this minimal erythema dose are sometimes required to produce this abnormal papular response and provide confirmatory evidence for the undoubted clinical photosensitivity.[1]

C. Actinic Prurigo

Because most commonly it affects females, lasts many years, is often associated with a normal action spectrum for erythema and has unknown aetiology, actinic prurigo is often included within the classification of Polymorphic Light Eruption. In the only case of this type reported from Japan the typical clinical eruption was reproduced by high exposure to UV-B given either as single or repeated doses but not with subminimal erythema dose exposures.[2] The typical lesions could also be elicited with CO_2 snow and this was taken to partly explain the incidence of actinic prurigo eruptions which occur in winter, and on covered sites.

There are, however, distinguishing features to support the view[3] that despite its idiopathic nature it should be kept separate from the atypical polymorphic light eruption already defined. It differs in that it usually starts in childhood, affects both exposed and covered skin, can be present all the year round but there is often aggravation of the exposed sites during the sunshine months. The skin changes are those of a prurigo, in some instances forming lichenified plaques which, in the younger child, may be frankly eczematous; cheilitis is also common.[4] It would appear to be similar to, if not identical with, the hereditary polymorphic light eruption occurring in North American Indians[5] and also in various

1. Epstein, J. H. (1980). Continuing medical education. Polymorphic light eruption. *J. Am. Acad. Derm.* **3**, 32.
2. Aoki, T. and Fujita, M. (1980). Actinic prurigo: a case report with successful induction of skin lesions. *Clin. exp. Derm.* **5**, 47.
3. Calnan, C. D. and Meara, R. H. (1977). Actinic prurigo (Hutchinson's summer prurigo). *Clin. exp. Derm.* **2**, 356.
4. Birt, A. R. and Hogg, G. R. (1979). The actinic Cheilitis of hereditary polymorphic light eruption. *Archs Derm.* **115**, 699.
5. Birt, A. R. and Davis, R. A. (1975). Hereditary polymorphic light eruption of American Indians. *Int. J. Derm.* **14**, 105.

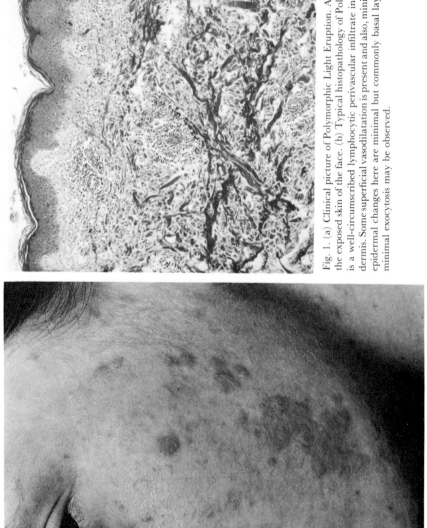

Fig. 1. (a) Clinical picture of Polymorphic Light Eruption. An erythematopapular reaction of the exposed skin of the face. (b) Typical histopathology of Polymorphic Light Eruption. There is a well-circumscribed lymphocytic perivascular infiltrate in both the superficial and middle dermis. Some superficial vasodilatation is present and also, minimal, sub-epidermal oedema. The epidermal changes here are minimal but commonly basal layer vacuolization, spongiosis and minimal exocytosis may be observed.

peoples of South America. Successful treatment with thalidomide[1] would suggest an immunological basis for the reaction in view of the ability of this drug to suppress severe reactions in leprosy.

D. Hydroa Vacciniforme

This is a reaction on exposed skin sites in which light appears to be involved, even though it is not usually possible to confirm this by means of currently available phototesting techniques. It is rare and presents usually as an acute skin reaction of the face and backs of the hands, with the formation of blisters which may reach a centimetre or more in diameter. This is followed by impetigo-like crusting and subsequent healing with depressed scars (Fig. 2). It is said to occur more commonly in male children[2] and to eventually clear after a period of years, but it occasionally develops for the first time in the adult.

The histological features are those of intraepidermal vesicle formation, presumably as a result of focal necrosis of the epidermal cells. The

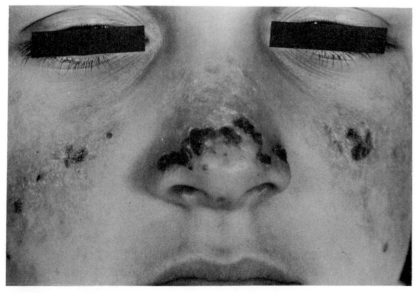

Fig. 2. Clinical picture of Hydroa Vacciniforme. The main features here are crusting and scarring over the accentuated exposed areas of the skin of the face.

1. Londono, F. (1973). Thalidomide in the treatment of actinic prurigo. *Int. J. Derm.* **12**, 326.
2. McGrae, J. D., Jr and Perry, H. O. (1963). Hydroa vacciniforme. *Archs Derm.* **87**, 124.

pathology also involves the directly subjacent dermis, with a cellular infiltrate of polymorphonuclear cells and lymphocytes extending deeply into the dermis with some necrosis and thrombosis of small vessels.[1, 5]

Although there are good clinical grounds for suspecting that the skin changes in hydroa vacciniforme are induced by exposure to light, phototesting has failed to produce clear-cut evidence of photosensitivity,[2] the action spectrum for erythema or abnormal responses being within normal limits, and, in some instances, the threshold for erythema in the UV-B wavelengths being in fact raised. Irradiation of the skin using multiples of the minimal erythema dose may produce abnormal responses.[1, 3, 4]

Abnormalities of amino acid metabolism do not appear to be a regular feature of this condition, although an association with Hartnup's disease has been described.[5] There has been an unconfirmed claim that there is defective DNA repair in the lymphocytes of patients with this disorder.[6]

E. Solar Urticaria

Although solar urticaria is a relatively uncommon photodermatosis, its importance lies in the fundamental mechanisms involved in its production. An urticarial weal as a manifestation of an abnormal reaction to light can sometimes be seen as part of the reaction in polymorphic light eruption. A minority of subjects with polymorphic light eruption experience immediate urtication associated with a delayed papular or an oedematous blotchy erythema. Also in some instances an immediate urtication can be demonstrated on phototesting which progresses to a delayed erythema with or without a papular element.

The diagnostic term "solar urticaria" indicates a monomorphic response in which an urticarial weal develops within a relatively short period (5–20 min) after exposure to sunshine. It should be appreciated that the patient's history may be suggestive of a sudden onset of erythema rather than an urticaria. It is only when such a subject is subsequently phototested and an immediate urtication clinically demonstrated that a definitive diagnosis of solar urticaria can be made.

Urticarial lesions may result from the presence in the skin of

1. Bickers, D. R., Demar, L. K., DeLeo, M. D., Poh–Fitzpatrick, M. B., Aronberg, J. M. and Harber, L. C. (1978). Hydroa vacciniforme. *Archs Derm.* **114**, 1193.
2. Macrae, J. D., Jr and Perry, H. O. (1963). Hydroa vacciniforme. *Archs Derm.* **87**, 124.
3. Schiff, M. and Jillson, P. F. (1960). Photoskin tests in hydroa vacciniforme. *Archs Derm.* **82**, 812.
4. Ramsay, C. (1972). Hydroa vacciniforme. *Br. J. Derm.* **87**, 395.
5. Ashurst, P. J. (1969). Hydroa vacciniforme occurring in association with Hartnup disease. *Br. J. Derm.* **81**, 486.
6. Giannelli, F. (1980). DNA repair in human diseases. *Clin. exp. Derm.* **5**, 119.

photoactive substances such as porphyrins or dyes which on exposure to appropriate wavelength irradiation produce the cutaneous reaction. However, such an association should be readily detected and the correct diagnosis made.

The sparing of some exposed skin sites is a feature common to both solar urticaria and to polymorphic light eruption. In polymorphic light eruption often only one area such as the face is spared, whereas in solar urticaria all the normally exposed skin sites may remain unaffected whilst the urticarial wealing only occurs on normally covered areas such as the limbs and trunk. However, in some mild examples of polymorphic light eruption the maximal affection is confined to sites normally covered by clothes as in the case of solar urticaria. This feature, together with the ability to improve both conditions with phototherapy[1,2,3] emphasizes clinical similarities between classical polymorphic light eruption and classical solar urticaria. As mentioned above, the reason for the involvement of skin not directly exposed to light may be due to the penetration of the clothing by the responsible wavelengths. Diagnostic difficulties may arise when the urticaria results from exposure to heat rays, but this possibility can easily be resolved by appropriate phototesting. The action spectrum determined by phototesting is often broad, UV-B, UV-A, and visible radiation all being involved in the production of the urticarial reaction.

1. Mechanisms in Solar Urticaria

The mechanisms involved in urticaria are complex and the reader is referred to Ryan and to Greaves in this series (Vols 2 and 7). The monograph by Warin with Champion[4] also provides much useful information. Solar urticaria is equally as complex and the mechanisms appear also to vary. The early classification of this disorder based on wavelength responsible for the wealing[5] might be useful in the elucidation of mechanisms involved provided the specific radiation absorbing chemicals responsible for the different action spectra could be identified. However, as early as 1939 an immunological basis for the skin

1. Ramsay, C. A. (1977). Solar urticaria treatment by inducing tolerance to artificial radiation and natural light. *Archs Derm.* **113**, 1222.
2. Van der Leun, J. C. (1980). Personal communication.
3. Morison, W. L., Momtaz, K., Mosher, D. B. and Parrish, J. A. (1982). UV-B phototherapy in the prophylaxis of polymorphic light eruption. *Br. J. Derm.* **106**, 231.
4. Warin, R. P. and Champion, R. H. (1974). 'Urticaria'. W. B. Saunders, London.
5. Blum, H. F. (1964). 'Photodynamic Action and Diseases caused by Light'. Hafner Publishing Company, New York.

reactions in solar urticaria was suspected,[1, 2, 3, 4] and the more recent classification formulated by Harber and his colleagues[5, 6] depends on both proven immunological involvement and wavelength dependence. The classifications of various groups of workers are shown in Table 3. Such classification has simplified the presentation of the individual patient data scattered throughout the literature, and it is also useful in that new cases can be fitted into the general pattern of the disease process. However, in terms of the mechanisms involved, it tends to emphasize the complexities. Drug and chemical induced photosensitized urticaria are quite properly excluded from this classification. In addition, because it is restricted to the urticarial reactions of erythropoietic protoporphyria in which the absorbing chromophore is known, and because the condition is more appropriately discussed in relation to the photosensitive porphyrias, the Type VI reaction should perhaps be withdrawn from the classification. When these are excluded, the trigger mechanism of Solar Urticaria, whether of Types I, II, III, IV or V, is unknown. This implies that the substance within the skin which absorbs radiation to initiate the urticarial process has not been identified.

The second step in the urticarial process appears to vary with the different types. Type I gave positive, passive, and reverse passive, transfer tests, and a preliminary attempt to characterize the serum factor responsible for the antigen–antibody reaction showed it to be heat labile and associated with both albumin and globulin.[7, 8, 9] Further studies of Type I have used more sophisticated protein analysis and have shown the activity to be associated with globulin, mainly of the IgE fraction,[10] and the wavelength responsible in this type appears to be restricted to the UV-B. The UV-induced change in the protein molecular structure produces an antigen against which the patient's antibodies react. At the

1. Epstein, S. (1939). Allergische Lichterdermatosen. *Dermatologica* **80**, 291.
2. Rajka, E. (1942). Passive transfer in light urticaria. *J. Allergy* **13**, 327.
3. Epstein, S. (1956). Urticarial Hypersensitivity to Light. *In* 'Allergic Dermatoses', pp. 51–67. J. B. Lippincott Co., Philadelphia.
4. Illig, I. (1963). Untersuchungen zur Pathogenese der Lichturticaria. *Arch. f klin. u exp. Derm.* **217**, 82.
5. Harber, L. C., Holloway, R. M., Wheatley, V. R. and Baer, R. L. (1963). Immunologic and biophysical studies in solar urticaria. *J. invest. Derm.* **41**, 439.
6. Harber, L. C. and Baer, R. L. (1969). Classification and characteristics of photoallergy. *In* 'The Biologic Effects of Ultraviolet Radiation (with Emphasis on Skin)' (Ed., Urbach, F.), pp. 519–525. Pergamon Press, Oxford.
7. Beal, P. L. (1948). Studies in solar urticaria. *J. invest. Derm.* **11**, 415–433.
8. Harber, L. C., Holloway, R. M., Wheatley, V. R. and Baer, R. L. (1963). Immunologic and biophysical studies in solar urticaria. *J. invest. Derm.* **41**, 439–443.
9. Sams, W. M., Jr, Epstein, J. E. and Winkelmann, R. K. (1969). Solar urticaria, investigation of pathogenic mechanisms. *Archs Derm.* **99**, 390–397.
10. Sams, W. M., Jr (1970). Solar urticaria: studies of the active serum factor. *J. Allergy* **45**, 295–301.

Table 3

Classification of solar urticaria

Urticaria type	Action spectrum	Passive transfer	Reverse passive transfer	Mechanism
		Harber and Baer (1969)[1]		
I	285–320 nm	+	+	Allergic
II	320–400 nm	−	−	Unknown—no serum factor demonstrated
III	400–500 nm	−	−	Unknown—no serum factor demonstrated
IV	400–500 nm	+	−	Unknown—probably allergic
V	280–500 nm	−	−	Unknown—no serum factor demonstrated
VI	400 nm	−	−	Protoporphyrin in photo-toxic reaction

Types VII and VIII are normally included but appear to be here urticaria, one being mediated as Cholinergic urticaria

Urticaria type	Action spectrum	Passive transfer	Reverse passive transfer	Mechanism
		Epstein (1971)[2]		
I	370 nm	+	+	Allergic
II	370 nm	−	−	Unknown—no serum factor demonstrated
III	400–500 nm	+ sometimes	−	Possibly allergic in some patients
IV	280–700 nm (multiple wavebands)	+ in one case	−	Possibly allergic in one case

Urticaria type	Action spectrum			
		Ive, Lloyd and Magnus (1965)[3]		
I	180–315 nm			
II	315–700 nm			
III	400–700 nm			
IV	250–700 nm (broad band)			

1. Harber, L. C. and Baer, R. L. (1969). Classification and characteristics of photoallergy. In 'The Biologic Effects of Ultraviolet Radiation (with emphasis on skin)' (Ed., Urbach, F.), pp. 519–525. Pergamon Press, Oxford.
2. Epstein, J. H. (1971). Adverse cutaneous reactions to the sun. In 'Year Book of Dermatology' (Eds, Malkinson, F. D. and Pearson, R. W.), pp. 4–43. Year Book Publishers, Chicago.
3. Ive, H., Lloyd, J. and Magnus, I. A. (1965). Action spectra in idiopathic solar urticaria. Br. J. Derm. **77**, 229.

present time it is suggested that immunological involvement is restricted to Types I and IV solar urticaria. Even in Type IV this is only tentative because only passive transfer tests have been successful.

The chromophore involved in the visible-radiation-induced urticaria merits little discussion here since there is no abnormality of porphyric metabolism in these patients. It is also possible that the ordinary passive transfer test, in which serum from a patient with solar urticaria is injected into the skin of a normal subject and the site then irradiated, may produce a reaction due to simple phototoxicity. However, in typical Type IV patients, Horio[1] showed that irradiation of the isolated patients' sera produced reactions when injected intradermally into the solar urticaria patients, but not in normal subjects. This would appear to support an immunological, rather than phototoxic, mechanism.

The skin reaction obtained in solar urticaria appears to be in the classic triple response of vasodilatation, weal and flare associated with "H" substances or histamine. Although the Coombs and Gell[2] Type I antigen–antibody reactions resulting in urticaria are associated primarily with the release of mast cell mediators of which histamine appears to be the main active component, histamine itself is not invariably associated with the reactions of solar urticaria. In one study, five out of eight patients had solar urticarial reactions which could be inhibited by antihistamines. In three of these the reactions were also abolished by prior treatment with 48/80 which depletes the skin histamine.[3] It is not possible to classify these patients in any particular solar urticaria type, the involvement of histamine or its non-involvement, being associated equally in the wavelength groups specified. In studies of Type I solar urticaria patients, using skin perfusion techniques, no histamine was detected and anti-histamine administration had little effect on this, or on the Type IV solar urticaria studies.[4] Because of the potential hazard of hepatitis associated with passive transfer tests, these have not been done in sufficient number to unequivocally identify the involvement of immunological mechanisms with specific wavelength dependence. Moreover, where histamine has been shown to play a part in the reactions, immunological studies have

1. Horio, T. (1978). Photoallergic urticaria induced by visible light. *Archs Derm.* **114**, 1761–1764.
2. Coombs, R. R. A. and Gell, P. G. H. (1953). *In* 'Clinical Aspects of Immunology' (Eds, Gell, P. G. H. and Coombs, R. R. A.). Blackwell Scientific Publications, Oxford.
3. Ive, H., Lloyd, J. and Magnus, I. A. (1965). Action spectra in idiopathic solar urticaria. *Br. J. Derm.* **77**, 229–243.
4. Sams, W. M., Jr, Epstein, J. E. and Winkelmann, R. K. (1969). Solar urticaria, investigation of pathogenetic mechanisms. *Archs Derm.* **99**, 390–397.

not been done; where immunologic studies have been done and mediators looked for, histamine appears to play no role.

An urticarial reaction due to photodynamic action with substances such as the porphyrins may be inhibited by restricting the circulation, thereby lowering the oxygen tension in the skin below that required for the photochemistry. In solar urticaria, a temporary inhibition of the wealing may be obtained in this way but the weal appears when the circulation is restored.[1, 2] This result may be interpreted as evidence for the involvement of circulating elements in the evolution of the urticarial reaction. However, it is possible that the physiological processes of wealing may be blocked by restricting the circulation and this aspect of the evidence for an immunological basis for solar urticaria remains equivocal. This point is stressed in the discussion of one case in which a major feature was an increase in dermal mast cells and histamine mediation was inferred from the inhibition of wealing obtained with antihistamine administration.[3] In this case, no involvement of the complement system was detected but, as reported for another group of patients,[4] there was a transient fibrin deposition. However, decreased fibrinolysis following irradiation is not a feature of solar urticaria.[5] No evidence of mast cell degranulation or histamine release *per se* was presented, but both effects have been observed in varying degrees in four patients with differing action spectra for wealing.[6]

The apparent tachyphylaxis demonstrated with 48/80 injections probably stems from mediator depletion rather than any change in vascular responsiveness and is not produced equally in all patients.[7] The tolerance induced by controlled exposure to radiation is probably a

1. Ive, H., Lloyd, J. and Magnus, I. A. (1965). Action spectra in idiopathic solar urticaria. *Br. J. Derm.* **77**, 229–243.
2. Ramsay, C. A., Scrimenti, R. J. and Crimps, D. J. (1970). Ultraviolet and visible action spectrum in a case of solar urticaria. *Archs Derm.* **101**, 520–523.
3. Baart de la Faille, H., Bottier, P. B. and Baart de la Faille-Kuyper, E. H. (1975). Solar urticaria: a case with possible increase of skin mast cells. *Br. J. Derm.* **92**, 101–107.
4. James, M. P., Eady, R. A. J., Kennedy, A. R. and Gunner, D. B. (1980). Physical urticaria: a microscopical study to evaluate the role of the mast cell. *Br. J. Derm.* **102**, 735.
5. Grice, K., Ryan, T. J. and Magnus, I. A. (1970). Fibrinolytic activity in lesions produced by monochromator ultraviolet irradiation in various photodermatoses. *Br. J. Derm.* **83**, 637–649.
6. Hawk, J. L. M., Eady, R. A. J., Challoner, A. V. J., Kobza-Black, A., Keahy, T. H. and Greaves, M. W. (1980). Elevated blood histamine levels and mast cell degranulation in solar urticaria. *Br. J. clin. Pharmac.* **9**, 183–186.
7. Magnus, I. A. (1976). Solar urticaria. *In* 'Dermatological Photobiology', pp. 202–210. Blackwell Scientific Publications, Oxford.

similar phenomenon.[1] Further research into the mechanisms of solar urticaria may well be facilitated by the ability to abolish the response in this controlled fashion.

F. Photosensitivity Dermatitis and Actinic Reticuloid

Photosensitivity dermatitis is by far the commonest photodermatosis to affect the male. It is rarely seen in females, being recorded in only 5·2% of 232 cases studied over a 12-year period.[2, 3] This is in sharp contrast to the sex incidence in polymorphic light eruption where females predominate.

Histologically the reaction is that of an eczema (Fig. 3), showing spongiosis, with epidermal vesiculation and patchy parakeratosis and exudation. In the chronic state there is thickening and lichenification of the epidermis and hyperkeratosis. The chronic state is commonly seen interspersed with acute or sub-acute episodes. The dermal changes are similar to those seen in a non-light sensitive chronic eczema with perivascular infiltrate of lymphocytes and histiocytes mainly in the superficial zone. When the cutaneous reaction is particularly severe there are pseudo-lymphomatous changes like those seen in actinic reticuloid.[4, 5]

The eruption usually occurs on the exposed sites, but it can also appear on covered skin, either as a result of penetration of thin fabrics by the responsible wavelengths, or as part of a general spreading of the eczematous response. An important aspect of this type of photosensitivity is an associated contact allergic sensitivity of cell mediated type in which the responsible chemical substance may also be photoactive.

In some subjects the cause of the photosensitivity is unexplained, and these are referred to as the "idiopathic" cases. Other subjects can apparently develop a similar state after some years of what may have been either a constitutional eczema or a contact eczema triggered off by factors which have acted either as primary irritants or as allergic sensitizers.

In some instances contact allergens such as tetrachlorsalicylanilide or chlorpromazine, which can also produce a photocontact reaction of either photoallergic or phototoxic type, are responsible. It is likely

1. Ramsay, C. A. (1977). Solar urticaria treatment by inducing tolerance to artificial radiation and natural light. *Archs Derm.* **113**, 1222.
2. Frain-Bell, W. (1979). Dowling Oration. What is that thing called light? *Clin. exp. Derm.* **4**, 1.
3. Frain-Bell, W. and Johnson, B. E. (1979). Contact allergic sensitivity to plants and the photosensitivity dermatitis and actinic reticuloid syndrome. *Br. J. Derm.* **101**, 503.
4. Ive, F. A., Magnus, I. A., Warin, R. P. and Wilson-Jones, E. (1969). 'Actinic Reticuloid'; chronic dermatosis associated with severe photosensitivity and the histological resemblance to lymphoma. *Br. J. Derm.* **81**, 469.
5. Frain-Bell, W., Lakshmipathi, T., Rogers, J. and Willock, Joyce (1974). The syndrome of chronic photosensitivity dermatitis and actinic reticuloid. *Br. J. Derm.* **91**, 617.

therefore that a number of factors are involved in the development of a photosensitivity reaction of this type. Such an interpretation highlights the importance of directing investigations towards a study of both the photosensitivity and the contact allergic sensitivity features.

It has been appreciated for some time now, and particularly since the halogenated salicylanilide outbreak of the early 1960s[1,2,3,4] that some individuals who develop photocontact dermatitis only experience a relatively short-lived skin reaction in which the dermatitis settles quickly with treatment, and in the absence of further contact with the responsible substance the temporary state of photosensitivity disappears and does not recur.

It is equally apparent that there are a number of individuals who, having had a similar onset, progress to a state of chronic photosensitivity in which their skin continues to react abnormally to light for months or even years.[2,5]

It has been suggested that in salicylanilide photocontact dermatitis certain wavelengths of ultraviolet radiation alter the photoactive substance forming a photoproduct which can trigger off a contact allergic cell mediated immunological response.[6,7] This secondary allergic response can then continue without the necessity for further exposure to light. It would also seem that a state of persistent light reaction can occur in the absence of any further contact with the responsible photoactive substance, the suggested reason for this being that minute amounts of the responsible substance remain in the skin and continue to be altered by exposure to light.[8]

It is also possible that the ability of the skin to react to light persists because of the presence of cross photosensitizers, or that other photoactive substances are unwittingly introduced during treatment. Again, an

1. Wilkinson, D. S. (1961). Photodermatitis due to tetrachlorsalicylanilide. *Br. J. Derm.* **73**, 213.
2. Wilkinson, D. S. (1962). Further experience with halogenated salicylanilides. *Br. J. Derm.* **74**, 295.
3. Harber, L. C., Harris, H. and Baer, R. L. (1966). Photoallergic contact dermatitis. *Archs Derm.* **94**, 255.
4. Herman, P. S. and Sams, W. M. (1972). 'Soap Photodermatitis. Photosensitivity to halogenated salicylanilides'. Charles C. Thomas, Springfield, Illinois.
5. Harber, L. C. and Baer, R. L. (1972). Special Review Article. Pathogenic mechanisms of drug-induced photosensitivity. *J. invest. Derm.* **58**, 327.
6. Willis, I. and Kligman, A. M. (1968). The mechanism of photoallergic contact dermatitis. *J. invest. Derm.* **51**, 378.
7. Morikaway, F., Nakayama, Y., Fukuma, M., Hamano, M., Yokoyama, Y., Nagura, T., Ishihara, Y. and Toda, K. (1974). Techniques for evaluation of phototoxicity and photoallergy in laboratory animals and man. *In* 'Sunlight and Man' (Ed., Fitzpatrick, T. B.), p. 529. Tokyo University Press, Tokyo.
8. Willis, I. and Kligman, A. M. (1968). The mechanism of persistent light reaction. *J. invest. Derm.* **51**, 385.

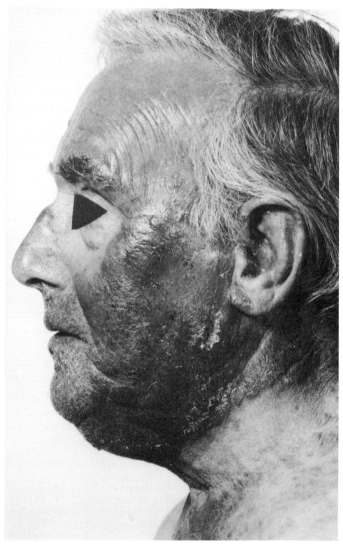

Fig. 3a. Clinical appearance of Photosensitivity Dermatitis. Sub-acute dermatitis is typical with a characteristic cut-off at the collar line and relative sparing of the peri-orbital skin.

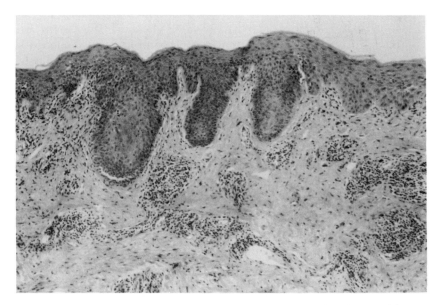

Fig. 3b. Typical histopathology of Photosensitivity Dermatitis. There is a dense, mainly peri-vascular infiltrate of lymphocytes and histiocytes, and some fibrosis, mostly confined to the middle and upper dermis. The epidermal changes are those of a regular acanthosis with focal spongiosis and lymphocytic exocytosis.

individual predisposed to the development of persistent light reaction may produce substances in his skin which absorb UVR or visible radiation and enable the photosensitivity reaction to continue.[1] The dermatitis reaction could also be maintained in response to exposure to one or more contact allergens in addition to a broad spectrum of environmental radiation.

Recent studies of the sesquiterpene lactone content of oleoresins extracted from plants of the Compositae family would suggest that there is a connection between a cell mediated contact allergic sensitivity to this group of substances[2] and other environmental contactants, including colophony and various fragrance materials resulting in a state of persistent light reaction and the clinical state of photosensitivity

1. Kochevar, I. E. (1979). Photoallergic responses to chemicals. *Photochem. Photobiol.* **30**, 437.
2. Frain-Bell, W. and Johnson, B. E. (1979). Contact allergic sensitivity to plants and the photosensitivity dermatitis and actinic reticuloid syndrome. *Br. J. Derm.* **101**, 503.

dermatitis.[1] It may well be, therefore, that an individual who has developed an allergic sensitivity to such chemical substances will continue to produce a contact eczematous response following exposure to the offending substances but in addition will also produce a photo-sensitivity reaction of persistent light reaction type because of the photoactive ability of the contact allergen or chemically related substances.

Action spectrum studies on photosensitivity dermatitis demonstrate involvement of the ultraviolet wavelengths along with a spread into the visible range in some cases.[2] Although the severity of photosensitivity is usually marked throughout the . UV from 290–400 nm, there is an extreme UV-B photosensitivity in some instances, so much so that the minimal response dose at 305 nm peak (± 5 nm) cannot be determined using conventional monochromator irradiation techniques. This broad action spectrum often narrows over a period of years; a change associated with clinical improvement.

Reference has been made to the histological changes observed in subjects with persistent light reaction of the photosensitivity dermatitis type which simulate those seen in cutaneous lymphoma, giving rise to the term "actinic reticuloid"[3] (Fig. 4). At that time it was considered that these skin changes might indicate a progression from a benign response to one with malignant potential. This question has yet to be finally resolved, and cutaneous reticulosis has been reported in association with actinic reticuloid. Nevertheless, the general concensus of opinion is that this pseudolymphomatous change is in most, if not all, instances a benign reaction. It merges clinically, histologically, and photobiologically with the features of photosensitivity dermatitis.[2,4] Moreover, a reversal of one of the original cases of actinic reticuloid to the relatively simple photosensitivity dermatitis has been reported.[5] The subsequent reporting of contact allergy to multiple allergens, and in particular to Compositae oleoresins in actinic reticuloid, adds support to the view that photo-

1. Addo, H. A., Ferguson, J., Johnson, B.E. and Frain-Bell, W. (1982). The relationship between exposure to fragrance materials and persistent light reaction in the photosensitive dermatitis with actinic reticuloid syndrome. *Br. J. Derm.* **107**, 261.
2. Frain-Bell, W. (1979). Dowling Oration. What is that thing called light? *Clin. exp. Derm.* **4**, 1.
3. Ive, F. A., Magnus, I. A., Warin, R. P. and Wilson Jones, E. (1969). 'Actinic Reticuloid'; chronic dermatosis associated with severe photosensitivity and histological resemblance to lymphoma. *Br. J. Derm.* **81**, 469.
4. Frain-Bell, W., Lakshmipathi, T., Rogers, J. and Willock, Joyce (1974). The syndrome of chronic photosensitivity dermatitis and actinic reticuloid. *Br. J. Derm.* **91**, 617.
5. Magnus, I. A. and Hawk, J. L. M. (1978). Resolution of actinic reticuloid with transition to photosensitive eczema. *Jl R. Soc. Med.* **71**, 608.

sensitivity dermatitis and actinic reticuloid are the same syndrome with differing degrees of intensity of the cutaneous reaction.

Over a period of time there is a tendency for many of those with photosensitivity dermatitis to show improvement although complete remission is rare. Some subjects who are virtually free from clinical signs or are significantly improved, nevertheless have an abnormal erythema action spectrum as determined by phototesting the normally non-exposed skin of the back.

There is said to be a separate entity where the action spectrum is confined to the UV-B wavelengths,[1] and this has been named photo-sensitive eczema. This is probably not a separate disorder. Any difference may be due to variations in phototesting techniques, and in any event the epidermal reaction of "photosensitive dermatitis" is of an eczematous character.

A relationship between contact sensitivity and photosensitivity of apparently unknown aetiology has also been described in patients with chromium dermatitis. The intensity of patch test reactions to potassium dichromate was increased by exposure to sub-minimal erythema dose exposures of solar simulating radiation in almost half the patients tested.[2] Light sensitivity is supposedly common in patients who react to chromium,[3,4] and the increased intensity of patch test reaction obtained was best illustrated in patients who presented with a history of light sensitivity. Phototoxicity due to potassium dichromate has not as yet been demonstrated.[4,5]

It may be that the repeated stimulus to the lymphoid cells by multiple allergens is responsible for the cellular infiltrate noted in actinic reticuloid. It may also be that in the rare cases in which a frank reticulosis develops, the sequence of events is similar to that which has been postulated for the development of mycoses fungoides from a relatively benign reactive phase. However, the part played by light in these reactions is obscure. It is intriguing that cutaneous photosensitivity has been reported in patients with a variety of reticuloses and in particular mycoses fungoides.[6] This has been detected both as clinical photo-sensitivity, confirmed by the demonstration of an abnormal action

1. Ramsay, C. A. and Black, A. K. (1973). Photosensitive eczema. *Trans. St. John's Hosp. Dis. Skin.* **59**, 152.
2. Wahlberg, J. E. and Wennersten, G. (1977). Light sensitivity and chromium dermatitis. *Br. J. Derm.* **97**, 411.
3. Tronnier, H. (1970). Zur Lichtempfindlichkeit von Ekzematikern (unter besonderer Berucksichtigung des Chromat-Ekzems). *Arch. Klin. Exp. Derm.* **237**, 494.
4. Feuerman, E. (1971). Chromates as the cause of dermatitis in housewives. *Dermatologica* **143**, 292.
5. Wennersten, G. (1977). Photodynamic aspects of some metal complexes. *Acta derm.* **57**, 519.
6. Volden, G. and Thune, P. O. (1977). Light sensitivity in mycoses fungoides. *Br. J. Derm.* **97**, 297.

spectrum for erythema, and also by an abnormal action spectrum in those in which photosensitivity was not suspected on clinical grounds.

There is some evidence for an abnormality of tryptophan metabolism in actinic reticuloid.[1] Kynurenic acid, a tryptophan derivative, has been identified as a crystalline deposit in the vicinity of eccrine sweat glands in the skin of an actinic reticuloid patient.[2] Because the inflammatory cells involved in the photosensitivity reaction in this patient appeared to accumulate in the same location, the authors suggested that kynurenic acid might be the photosensitizer. The role for kynurenic acid in the photosensitivity associated with actinic reticuloid, or any other condition, remains to be confirmed, but it is certainly an effective phototoxic agent *in vitro*.[3,4]

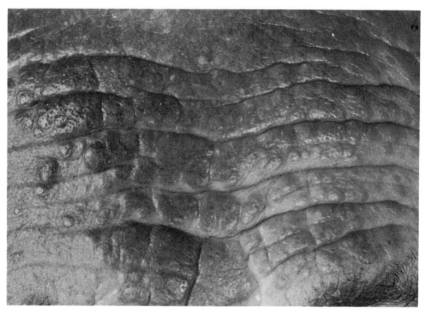

Fig. 4a. Clinical appearance of Actinic Reticuloid in forehead skin. Pseudolymphoma, nodule and plaque formation are present with sparing of the skin creases.

1. Binazzi, M. and Calandra, P. (1971). Actinic Reticuloid; Pathogenic Aspects. *Arch. Dermatol. Forsch.* **241**, 391.
2. Swanbeck, G. and Wennersten, G. (1973). Evidence of kynurenic acid as a possible photosensitiser in actinic reticuloid. *Acta derm-venereol. (Stockholm)* **53**, 109.
3. Swanbeck, G. and Wennersten, G. (1974). Photohaemolytic activity of Tryptophan at Phenylalamine metabolites. *Acta derm-venereol. (Stockholm)* **54**, 99.
4. Nilsson, R., Swanbeck, G. and Wennersten, G. (1975). Primary mechanisms of Erythrocyte photolysis induced by Biological sensitizers and Phototoxic Drugs. *Photochem. Photobiol.* **22**, 183.

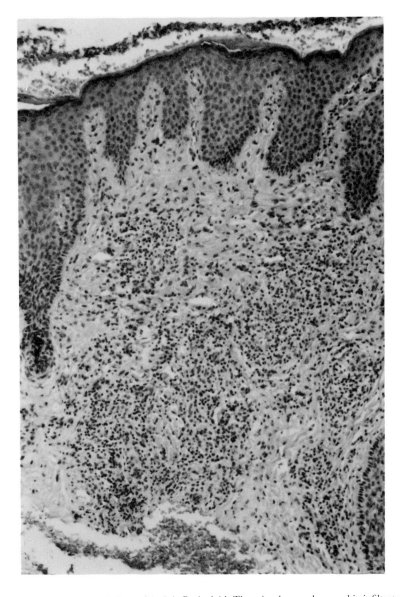

Fig. 4b. Typical histopathology of Actinic Reticuloid. There is a heavy pleomorphic infiltrate, consisting of lymphocytes, histiocytes, occasional plasma cells and atypical monocytes, throughout the whole of the dermis. Abnormal mitotic figures may be seen. The epidermis shows mainly acanthosis and some parakeratosis.

II. THE EFFECT OF SOLAR RADIATION ON CERTAIN DERMATOSES

A. The Photobiology of Lupus Erythematosus

It is known that exposure to sunlight is detrimental to some cases of cutaneous and systemic lupus erythematosus. However, the majority react abnormally to UVR as shown by their response to sunburn erythema, or by aggravation of the cutaneous lesions, or both. It has been suggested that such aggravation is more likely to occur in disseminated discoid lupus erythematosus and in systemic lupus erythematosus rather than in the more commonly seen fixed localized discoid variety.[1] Occasionally the reaction is urticarial, and erythema multiforme and vesiculo-bullous reactions have also been described; whether or not these can be UV-induced is less clear. Clinical photosensitivity has been variably reported up to a maximum of 50% of cases.[2,3]

The techniques used to study the photobiological aspects of lupus erythematosus have been directed towards the confirmation of a history of clinical photosensitivity. This included the determination of their action spectrum for erythema and relating it to that found in normal non-light sensitive subjects, and the irradiation of the skin with short wavelength UV in an attempt to reproduce the clinical and histological changes of lupus erythematosus. This reproduction of the cutaneous lesions was achieved by Epstein et al., who biopsied 25 subjects following repeated UV exposures.[4] They were able to reproduce the histological changes commonly seen in chronic cutaneous lupus erythematosus by demonstrating hyperkeratosis, follicular and non-follicular keratin plugging, patchy oedema, a marked liquefaction degeneration of the epidermal basal layer, and at times irregular epidermal atrophy and also a consistent round cell infiltrate in the upper dermis with a tendency to perivascular distribution. These changes were noted in four of 21 patients with systemic lupus erythematosus and in one of those with discoid lupus erythematosus. None of the 16 patients without a history of clinical light sensitivity showed such an abnormal phototest response. The action spectrum for these changes was in the UV wavelength range below 320 nm and the reaction was not reproducible following irradiation with long wavelength UV. The effectiveness of this short wavelength UV

1. Baer, R. L. and Harber, L. C. (1965). Photobiology of Lupus Erythematosus. *Archs Derm.* **92**, 124.
2. Epstein, J. H. (1975). Photobiology of Lupus Erythematosus. *Cutis* **15**, 212.
3. Frain-Bell, W. (1979). Dowling Oration. What is that thing called light? *Clin. exp. Derm.* **4**, 1.
4. Epstein, J. H., Tuffanelli, D. L. and Dubois, E. I. (1965). Light sensitivity and lupus erythematosus. *Archs Derm.* **91**, 483.

action spectrum has been confirmed by others.[1,2,3] The clinical cutaneous change as a result of repeat irradiation simulated, although was not identical with, that seen in cutaneous lupus erythematosus.

A number of suggestions have been made as to the mechanism involved in the adverse reaction of the skin in lupus erythematosus to UVR. It has been suggested that the chronic inflammatory reaction makes individuals more susceptible to the action of light.[4] Others believe that it may be a type of Koebner response,[5] and there is some support for this view in that lesions of lupus erythematosus may also be produced by exposure to heat or freezing with liquid nitrogen.[6] The observation, however, that exposure to sunlight seems to precipitate systemic manifestations of lupus erythematosus in some individuals and also aggravates the cutaneous lesions would suggest that UVR has more than a non-specific effect. It has been suggested that UV-induced DNA damage may provide altered nuclear material which triggers off a hypersensitivity immune response.[7] The photoproducts of DNA which are probably dimers are known as "UV-DNA", and these are highly immunogenic.[8]

Antigenicity of altered DNA, subsequent to UV damage, is well recognized,[9] and it has been shown that experimental animals sensitized to UV-irradiated DNA deposit immunoglobulins at the dermo–epidermal interface following cutaneous irradiation.[10] Circulating anti-nuclear antibodies have been demonstrated in mice following cutaneous UV irradiation,[11] and although care must be taken in extrapolating the results of animal studies to man, it is reasonable to accept that cutaneous photo-damage may result in an additional antigen load to

1. Freeman, R. G., Knox, J. N. and Owens, D. W. (1969). Cutaneous lesions of lupus erythematosus induced by monochromatic light. *Archs Derm.* **100**, 677.
2. Cripps, D. J. and Rankin, J. (1973). Action spectra of lupus erythematosus and experimental immunofluorescence. *Archs Derm.* **107**, 563.
3. Frain-Bell, W. (1979). Dowling Oration. What is that thing called light? *Clin. exp. Derm.* **4**, 1.
4. Sapuppo, A. (1954). Cutaneous reactivity to ultraviolet rays in subjects with chronic discoid lupus erythematosus. *Minerva Derm.* **29**, 6.
5. Kestin, B. and Slatkin, M. (1953). Diseases related to light sensitivity. *Archs Derm.* **67**, 284.
6. Epstein, H. and Tuffanelli, D. L. (1974). Discoid lupus erythematosus. In 'Lupus Erythematosus' (Ed., Dubois, E. L.), edition 2, pp. 210–224. University of Southern California Press, Los Angeles.
7. Baer, R. L. and Harber, L. C. (1965). Photobiology of lupus erythematosus. *Archs Derm.* **92**, 124.
8. Levine, L., Seaman, E., Hammerschlag, E. and Van Vunakis, M. (1966). Antibodies to photoproducts of DNA irradiated with ultraviolet light. *Science* **153**, 1666.
9. Tan, E. M. and Stoughton, R. B. (1969). *In vivo* alterations of cellular DNA by ultraviolet light. *Proc. natn. Acad. Sci.* **62**, 708.
10. Natali, P. G. and Tan, E. M. (1973). Experimental skin lesions in mice resembling systemic lupus erythematosus. *Arthritis Rheum.* **16**, 579.
11. Ten Veen, J. H. and Lucas, C. J. (1970). Induction of antinuclear antibodies by ultraviolet irradiation. *Ann. rheum. Dis.* **29**, 556.

a patient with lupus erythematosus.[1] Patients with systemic lupus erythematosus have antibodies to UV-DNA and these may cross react with native DNA.[2] There is no correlation between degree of photosensitivity and UV-DNA antibody titre in these patients, but such antibodies were not detected in patients with other photodermatoses.[3] There is an UV-induced deposition of both UV-DNA and immunoglobulin at the dermo–epidermal junction in rabbits immunized with UV-DNA. Moreover, both native DNA and UV-DNA bind to the dermo–epidermal junction *in vitro*.[4] It is not clear why this reaction occurs in systemic lupus erythematosus but there may be a deficiency in repair of UV-DNA in these patients[5] which allows the persistence of the normally removed immunogenic photoproducts. The overall pathophysiological processes involved obviously differ from those of the better recognized repair deficient diseases. It has also been suggested that UV-induced lysosomal membrane injury may play a role in the lupus erythematosus reaction,[6] and this lysosomal photoreactivity has been proposed to be a feature common to both lupus erythematosus and porphyria cutanea tarda.[7] This might explain the co-existence of lupus erythematosus and porphyria in some subjects.[8, 9] There is some evidence[10] that the repeated irradiation of LE patients causing the morphological and histological changes already referred to, results in the immunoglobulin deposition at the dermo–epidermal junction, although this may not be seen until some months after the irradiation.

The deposition of fluorescein-conjugated anti-human immune globulins at the dermo–epidermal junction (the lupus band test (LBT)) may be demonstrated by fluorescence microscopy in over 90% of examined skin specimens from lesions in both systemic lupus erythematosus and chronic cutaneous lupus erythematosus. This fluorescent band is obtained in the

1. Epstein, J. H. (1975). Photobiology of lupus erythematosus. *Cutis* **15**, 212.
2. Davis, P., Russell, A. S. and Percy, J. S. (1976). Antibodies to UV light denatured DNA in systemic lupus erythematosus. *J. Rheum.* **3**, 375.
3. Davis, P. (1977). Antibodies to UV DNA and photosensitivity. *Br. J. Derm.* **97**, 197.
4. Davis, P. and Percy, J. S. (1978). Role of ultraviolet light and UV DNA in the induction of skin lesions in experimental animals. *Br. J. Derm.* **99**, 201.
5. Beighlie, D. J. and Teplitz, R. L. (1975). Repair of UV damaged DNA in systemic lupus erythematosus. *J. Derm.* **2**, 149.
6. Baer, R. L. and Harber, L. C. (1965). Photobiology of lupus erythematosus. *Archs Derm.* **92**, 124.
7. Voron, D. A. and Tonken, S. W. (1975). Lupus erythematosus coexisting with porphyria cutanea tarda: lysosomal photoreactivity as a common demoninator. *Cutis* **15**, 69.
8. Cram, D. L., Epstein, J. H. and Tuffanelli, D. L. (1973). Lupus erythematosus and porphyria. *Archs Derm.* **108**, 779.
9. Hetherington, G. W., Jetton, R. L. and Knox, J. M. (1970). The association of lupus erythematosus and porphyria. *Br. J. Derm.* **82**, 118.
10. Cripps, D. J. and Rankin, J. (1973). Action spectra of lupus erythematosus and experimental immunofluorescence. *Archs Derm.* **107**, 563.

normal skin of over half the patients with systemic lupus erythematosus, but is not found in normal skin of chronic cutaneous lupus erythematosus. Because the LBT is negative in affected skin from patients with polymorphic light eruption, it forms a useful additional test for differentiating this photodermatosis from the potentially more serious lupus erythematosus group.[1] The inclusions or cytoplasmic tubular aggregates (CTA) described by Gyorkey in 1969[2] in the renal endothelial cells in patients with systemic lupus erythematosus can be shown to increase following UV irradiation of the normal skin of patients with systemic lupus erythematosus and discoid lupus erythematosus.[3] Also, the incidence of the positive LBT varies with the site of skin biopsy: thus, patients with systemic lupus erythematosus with severe renal disease often have a positive LBT on both the buttock and the forearm skin, but if the systemic disease is less severe the LBT is negative, or, if positive, only on the exposed forearm skin.[4]

B. Photosensitivity in Psoriasis [5]

Exposure to sunlight tends to improve the skin changes in psoriasis (see phototherapy, page 2608). In a minority of subjects such exposure aggravates the condition and results in the appearance of psoriatic lesions on the exposed skin. This reaction to light occurs most often in fair complexioned individuals following sunburn erythema and as such appears to be an isomorphic reaction. Psoriasis may also occur in individuals who suffer from one or other of the photodermatoses such as polymorphic light eruption or photosensitivity dermatitis. However, in these circumstances the Koebner type of photosensitivity psoriatic reaction does not occur. This would support the view that when it occurs it is not a non-specific isomorphic response to UVR.

C. Lichen Planus

As in photosensitive psoriasis, where the lesions are produced on the exposed skin following sunburn erythema, classical lichen planus can be produced on exposed sites. In addition there is a form of lichen planus

1. Epstein, J. H. (1974). The use of fluorescent microscopy in the study of photocutaneous disorders. *In* 'Sunlight and Man' (Ed., Fitzpatrick, T. B.), p. 613. University of Tokyo Press, Tokyo.
2. Gyorkey, F., Min, K. W. and Sincovics, J. G. (1969). Systemic lupus erythematosus and myxovirus. *New Eng. J. Med.* **280**, 333.
3. Berk, S. H. and Blank, H. (1974). Ultraviolet light and cytoplasmic tubules in lupus erythematosus. *Archs Derm.* **109**, 364.
4. Ahmed, A. R. and Provost, T. T. (1979). Incidence of a positive lupus band test using sun-exposed and unexposed skin. *Archs Derm.* **115**, 228.
5. Bielicky, T. and Kvicalova, Eva (1964). Photosensitive Psoriasis. *Dermatologica* **129**, 339.

B. E. JOHNSON

which occurs in pigmented individuals in sub-tropical climates as a response to exposure to sunshine to which the label "actinic lichen planus" has been applied.[1,2,3,4] The condition, first clearly described by Dostrovsky and Sagher, has a number of features which differ from those of classical lichen planus. It occurs most commonly in children and young adults, and the itching, which is a prominent feature of classical lichen planus, is minimal or absent. The lesions appear, or become aggravated, following exposure to sunshine and the papules show pigmentation or depigmentation, or there may be granuloma annulare-like lesions. The histological changes often differ from those seen in classical lichen planus, there being a basophilic degeneration of the collagen in the upper dermis with a perivascular infiltration of lymphocytes. There is also a lymphocytic infiltration in the upper and middle dermis, with patchy liquefaction degeneration of the basal cells and follicular keratotic plugging in the thinned epidermis. Thus, it has some resemblance to lupus erythematosus.[5,6] Although it is most likely that this is a form of lichen planus, further studies of the pigmentary and photobiological features will help to clarify the nature of these lesions.

D. Cutaneous Lymphocytoma

It is known that some patients with cutaneous lymphocytoma have clinical photosensitivity.[7,8,9] There is also an uncommon but interesting association between the development of cutaneous lymphocytoma and polymorphic light eruption and solar urticaria.[10,11,12,13] Protection of the skin from the responsible wavelengths will minimize the photodermatoses and result in a reduction of the lymphocytoma.[13] It is of interest to contrast

1. Dostrovsky, A. and Sagher, R. (1949). Lichen planus in subtropical countries. *Archs Derm.* **59**, 308.
2. Zawahry, M. el (1963). 'Skin Diseases in Arabian countries. Milestones in Dermatology', Vols 1–3, 313.
3. Santoianni, P. (1965). Lichen planus actinicus (vel tropicus). *Minerva Dermatologica* **40**, 421.
4. Santoianni, P. (1974). II. Lichen actinicus. *G. ital. Derm.* **109**, 102.
5. Katzenellenbogen, I. (1962). Lichen planus Actinicus (Lichen Planus in Subtropical Countries). *Dermatologica* **126**, 10.
6. Almeyda, J. (1970). Lichen Planus Actinicus. *Br. J. Derm.* **82**, 426.
7. Epstein, S. (1935). Lymphocytoma der Haut mit Beteiligung der Conjunctiva bulbi. Beitrag zur Pathogenese der Lymphocytome. *Archiv für Derm und Syph. Bd.* **172/3**, 13.
8. Bettley, F. R. (1947). Miliary Lymphocytoma. *Br. J. Derm.* **59**, 70.
9. Alexander, J. O'D and Pasieczny, T. (1954). Follicular lymphoma of the skin. *Dermatologica* **109**, 1.
10. Wiskemann, A. (1957). Miliare Lymphocytome bei gleichzetig bestehenhenden chronisch polymorphen Lichtexanthem. *Hautarzt* **8**, 275.
11. Wiskemann, A. (1963). Lymphozytome bei Lichturtikaria. *Derm. Wschr.* **147**, 350.
12. Slepyan, A. H. (1958). Case Presentation. Chicago Dermatological Society, March 19th, 1958; quoted by Bluefarb (1960) p. 141.
13. Frain-Bell, W. and Magnus, I. A. (1971). A study of the photosensitivity factor in cutaneous lymphocytoma. *Br. J. Derm.* **84**, 25.

the histological picture of lymphocytoma with its monomorphic masses of dermal lymphocytes with the pleomorphic reaction seen in the highly reactive forms of photosensitivity dermatitis and the actinic reticuloid syndrome (see page 2506). This striking dermal lymphocyte response can develop as a result of phototesting in the absence of a previous lymphocytoma.[1] It may be that the cell mediated contact allergic reaction associated with photosensitivity dermatitis can modify the cellular infiltrate and thus allow for both the monomorphic and the polymorphic infiltrates. On the other hand, photosensitivity suspected on clinical grounds, in some cases of Jessner's lymphocytic infiltration,[2] is not usually confirmed by subsequent phototesting.[3]

E. Pemphigus Group of Conditions and Darier's Disease in Relation to UV Exposure

The fact that exposure to sunlight can result in the development or exacerbation of lesions in pemphigus erythematosus is well established.[4, 5, 6] Jacobs described a patient whose eruption was exacerbated by exposing the skin to sunlight and in whom the morphological and histological features of the condition could be reproduced by controlled exposure to the sunburn wavelengths of 280–320 nm UVR.[7] UV-induced acantholysis in pemphigus foliaceous has also been described, and this could be inhibited by the oral administration of chloroquine phosphate. A minimal erythema dose was sufficient to produce acantholysis in some subjects, but in others multiples of the MED were required. The action spectrum for the production of acantholysis in pemphigus is not known but window glass appears ineffective against this UV effect so that wavelengths greater than 320 nm may well be involved in addition to UV-B.[8] UV-induced acantholysis can also be demonstrated in Darier's Disease[9] and its bullous counterpart, benign familial chronic pemphigus

1. Miescher, G. (1957). Zur Histologie der lichtbedingten Reaktionen. *Dermatologica* **115**, 345.
2. Gottlieb, B. and Winkelmann, R. K. (1962). Lymphocytic infiltration of skin. *Archs Derm.* **86**, 106.
3. Frain-Bell, W. (1981). Unpublished Data.
4. Jacobson, C. and Pilsbury, D. M. (1952). Pemphigus erythematosus (Senear–Usher Syndrome). *Am. Archs Derm. Syph.* **66**, 661.
5. Miller, J. L. (1956). Senear–Usher pemphigus: pemphigus erythematosus. *Am. Archs Derm. Syph.* **73**, 300.
6. Pilsbury, D. M., Shelley, W. B. and Kligman, A. M. (1956). 'Dermatology', p. 791. W. B. Saunders Co., Philadelphia.
7. Jacobs, S. E. (1965). Pemphigus erythematosus and ultraviolet light. *Archs Derm.* **91**, 139.
8. Cram, D. L. and Winkelmann, R. K. (1965). Ultraviolet-induced acantholysis in pemphigus. *Archs Derm.* **92**, 7.
9. Preissman, M. (1945). Sur l'action provcatrice de la lumière dans la maladie de Darier. *Dermatologica* **91**, 28.

(Hailey–Hailey Disease).[1,2] In contrast to pemphigus, it is possible to induce acantholysis in Darier's disease with phenol, ethyl chloride spray, scarification, application of adhesives, and other physical agents including UVR.[3,4,5]

The mechanisms involved in the reproduction by UVR of lesions in these diseases are not well defined. In psoriasis, lichen planus, discoid lupus erythematosus, Hailey–Hailey disease, lesions may arise through the isomorphic or Koebner response and are most easily induced when the disease is in its florid state. A similar effect occurs in pemphigus vulgaris and in bullous pemphigoid when the skin is exposed to UVR.[6] Immuno-histochemical techniques appear to show an increase in the binding of IgG and complement in UV-irradiated normal skin of patients with pemphigus vulgaris and bullous pemphigoid preceding the development of clinical and histological changes.[6] This study gives some insight into the pathogenesis of the isomorphic response to UVR in bullous diseases in which antibody and complement activation is involved and may be relevant to the other diseases in this group.

F. Light Sensitivity and Secondary Plane Xanthoma

A case[7] was presented at the Royal Society of Medicine of an elderly male patient with photosensitivity dermatitis who had yellowish macules on the forehead. Histological examination showed an extensive xanthomatous infiltrate in the middle and upper dermis containing a mixture of lipids within histiocytic cells. He was extremely photosensitive in the sunburn wavelengths (300–320 nm), although details of the full action spectrum were not reported. Earlier Walker and Sneddon[8] had described four patients (one with actinic reticuloid) who developed plane xanthomata after a pre-existing erythrodermic state. Their interpretation

1. Chorzelski, T. (1962). Experimentally induced acantholysis in Hailey's Benign Pemphigus. *Dermatologica* **124**, 21.
2. Cram, D. L., Muller, S. A. and Winkelmann, R. K. (1967). Ultraviolet-induced acantholysis in familial benign chronic pemphigus. *Archs Derm.* **96**, 636.
3. Preissman, M. (1945). Sur l'action provocatrice de la lumière dans la maladie de Darier. *Dermatologica* **91**, 28.
4. Shelley, W. B., Arthur, R. P. and Pilsbury, D. M. (1959). A view of keratosis follicularis (Darier's Disease) as a neoplastic process. *Archs Derm.* **80**, 332.
5. Penrod, J. N., Everett, M. A. and McCreight, W. G. (1960). Observations on keratosis follicularis. *Archs Derm.* **82**, 367.
6. Cram, D. L. and Fukuyama, K. (1972). Immunohistochemistry of ultraviolet-induced pemphigus and pemphigoid lesions. *Archs Derm.* **106**, 819.
7. Marks, R. and Wilson-Jones, E. (1971). Light sensitivity and secondary plane xanthoma. *Br. J. Derm.* **85**, 297.
8. Walker, A. E. and Sneddon, I. B. (1968). Skin xanthoma following erythroderma. *Br. J. Derm.* **80**, 580.

was that lipidization can take place in areas of reticulo–endothelial cell hyperplasia. Three other examples of xanthomas developing as part of the skin response in the photosensitivity dermatitis and actinic reticuloid syndrome were described by James and Warin,[1] and reference was made to similar reports.[1,2,3] In none of these cases was there an abnormality of the plasma lipid levels, and this suggests that the production of xanthoma was probably due to local factors rather than to a systemic process. It would seem that the foam cells develop from dermal macrophages by the uptake of lipids.

However, other cases have shown abnormal plasma lipids and lipoprotein abnormality, and, although this type of cutaneous xanthoma is commonly associated with chronic photosensitivity, it is not invariable.[4] An increase in plasma lipids and lipoproteins would favour the production of cutaneous xanthoma; but this formation process is probably at cellular level and elevated plasma lipid levels are not essential for the accumulation of intracellular lipid.[1]

G. Pellagra[5,6]

Pellagra is a niacin deficiency disorder characterized by gastrointestinal disturbances, symmetrical skin lesions and encephalopathy. It is of interest to photobiologists because the majority of skin lesions are on exposed areas and appear to be precipitated by sunlight during spring and summer but improve during the winter.[7,8] The skin changes detected early in the course of the disease are an acute, burning erythema of exposed areas which may progress to blistering. The "V" area of the neck is particularly affected, and there is also desquamation, thickening and hyperpigmentation of the hands and arms.

Despite the marked association with exposure to sunlight, it is not

1. James, M. P. and Warin, A. P. (1978). Plane xanthoma developing in photosensitive eczema. A report of 3 cases with a discussion of a possible mechanism for lipid accumulation in plane xanthomas. *Clin. exp. Derm.* **3**, 307.
2. Sato, A., Tonahashi, Y., Maie, O. and Maruhama, Y. (1976). Xanthoma secondary to reticulohistiocyte infiltration. *Archs derm. Res.* **257**, 93.
3. Degos, R., Belaich, S., Foix, C. and Dubertret, L. (1975). Xanthomatisation des lésions cutanées au secours d'une actinoreticulose. *Bull. Soc. fr. Derm.* **82**, 5.
4. Walker, A. E. and Sneddon, I. B. (1968). Skin xanthoma following erythroderma. *Br. J. Derm.* **80**, 580.
5. Cairns, R. J. (1972). Metabolic and nutritional disorders. *In* 'Textbooks of Dermatology', 2nd edition (Eds, Rook, A., Wilkinson, D. S. and Ebling, F. J. G.), Vol. 2, p. 1831. Blackwell, Oxford.
6. Harris, S. (1941). 'Clinical Pellagra'. Mosby, St. Louis.
7. Spivak, J. L. and Jackson, D. L. (1977). Pellagra: an analysis of 18 patients and a review of the literature. *John Hopkins med. J.* **140**, 295.
8. Cripps, D. J. (1967). Diseases aggravated by sunlight. *Postgrad. Med.* **41**, 57.

possible to clearly define the photosensitivity in pellagra.[1] The acute state is not obviously related to a single exposure to sunlight and lesions cannot be elicited with controlled xenon arc or natural sunlight exposures, and strangely there is no abnormal photosensitivity on phototesting.[2]

Skin reactions to repeated UVR exposures in Bantu subjects with pellagra were not different from those in controls, although histological examination did reveal some slight changes in the superficial epidermis.[3]

Niacin is the dietary source of the nicotinamide required for cellular oxidation–reduction processes, but it is difficult to explain a chronic photosensitivity state on the grounds of such a deficiency. Isoniazid is a structural analogue of niacin and is used in the treatment of tuberculosis. This probably acts as a niacin antagonist and can induce pellagra, especially in patients with poor nutritional status.[4, 5, 6] Nicotinamide is a major metabolite of tryptophan, and when pellagra occurs as part of a general protein deficiency, as is seen in chronic alcoholism, the changes are attributed to this primary tryptophan deficiency.[7, 8] When pellagra occurs with the "carcinoid syndrome", it is also associated with nicotinamide deficiency secondary to an abnormal tryptophan metabolism in which the metabolic pathway is diverted towards 5-hydroxytryptamine.[9, 10]

III. ABNORMAL REACTIONS IN CERTAIN GENODERMATOSES

A. Xeroderma Pigmentosum

Xeroderma pigmentosum (XP) is essentially a multi-system disease

1. Magnus, I. A. (1976). 'Dermatological Photobiology'. Blackwell, Oxford.
2. Smeenk, G. and Hulsmans, H. A. M. (1969). Dermatological and biochemical anomolies in two patients with Pellagroid Syndrome. *Dermatologica* **138**, 295.
3. Findlay, G. H., Rein, L. and Mitchell, D. (1969). Reactions to light on the normal and pellagrous Bantu skin. *Br. J. Derm.* **81**, 345.
4. Harrison, R. J. and Feiwel, M. (1956). Pellagra caused by isoniazide. *Br. med. J.* **2**, 852.
5. Di Lorenzo, P. A. (1967). Pellagra-like syndrome associated with isoniazid therapy. *Acta dermvenereol. (Stockholm)* **47**, 318.
6. Comaish, J. S., Felix, R. H. and McGrath, H. (1976). Topically applied niacinamide in isoniazid-induced pellagra. *Archs Derm.* **112**, 70.
7. Spivak, J. L. and Jackson, D. L. (1977). Pellagra: an analysis of 18 patients and a review of the literature. *John Hopkins Med. J.* **140**, 295.
8. Parrish, J. A., White, H. A. D. and Pathak, M. A. (1979). Photomedicine. *In* 'Dermatology in General Medicine' (Eds, Fitzpatrick, T. B., Eisen, A. Z., Wolff, K., Freedburg, I. M. and Austen, K. F.), p. 975. McGraw Hill, New York.
9. Bridges, J. M., Gibson, J. B., Loughridge, L. W. and Montgomery, D. A. D. (1957). Carcinoid syndrome with pellagrous dermatitis. *Br. J. Surg.* **45**, 117.
10. Castiello, R. J. and Lynch, P. J. (1972). Pellagra and the carcinoid syndrome. *Archs Derm.* **105**, 574.

having cutaneous features as a major component.[1] This rare disorder has an incidence of 1 in 4 million and is often the result of a consanguinous marriage. It is inherited as an autosomal recessive, although a mild form with a suggested dominant inheritance has been reported.[2] It usually presents in early childhood as a heightened sensitivity to sunlight causing a sunburn type of reaction which can be severe, and differs from that occurring in normal subjects by its persistence. This type of sunburn reaction does not occur in all cases of XP, and this may reflect variations in the individual's cellular sensitivity to UVR and to varying degrees of ethnic skin pigmentation. Within a short time numerous freckles appear on sun-exposed sites and the skin becomes dry and scaly with telangiectasis and areas of hypopigmentation. Later, localized hyperkeratotic changes occur with the development of actinic keratoses. By this time there may be evidence of localized atrophy, the general picture being that of a rapid and premature ageing of the skin. Sooner or later, depending on the form of XP and the amount of sun exposure, malignant changes begin to appear. These are basal cell epithelioma, squamous cell epithelioma, and malignant melanoma. Keratoacanthoma can also develop (Fig. 5) and other tumours such as angiomas, fibromas and sarcomas have been reported. The eyes and eyelids may be similarly involved. Rarely these skin and eye changes are associated with a wide range of neurological symptoms in the de Sanctis–Cacchione syndrome.

A small number of subjects have similar skin changes but of a reduced severity and there is a delayed onset (Fig. 6). This form, originally called "Pigmented Xerodermoid",[3, 4] has since been shown to have the molecular defect of a variant form of XP which nevertheless can have clinical features just as severe as those seen in the classical type.[5, 6, 7]

Studies of XP skin reactions to controlled UVR exposure were first reported by Rothman,[8] who found little difference from normal in the

---

1. Hebra, F. and Kaposi, M. (1874). 'On Diseases of the Skin including the Exanthemata', Vol. 3, p. 252. The New Sydenham Society, London.
2. Anderson, T. E. and Begg, M. (1950). Xeroderma pigmentosum of mild type. *Br. J. Derm.* **62**, 402.
3. Jung, E. G. (1970). New form of molecular defect in xeroderma pigmentosum. *Nature* **228**, 361.
4. Jung, E. G. (1971). Das pigmentierte Xerodermoid. Ein Defekt der Rekombinationserholung von UV-Schaden. *Archs derm. Res.* **241**, 33.
5. Burk, P. G., Lutzner, M. A., Clarke, D. D. and Robbins, J. H. (1971). Ultraviolet-stimulated Thymidine Incorporation in Xeroderma Pigmentosum Lymphocytes. *J. Lab. clin. Med.* **77**, 759.
6. Cleaver, J. E. (1972). Xeroderma pigmentosum: variants with normal DNA repair and normal sensitivity to ultraviolet light. *J. invest. Derm.* **58**, 124.
7. Fischer, E., Jung, E. G. and Cleaver, J. E. (1980). Pigmented Xerodermoid and XP-variants. *Archs derm. Res.* **269**, 329.
8. Rothman, S. (1923). Untersuchungen über Xeroderma pigmentosum. *Arch. für derm. Syph.* **144**, 440.

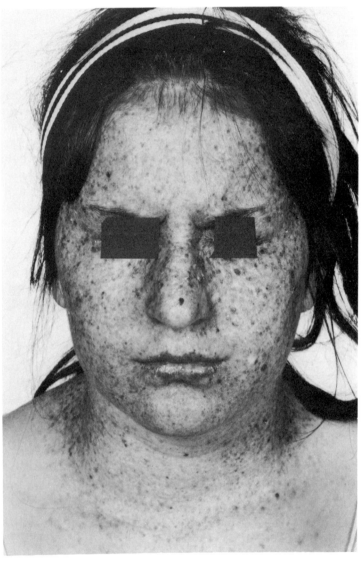

Fig. 5. Classical Xeroderma Pigmentosum. There is typically a universal affection of the exposed skin of the face and neck with premalignant and malignant changes. Some sparing of the normally covered skin is evident.

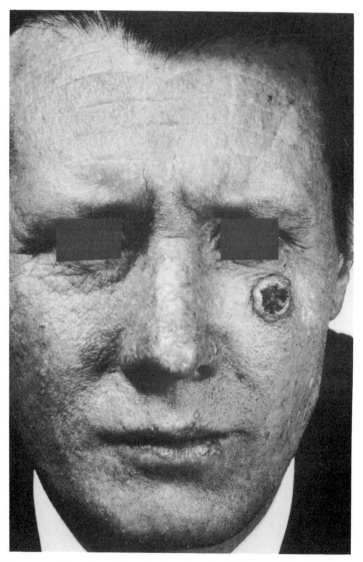

Fig. 6. Xeroderma Pigmentosum Variant. There is universal dryness of the skin of the face with scarring, particularly well seen over the bridge of the nose. A spontaneously resolving keratoacanthoma, typical of this condition, is present on the skin of the left cheek.

initial stages of the reaction. However, he noted a delay in the resolution of the erythema and a greater intensity of the subsequent pigmentation. The persistence of erythema with marked pigmentation, following acute reactions which were sometimes of less than normal intensity, were characteristic of the phototest.[1] The wavelength dependence for these reactions was probably the same as for sunburn in that a window glass filter prevented their occurrence.[1]

A second, possibly more significant characteristic of the XP skin reaction to UVR is the delay in its development following exposure to UV-B. The exposure dose of wavelengths around 300 nm required to produce erythema in XP was less than that for normal skin, but whereas in the latter the erythema was present some 3 h after the exposure, it was not observed in XP skin until 24 h.[2] These observations have been confirmed and examined in detail by minimal erythema dose (MED) determinations with monochromatic radiation.[3,4,5] When the MED to 290–320 nm of these patients is observed at 24 h, it varies little from normal. The MED at 24 h may be higher for XP than for normal skin.[6] However, whereas the normal skin reaction has disappeared by 72 h, in XP not only is there a persistent erythema, but also reactions to lower doses begin to appear. The true MED for XP skin is, therefore, lower than that for normal skin but only as an abnormally delayed response. Action spectrum studies have shown that for most cases of XP the reactions to 250, 260, and 270 nm radiation are normal.[5,6] It seems, therefore, that the abnormal reactions, some of which were papular,[5] are produced by the sunburn wavelengths, but in some cases this active range may extend into the UV-A as far as 340 nm.[4]

It is widely accepted that DNA is the primary target for the biologic effects of UVR in bacteria and higher organism cells in culture (see page 2439). The most important photoproducts are pyrimidine dimers, and it is clear that the genetic and metabolic integrity of the cell is maintained because repair mechanisms are available to make good these photo-

1. Lynch, F. W. (1934). Xeroderma pigmentosum. A study in sensitivity to light. *Archs Derm.* **29**, 858.
2. Zoon, J. J. (1936). Untersuchungen über die Empfindlichkeit der Haut für ultraviolette Strahlen bei 2 Patienten mit Xeroderma pigmentosum. *In* 'Dritter International Kongress für Lichtforschung', Wiesbaden, p. 298.
3. Rottier, P. B. (1956). Ultraviolet radiation and skin: some facts and some problems. *In* 'Proceedings of the 1st International Photobiology Congress', Amsterdam, p. 186.
4. Cripps, D. J., Ramsay, C. A. and Ruch, D. M. (1971). Xeroderma pigmentosum: abnormal monochromatic action spectrum and autoradiographic studies. *J. invest. Derm.* **56**, 281.
5. Ramsay, C. A. and Gianelli, F. (1975). The erythemal action spectrum and deoxyribonucleic acid repair synthesis in xeroderma pigmentosum. *Br. J. Derm.* **92**, 49.
6. Johnson, B. E. (1973). Unpublished observation.

chemical lesions. Repair deficient bacteria are many times more sensitive than normal to the mutagenic and lethal effects of UVR.[1] "Excision repair" is the best known of these repair mechanisms. It involves recognition of the dimer induced strand distortion, endonuclease incision into the strand, removal of the dimer and neighbouring bases by exonuclease action and the resulting gap is then filled by a polymerase directed new DNA synthesis. A ligase completes the repair process by joining the newly formed DNA into the parent strand (see Fig. 8, Chapter 80). This gap filling by newly formed DNA is known as repair replication or unscheduled DNA synthesis (UDS). The description of excision repair given here is important because Cleaver[2] first reported that, while normal fibroblasts in culture performed repair replication after UV-irradiation, those from an XP patient were much less efficient and in a case of De Sanctis–Cacchione syndrome there was no repair at all. Although an enzyme deficiency was suspected, its nature was uncertain, nor was it known whether the same deficiency was present in all forms of the disease. Because thymine dimers were not removed from the DNA of UV-irradiated XP cells as from normal cells, and because repair appeared normal when the damage to DNA involved breakage by X-rays, it was suggested that the defect occurred in the early stages of the repair mechanism. It was suggested that the endonuclease step was specifically involved[3, 4] and this has since been confirmed in many XP cases.[5, 6]

The defect in excision repair has been detected in the cells throughout the epidermis of XP patients as well as in the dermal fibroblasts.[7] Similar findings have been reported for epidermis irradiated *in vitro*,[8, 9] and also

1. Hanawalt, P. C. and Setlow, R. B. (Eds) (1975) 'Molecular Mechanisms for Repair of DNA', Parts A and B, Plenum Press, New York.
2. Cleaver, J. E. (1968). Defective repair replication of DNA in Xeroderma pigmentosum. *Nature* **218**, 652.
3. Cleaver, J. E. (1969). Xeroderma pigmentosum: a human disease in which the initial stage of DNA repair is defective. *Proc. natn. Acad. Sci. USA* **63**, 428.
4. Setlow, R. B., Regan, J. D., German, J. and Carrier, W. L. (1969). Evidence that xeroderma cells do not perform the first step in repair of ultraviolet damage to their DNA. *Proc. natn. Acad. Sci. USA* **64**, 1035.
5. Fornace, A. J., Kohn, K. W. and Kahn, H. E. (1976). DNA single-strand breaks during repair of UV damage in human fibroblasts and abnormalities of repair in xeroderma pigmentosum. *Proc. natn. Acad. Sci. USA* **73**, 39.
6. Cook, P. R., Brazell, I. A., Pawsey, S. A. and Gianelli, F. (1978). Changes induced by ultraviolet light in superhelical DNA of lymphocytes from subjects with xeroderma pigmentosum and normal controls. *J. Cell Sci.* **29**, 117.
7. Epstein, J. H., Fukuyama, K., Reed, W. R. and Epstein, W. L. (1970). Defect in DNA synthesis in skin of patients with xeroderma pigmentosum demonstrated *in vivo*. *Science* **168**, 1477.
8. Robbins, J. H., Levis, W. R. and Miller, A. E. (1972). Xeroderma pigmentosum epidermal cells with normal UV-induced thymidine incorporation. *J. invest. Derm.* **59**, 402.
9. Jung, E. G. and Bantle, K. (1971). Xeroderma pigmentosum and pigmented xerodermoid. *Birth Defects* **7**, 125.

for peripheral blood lymphocytes[1] and conjunctival cells.[2] There seems little doubt that in these patients all cell types throughout the body are affected. Normal repair replication occurs in dorsal root ganglion cells irradiated in culture,[3] and the deficiency of repair in these ganglion cells and in other neurons of XP patients is perhaps related to the neurological disturbance that occurs in this condition. Although the damage cannot be due to UV radiation, chemical damage requiring the same type of repair may well be defective. Carcinogens, such as 4-nitroquinoline-1-oxide, N-acetoxy-2-acetylaminofluorene, and 1,3-bis(2-chloro-ethyl)-1-nitrosourea, cause such damage, and it is postulated that a similar form of chemical damage may occur during foetal and post-embryonic life which is repaired in normal subjects, but only partially or not at all in XP patients.[4]

As more patients with XP were examined for defective repair mechanisms, data accumulated confirming Cleaver's original observation that the extent of excision repair deficiency may vary in different patients. Also *in vitro* studies of repair replication, loss of dimers from cellular DNA,[5] mutation induction, cell survival, and colony formation following UV-irradiation have all revealed a variation between individual patients.[6, 7] The ability of fibroblasts in culture to restore the activity of UV-inactivated viruses (host–cell reactivation) is probably part of the same general pattern.[8]

The possibility of genetic variation within the XP spectrum is suggested by the clinical sub-grouping depending on the presence or absence of neurological disturbance. That there is a complex genetic basis for the variation in the levels of the defect in excision repair is

1. Burk, P. G., Lutzner, M. A., Clarke, D. D. and Robbins, J. H. (1971). Ultraviolet-stimulated Thymidine Incorporation in Xeroderma Pigmentosum Lymphocytes. *J. Lab. clin. Med.* **77**, 759.
2. Newsome, D. A., Kraemer, K. H. and Robbins, J. H. (1973). Conjunctival cell cultures and the DNA repair defect in xeroderma pigmentosum (abs.). *Clin. Res.* **21**, 481.
3. Sanes, J. R. and Okun, L. M. (1972). Induction of DNA synthesis in cultured neurons by ultraviolet light or methyl methane sulfonate. *J. Cell Biol.* **53**, 587.
4. Andrews, A. D., Barrett, S. F. and Robbins, J. H. (1978). Xeroderma pigmentosum neurological abnormalities correlate with colony-forming ability after ultraviolet radiation. *Proc. natn. Acad. Sci. USA* **75**, 1984.
5. Cleaver, J. E. and Bootsma, D. (1975). Xeroderma pigmentosum: Biochemical and genetic characteristics. *Ann. Rev. Genet.* **9**, 19.
6. Setlow, R. B. (1978). Repair deficient human disorders and cancer. *Nature* **271**, 713.
7. Kraemer, K. H., Andrews, A. D., Barrett, S. F. and Robbins, J. H. (1976). Colony-forming ability of ultraviolet-irradiated xeroderma pigmentosum fibroblasts from different DNA repair complementation groups. *Biochim. biophys. Acta* **442**, 147.
8. Day, R. (1975). The use of human adenovirus 2 in the study of the xeroderma DNA-repair defect. *In* 'Molecular Mechanisms for Repair of DNA' (Eds, Hanawalt, P. C. and Setlow, R. B.), p. 747. Plenum Press, New York.

indicated by the results of cell fusion studies.[1,2] When fibroblasts from two XP patients are fused together, the resulting binucleate cell may exhibit the same level of repair as before. In this case, there is no complementation of the metabolic defect, the two patients are then considered to carry the same genetic defect and are assigned to the same complementation group. However, when the defect is not apparent after fusion, the cells are said to complement each other, the genetic defects differ and the patients are considered to belong to different complementation groups. Seven such groups have been described for XP,* labelled A to G, but the majority of reported cases belong to groups A, C, and D. In Europe and North America, group C is predominant,[3] whilst in Japan most cases belong to group A.[4] The solitary case assigned to group B also presented with Cockayne's syndrome,[5] and this emphasizes the difficulty in interpreting both the genetic and clinical aspects.[6]

The different groups may have different levels of residual repair activity, but in each case the defect occurs at the incision stage.[7,8,9] The simple hypothesis of a single gene defect resulting in a single enzyme deficiency obviously cannot be valid. However, within the complex nucleoprotein structure of human chromatin, the initial step in excision-repair may itself be a series of processes under genetic control and the complementation groups may represent different mutations acting at different stages.[10] This is supported by the fact that UV-irradiated,

1. De Weerd-Kastelein, E. A., Keijzer, W. and Bootsma, D. (1972). Genetic heterogeneity of xeroderma pigmentosum demonstrated by somatic cell hybridization. *Nature New Biol.* **238**, 80.

2. Gianelli, F. (1978). Xeroderma pigmentosum and the role of DNA repair in oncogenesis. *Bulletin du Cancer* **65**, 323.

3. Robbins, J. H. (1978). Significance of repair of human DNA: Evidence from studies of xeroderma pigmentosum. *J. natn. Cancer Inst.* **601**, 645.

4. Takebe, H., Miki, Y., Kozuka, T., Furuyama, J.-I., Tanaka, K., Sasaki, M. S., Fujiwara, Y. and Akiba, H. (1977). DNA repair characteristics and skin cancers of xeroderma pigmentosum patients in Japan. *Cancer Res.* **37**, 490.

5. Robbins, J. H., Kraemer, K. H., Lutzner, M. A., Festoff, B. W. and Coon, H. (1974). Xeroderma pigmentosum: An inherited disease with sun sensitive multiple cutaneous neoplasms, and abnormal DNA repair. *Ann. intern. Med.* **80**, 221.

6. Friedburg, E. C. (1978). Xeroderma pigmentosum: Recent studies on repair defects. *Archs Pathol. Lab. Med.* **102**, 3.

7. Paterson, M. C. (1978). Use of purified lesion-recognising enzyme monitor DNA repair *in vivo. Adv. Rad. Biol.* **7**, 1.

8. Tanaka, K., Sekiguchi, M. and Okada, Y. (1975). Restoration induced unscheduled DNA synthesis of xeroderma pigmentosum concomitant treatment with bacteriophage T4 endonuclease virus. *Proc. natn. Acad. Sci. USA* **72**, 4071.

9. Fornace, A. J., Kohn, K. W. and Kahn, H. E. (1976). DNA single-strand breaks during repair of UV damage in human fibroblasts and abnormalities of repair in xeroderma pigmentosum. *Proc. natn. Acad. Sci. USA* **73**, 39.

10. Cleaver, J. E. (1978). Xeroderma pigmentosum: Genetic and environmental influences in skin carcinogenesis. *Int. J. Derm.* **17**, 435.

*This number has recently increased.

purified DNA, as well as endonuclease incized DNA, is repaired equally well by cell free extracts from normal and XP cell lines, so the required enzyme would appear to be present. However, the XP extract is unable to repair UV-irradiated chromatin, and it is postulated that in XP chromatin there is a non-enzymatic defect in addition to, or in place of, a primary enzyme defect.[1]

The extent of excision repair in the major complementation groups is shown in Table 4 along with the associated clinical manifestations. There does appear to be a variation according to complementation groups, not only in the extent of the repair defect but also in the severity of the clinical disease. A relationship between the extent of the skin damage and the

Table 4

Xeroderma pigmentosum

Table of XP complementation groups showing relationship between unscheduled DNA synthesis (UDS) defect, skin lesions and neurological symptoms

Complementation group	UDS (% of control)	Skin lesions	Neurological symptoms
A	Most less than 5	+++ to + (varies with extent of defect)	+++ to nil (varies with extent of defect)
B	3–7	++	+++
C	5–30	++ to + (varies with extent of defect)	nil
D	2–10 Higher figures in USA series	++	++
E	40–50	+	nil

Data from Bootsma, D. (1977). Defective DNA repair and cancer. *In* 'Research in Photobiology' (Ed. Castellani, A.), p. 455. Plenum Press, New York.

repair defect would be a strong argument for an association between this defect and the development of malignant change, and there is some support for this both in Europe and Japan.[2] However, the relatively

1. Friedberg, E. C., Cook, K. H., Mortelmans, K. and Rude, J. (1977). Studies on the enzymology of excision repair in extracts of mammalian cells. *In* 'Research in Photobiology' (Ed., Castellani, A.), p. 299. Plenum Press, New York.
2. Bootsma, D. (1977). Defective DNA repair and cancer. *In* 'Research in Photobiology' (Ed., Castellani, A.), p. 455. Plenum Press, New York.

severe clinical condition in group D is associated with relatively high levels of residual repair in the United States series, and although this may be due to some anomaly,[1] the relationship remains obscure.[2] Similar difficulties are encountered in relating the history of clinical photosensitivity and the results of phototesting to the degree of repair deficiency although an apparent relationship can be demonstrated. The neurological abnormalities in XP do however appear to correlate well with the extent of the repair defect as judged by loss of colony formation in UV-irradiated fibroblasts.[3] The correlation between skin manifestations and reduced repair is complicated by different degrees of natural pigmentation of the patient and differences in sun-exposure. A similar difficulty is met in attempts to determine an increased incidence of non-melanoma skin cancer in XP family heterozygotes. None the less, there does appear to be an increase,[4] and XP heterozygotes may have a reduced repair capability.[1]

Where the clinical manifestations of XP occur with apparently normal excision repair and normal cell sensitivity to UVR, another molecular defect has been suspected.[5, 6, 7] It is now clear that this variant form of XP, including the Pigmented Xerodermoid of Jung,[5] is deficient in some form of repair which takes place in daughter strand DNA after normal semi-conservative replication.[8] This post replication repair (PRR) process has not been fully elucidated, and various schemes are proposed to account for the experimental results obtained.[9, 10] In PRR synthesis of DNA, the

1. Giannelli, F. (1980). DNA repair in human diseases. *Clin. exp. Derm.* **5**, 119.
2. Pawsey, S. A., Magnus, I. A., Ramsay, C. A., Benson, P. F. and Giannelli, F. (1979). Clinical, genetic and DNA repair studies on a consecutive series of patients with xeroderma pigmentosum. *Q. J. Med., New Series XLVIII* **190**, 179.
3. Andrews, A. D., Barrett, S. F. and Robbins, J. H. (1978). Xeroderma pigmentosum neurological abnormalities correlate with colony-forming ability after ultraviolet radiation. *Proc. natn. Acad. Sci. USA* **75**, 1984.
4. Swift, M. and Chase, C. (1979). Cancer in families with xeroderma pigmentosum. *J. natn. Cancer Inst.* **62**, 1415.
5. Jung, E. G. (1970). New form of molecular defect in xeroderma pigmentosum. *Nature* **228**, 361.
6. Burk, P. G., Lutzner, M. A., Clark, D. D. and Robbins, J. H. (1971). Ultraviolet-stimulated thymidine incorporation in xeroderma pigmentosum lymphocytes. *J. Lab. clin. Med.* **77**, 759.
7. Cleaver, J. E. (1972). Xeroderma pigmentosum: Variants with normal DNA repair and normal sensitivity to ultraviolet light. *J. invest. Derm.* **58**, 124.
8. Lehmann, A. R. (1976). Post-replication repair of DNA in mammalian cells: a discussion on the mechanisms and biological importance. *In* 'Radiation and Cellular Control Processes' (Ed., Keifer, J.), p. 147. Springer-Verlag, Berlin.
9. Lehmann, A. R., Kirk-Bell, S., and Arlett, C. F. (1977). Post-replication repair in human fibroblasts. *In* 'Research in Photobiology' (Ed., Castellani, A.), p. 293. Plenum Press, New York.
10. Fujiwara, Y. and Kondo, T. (1974). Post replication gap-filling repair in ultraviolet-irradiated mouse L cells. *In* 'Sunlight and Man' (Ed., Fitzpatrick, T. B.), p. 91. University of Tokyo Press, Tokyo.

replication bypasses an abnormality such as a thymine dimer and leaves a gap in the daughter strand which has to be filled later. It is the details of this "gap-filling" process which are uncertain, and it is suggested that this kind of delayed repair is liable to error. In classical XP where error-free excision repair is deficient, errors may contribute to mutation induction. A difference in the repair defect may be the reason why the clinical manifestations of the disease are slight in some variant patients and are delayed in onset. However, some variants are clinically indistinguishable from classic XP, and it is possible that the variant type may also be an heterogenous group like the classic form.[1]

Although the importance of photoreactivation in mammalian cells is not generally accepted,[2,3,4] it is nevertheless deficient in XP.[5] A picture of typical repair deficiency in XP presented by Setlow[6] is a repair level of about 50% of normal; the failure is brought about by a combination of a deficiency in all three repair processes.

There is no direct relationship between the molecular defect and the abnormal UV-induced skin reactions in XP. It may be that the delayed and persistent inflammatory response to sunburn wavelengths is simply a manifestation of cell death.

At any given level of cell survival after UV-irradiation, the mutation rate in various XP strains is the same as in normal cells,[7] although variants may be more susceptible to the mutagenic rather than the lethal effects.[8] It has therefore been suggested that the difference between the reactions of classical XP and normals is quantitative rather than qualitative. This is patently not so for the acute skin responses but may be more relevant in relation to the long-term changes in chronically exposed

1. Fischer, E., Jung, E. G. and Cleaver, J. E. (1980). Pigmented xerodermoid and XP-Variants. *Archs derm. Res.* **269**, 329.
2. Sutherland, B. M. and Oliver, R. (1976). Culture conditions affect photoreactivating enzyme levels in human fibroblasts. *Biochim. biophys. Acta* **442**, 358.
3. Mortelmans, K., Cleaver, J. E., Friedberg, E. C., Paterson, M. C., Smith, B. P. and Thomas, G. H. (1977). Photoreactivation of thymine dimers in UV-irradiated human cells; unique dependence on culture conditions. *Mutation Res.* **44**, 433.
4. Giannelli, F. (1980). DNA repair in human diseases. *Clin. exp. Derm.* **5**, 119.
5. Sutherland, B. M., Oliver, R., Fuselier, C. O. and Sutherland, J. C. (1976). Photoreactivation of pyrimidine dimers in the DNA of normal and xeroderma pigmentosum cells. *Biochemistry* **15**, 402.
6. Setlow, R. B. (1978). Repair deficient human disorders and cancer. *Nature* **271**, 713.
7. Maher, V. M. and McCormick, J. J. (1976). Effect of DNA repair on the cytotoxicity and mutagenicity of UV irradiation and of chemical carcinogens in normal and xeroderma pigmentosum cells. *In* 'Biology of Radiation Carcinogenesis' (Eds, Yuhas, J. M., Tennant, R. W. and Regan, J. B.), p. 129. Raven, New York.
8. Maher, V. M., Oullette, L. M., Curren, R. D. and McCormick, J. J. (1976). Frequency of ultraviolet light-induced mutations is higher in xeroderma pigmentosum variant cells than in normal human cells. *Nature* **261**, 593.

skin. Epidemiologic and experimental animal studies have established a relationship between the exposure of skin to sunlight and the development of cancer. There is direct evidence, albeit in fish, that the UV-induced-pyrimidine-dimers lead to malignant transformation.[1] Deficiencies in the repair of these lesions, either by excision or post replication processes, are associated with the increased UV-carcinogenesis in XP. This may result from the greater and more rapid accumulation of UV-induced mutations in accord with the somatic mutation hypothesis of carcinogenesis.[2, 3] Giannelli[2] has pointed out that these changes would also favour viral transformation of host cells.

The UVR-stimulated induction of suppressor T lymphocytes play a part in UV-carcinogenesis by inhibiting the rejection of putative cancer cell clones.[4] However, it is likely that the original UV-induced cellular lesions are important and the persistence of these lesions in XP would be expected to lead to an increase in the rate at which potentially malignant cells are produced.

The persistence of UV-induced mutation may also be postulated as the cause of the increased freckling so characteristic of XP. The even distribution of the pigment throughout the individual freckles has led to the suggestion that each one has been derived from a single melanocyte mutation.[5]

There is no doubt that XP is a life-threatening disease unless appropriate prophylactic measures are taken. It is now apparent that when early diagnosis is made, avoidance of sunlight and the application of efficient sunscreens may allow some XP patients to pass the early stages of childhood without developing malignancy, or with a greatly reduced chance of further skin damage if such protection is not initiated until skin changes have already occurred.[6, 7]

1. Hart, R. W., Setlow, R. B. and Woodhead, A. D. (1977). Evidence that pyrimidine dimers in DNA can give rise to tumours. *Proc. natn. Acad. Sci. USA* **74**, 5574.
2. Trosko, J. E. and Chu, E. (1975). The role of DNA repair and somatic mutation in carcinogenesis. *In* 'Advances in Cancer Research' (Eds, Klein, G. and Weinhouse, S.) Vol. 5, p. 391. Academic Press, London, Orlando and New York.
3. Giannelli, F. (1978). Xeroderma pigmentosum and the role of DNA repair in oncogenesis. *Bull. Cancer* **65**, 325.
4. Kripke, M. L. (1980). Immunologic effects of UV radiation and their role in photo-carcinogenesis. *In* 'Photochemical and Photobiological Review' (Ed., Smith, K. C.) Vol. 5, p. 257. Plenum Press, New York.
5. Burnet, F. M. (1970). Differentiation and somatic mutation. *In* 'Immunologic Surveillance', p. 50. Pergamon Press, New York.
6. Robbins, J. H., Kraemer, K. H., Lutzner, M. A., Festoff, B. W. and Coon, H. G. (1974). Xeroderma Pigmentosum. An inherited disease with sun sensitivity, multiple cutaneous neoplasm, and abnormal DNA repair. *Ann. intern. Med.* **80**, 221.
7. Goldstein, N. and Hay-Roe, V. (1975). Prevention of skin cancer with a PABA in Alcohol sunscreen in Xeroderma pigmentosum. *Cutis* **15**, 61.

It is obviously of paramount importance that the existence of a repair defect is determined as early as possible, especially in those families where an XP child has already been born. This may now be carried out prenatally, the repair function of cells obtained by aminocentesis being examined by standard methods.[1] This allows both genetic counselling and the planning of the lifetime protective regimen required to minimize the serious effects of exposure to UV.

B. Hereditary Syndromes

Recognition of the association between a genetically based molecular defect in the repair of UV-damaged DNA and the clinical manifestations of XP has led to investigations of DNA repair in other conditions which exhibit photosensitivity or have an increased incidence of cancer.

Normal repair mechanisms have been reported in lupus erythematosus and dyskeratosis congenita;[2] oculo–cutaneous albinism:[3] Fanconi's anaemia, Mendes da Costa syndrome, parakeratosis of Mihelli, and disseminated superficial actinic parakeratosis;[4] basal cell naevus syndrome;[3, 4, 5] and progeria.[2, 3, 4, 5] Miscellaneous conditions also shown to have normal repair levels include malignant melanoma, multiple basal cell carcinomas, multiple cancers, psoriasis, and solar urticaria.[4]

Although reservations may be expressed concerning the methods of investigations,[6] cells from patients with solar keratoses appear to have lower than normal levels of unscheduled DNA synthesis following exposure to UVR.[7, 8, 9] It is not clear whether an abnormal erythema response, similar to that seen in XP, occurs in subjects with solar keratoses. Nor is there any evidence that this test can be used to predict a

1. Ramsay, C. A., Coltart, T. M., Blunt, S., Pawsey, S. A. and Giannelli, F. (1974). Prenatal diagnosis of xeroderma pigmentosum: report of first successful case. *Lancet* **2**, 1109.
2. Cleaver, J. E. (1970). DNA damage and repair in light-sensitive human skin disease. *J. invest. Derm.* **54**, 181.
3. Jung, E. G. (1970). Investigations on dark repair in various light sensitive inherited disorders. *Humangenetik* **9**, 191.
4. Lehmann, A. R., Kirk-Bell, S., Arlett, C. F., Harcourt, S. A., de Weerd-Kastelein, E. A., Keijzer, W. and Hall-Smith, P. (1977). Repair of ultra violet light damage in a variety of human fibroblast cell strains. *Cancer Res.* **37**, 904.
5. Epstein, W. L., Fukuyama, K. and Epstein, J. H. (1971). Ultraviolet light, DNA repair and skin carcinogenesis in man. *Fedn. Proc.* **30**, 1766.
6. Giannelli, F. (1980). DNA repair in human diseases. *Clin. exp. Derm.* **5**, 119.
7. Lambert, B., Ringborg, U. and Swanbeck, G. (1976). Ultraviolet induced DNA repair synthesis in lymphocytes from patients with actinic keratosis. *J. invest. Derm.* **67**, 594.
8. Abo-Darub, J. M., Mackie, R. and Pitts, J. D. (1978). DNA repair deficiency in lymphocytes from patients with actinic keratosis. *Bull. Cancer* **65**, 357.
9. Sbano, E., Andreassi, L., Fimiani, M., Valentino, A. and Baiocchi, R. (1978). DNA-repair after UV-irradiation in skin fibroblasts from patients with actinic keratosis. *Archs derm. Res.* **262**, 55.

greater than normal tendency to develop solar keratoses or skin cancer.

In a number of the rare hereditary syndromes, photosensitivity has been recorded, but in the past this has been based on clinical grounds. It is probable that exposure to sunlight does play a part in the production of at least some of the skin changes seen in these syndromes, even though on conventional phototesting both the action spectrum for erythema and the responses obtained appear normal.

It is uncertain whether the Rothmund–Thomson syndrome, Cockayne syndrome, ataxia telangiectasis and dyskeratosis congenita are separate entities or whether in fact they are variants of the same basic abnormality. Nevertheless, there is a similarity in the clinical presentation of the Bloom's, Cockayne, and Rothmund–Thomson syndromes.

1. Bloom's Syndrome

Bloom's syndrome, a genodermatosis inherited as an autosomal recessive gene, is most prevalent amongst Jews. Males are most often affected: they are of small stature and have a telangiectatic erythema of the face which starts in infancy and is associated with an apparent "sensitivity" to sunlight.[1, 2, 3]

The erythema favours the light exposed areas of the face but may occasionally involve the skin of the forearms and the backs of the hands. There is a tendency for this to fade after puberty. Blistering and crusting may follow exposure to sunlight, but although photosensitivity has been confirmed in two reports by the demonstration of a lowered threshold for UV-erythema,[4, 5] other investigators were unable to elicit this response and concluded that any photosensitivity was restricted to the already damaged telangiectatic regions.[1]

An immunological deficiency may be present and there is also a tendency to develop leukaemia. Numerous structural abnormalities of the chromosomes have been observed, but a 10-fold increase above the

1. Bloom, D. (1966). The syndrome of congenital telangiectatic erythema and stunted growth. *J. Pediat.* **68**, 103.
2. Landau, J. W., Sasaki, M. S., Newcomer, V. D. and Norman, A. (1966). Bloom's syndrome. *Archs Derm.* **94**, 687.
3. German, J. (1974). Bloom's syndrome II. The prototype of human genetic disorders predisposing to chromosome instability and cancer. *In* 'Chromosomes and Cancer' (Ed., German, J.), p. 601. Wiley, New York.
4. Katzenellenbogen, I. and Laron, Z. (1960). A contribution to Bloom's syndrome. *Archs Derm.* **82**, 609.
5. Fitzpatrick, T. B., Pathak, M. A., Magnus, I. A. and Curwen, W. L. (1963). Abnormal reactions of man to lights. *Ann. Rev. Med.* **14**, 195.

normal level of spontaneous sister chromatid exchanges appears to be the characteristic defect.[1, 2, 3]

It has been suggested that the chromosomal abnormalities in Bloom's syndrome reflect not only some form of repair defect but also a defect in normal replication.[4] Although there is a moderately increased sensitivity in UVR in fibroblasts *in vitro*,[5] there is no defect in the dark repair system,[6, 7] and pyrimidine dimer excision daughter-strand repair, and the rejoining of single strand breaks are normal.[5] Despite this there is some evidence that a part of the complex polymerase dependent repair system for gamma ray-induced changes in DNA may be deficient in fibroblasts of Bloom's syndrome.[8]

2. Cockayne's Syndrome

Cockayne's syndrome is another rare, recessively inherited disorder presenting with cutaneous photosensitivity but without greater than normal cancer incidence. Affected individuals are characteristically dwarfed and mentally retarded with microcephaly, the sunken eyes are emphasized by their relatively large ears and nose.[9, 10, 11] The "photosensitivity" presents during the first year of life as an erythema of the skin of the face, particularly over the butterfly area of the cheeks; subsequently there is hyperpigmentation, atrophy and loss of subcutaneous fat leading to the appearance of premature ageing.[12]

Spontaneous sister chromatid exchange levels are normal in Cockayne syndrome. However, greater than normal increases in sister chromatid

1. Chaganti, R. S. K., Schonberg, S. and German, J. (1974). A many-fold increase in sister chromatid exchanges in Bloom's syndrome lymphocytes. *Proc. natn. Acad. Sci. USA* **71**, 4508.
2. Giannelli, F. (1980). DNA repair in human diseases. *Clin. exp. Derm.* **5**, 119.
3. Setlow, R. B. (1978). Repair deficient human disorders and cancer. *Nature* **271**, 713.
4. Hand, R. and German, J. (1975). A retarded rate of DNA chain growth in Bloom's syndrome. *Proc. natn. Acad. Sci. USA* **72**, 758.
5. Giannelli, F., Benson, P. F., Pawsey, S. A. and Polani, P. E. (1977). Ultraviolet light sensitivity and delayed DNA-chain maturation in Bloom's syndrome fibroblasts. *Nature* **265**, 466.
6. Cleaver, J. E. (1970). DNA damage and repair in light sensitive human skin disease. *J. invest. Derm.* **54**, 181.
7. Jung, E. G. (1970). Investigations on dark repair in various light sensitive inherited disorders. *Humangenetik* **9**, 191.
8. Inoue, T., Hirano, K., Yokoiyama, A., Mada, T. and Kato, H. (1977). DNA repair enzymes in ataxia telangiectasia and Bloom's syndrome fibroblasts. *Biochim. biophys. Acta* **479**, 497.
9. Cockayne, E. A. (1936). Dwarfism with retinal atrophy and deafness. *Arch. Dis. Childhood* **11**, 1.
10. Cockayne, E. A. (1946). Cas reports: dwarfism with retinal atrophy and deafness. *Arch. Dis. Childhood* **21**, 52.
11. MacDonald, W. B., Fitch, K. D. and Lewis, I. C. (1960). Cockayne's syndrome: An heredofamilial disorder of growth and development. *Pediatrics* **25**, 997.
12. Schmickel, R. D., Chu, E. H. Y., Trosko, J. E. and Chang, C. C. (1977). Cockayne syndrome: a cellular sensitivity to ultraviolet light. *Pediatrics* **60**, 135.

exchange were obtained following UV-irradiation of Cockayne synd-rome cells but, as with XP groups B and E, the difference was not statistically significant, unlike the results with XP groups, A, C, and D.[1] Cells from patients with Cockayne syndrome are more than normally sensitive to UVR as judged by colony forming ability after exposure,[2, 3] but have normal sensitivity towards X-rays[2] so that their radiation sensitivity resembles that of XP. However, although a defect in excision repair was at one time suspected,[4] both dimer excision and repair replication appear normal in Cockayne syndrome.[2, 3] The only decreased repair replication reported in this disorder was in a patient who also had XP, complementation group B.[5]

Both ataxia telangiectasia and Fanconi anaemia cells exhibit multiple chromosome abnormalities and may be more sensitive to radiation damage than normal.[6, 7] However, although photosensitivity may play a part in the long-term cutaneous changes in ataxia telangiectasia[7] and repair mechanisms for various DNA damaging agents are possibly deficient in both diseases, no clearly defined relationship between deficiencies and the clinical manifestations has been established.[8, 9]

3. Rothmund–Thomson Syndrome

In the Rothmund–Thomson syndrome (poikiloderma congenitale)[10, 11] the inheritance is typically recessive, and the affected individual is small

1. Cheng, W.-S., Tarone, R. E., Andrews, A. D., Whang-Peng, J. S. and Robbins, J. H. (1978). Ultraviolet light-induced sister chromatid exchanges in Xeroderma pigmentosum and in Cockayne's syndrome lymphocyte cell lines. *Cancer Res.* **38**, 1601.
2. Schmickel, R. D., Chu, E. H. Y., Trosko, J. and Chang, C. C. (1977). Cockayne syndrome: a cellular sensitivity to ultraviolet light. *Pediatrics* **60**, 135.
3. Andrews, A. D., Barrett, S. F., Yoder, F. W. and Robbins, J. H. (1978). Cockayne's syndrome fibroblasts have increased sensitivity to ultraviolet light but normal rates of unscheduled DNA synthesis. *J. invest. Derm.* **70**, 237.
4. Schmickel, R. D., Chu, E. H. Y. and Trosko, J. (1975). The definition of a cellular defect in two patients with Cockayne syndrome. *Pediat. Res.* **9**, 317.
5. Kraemer, K. H. (1980). Xeroderma pigmentosum. A prototype disease of environmental-genetic interaction. *Archs Derm.* **116**, 541.
6. Cleaver, J. E. (1977). Human diseases with *in vitro* manifestations of altered repair and replication of DNA. *In* 'Genetics of Human Cancer' (Eds, Mulvihill, J. J., Miller, R. W. and Fraumeni, J. F., Jr), p. 355. Raven Press, New York.
7. Setlow, R. B. (1978). Repair deficient human disorders and cancer. *Nature* **271**, 713.
8. Reed, W. B., Epstein, W. L., Boder, E. and Sedgwick, R. (1966). Cutaneous manifestations of Ataxia-telangiectasia. *J. Am. med. Ass.* **195**, 126.
9. Inoue, T., Hirano, K., Yokoiyama, A., Kada, T. and Kato, H. (1977). DNA repair enzymes in Ataxia telangiectasia and Bloom's syndrome fibroblasts. *Biochim. biophys. Acta* **479**, 497.
10. Rook, A., Davis, R. and Stevanovic, D. (1959). Poikiloderma congenitale Rothmund–Thomson syndrome. *Acta derm-venereol.* **39**, 392.
11. Rook, A. (1972). Genetics in Dermatology. *In* 'Textbook of Dermatology', 2nd Edition (Eds, Rook, A., Wilkinson, D. S. and Ebling, F. J. G.), p. 91. Blackwell Publications, Oxford.

in stature with poikilodermatous changes of both exposed and covered skin (Fig. 7). Early skin changes are an erythema of the exposed areas developing within the first 2 months of life. Again, there is clinical evidence of an abnormal reaction to sunlight which may be severe, with blistering, but this was not confirmed in two cases phototested, and the

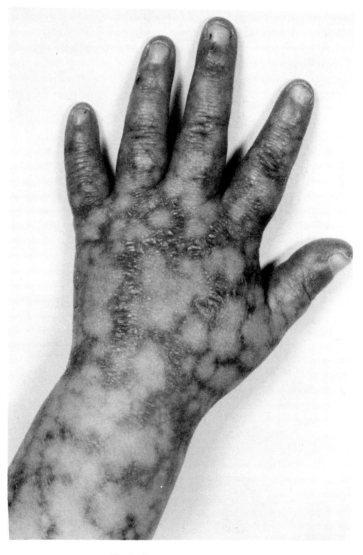

Fig. 7. Congenital Poikiloderma.

action spectrum for erythema appeared to be normal.[1] Presumably, as in Bloom's syndrome, the abnormal reaction to light involves mechanisms other than those of erythema production. There are three reports that excision repair processes in cells from Rothmund–Thomson syndrome patients are normal,[1,2,3] and both excision and post replication repair studies have yielded normal results for cells from one other patient.[4]

4. Hartnup's Disease[5]

Skin changes similar to those seen in pellagra occur in Hartnup's Disease, which takes its name from the family in which it was first described.[2] Since then genetic studies of the 53 reported cases have shown it to be a familial disease with a rare autosomal inherited abnormality of amino acid transport.

The clinical features appear to be related specifically to malabsorption of tryptophan so that there is a biochemical, as well as a clinical, similarity to pellagra. Thus, when pellagrinous skin changes are observed without a significant dietary deficiency, a diagnosis of Hartnup's disease should be considered. This may be confirmed by the characteristic urinary amino acid pattern in which the monoaminomonocarboxylic amino acids, alanine, asparagine, glutamine, histidine, isoleucine, leucine, phenylalanine, threonine, tryptophan, tyrosine, and valine are excreted in up to 10 times the normal quantities. In addition, greater than normal amounts of indican, indolic acids and related bacterial breakdown products of tryptophan may be detected because the amino acid is exposed to colonic bacteria rather than being absorbed higher in the alimentary tract.

As with pellagra, the apparent photosensitivity is attributed to nicotinamide-deficiency. Vitamin B administration usually controls the skin reactions[7] but is not effective in all cases.

1. Frain-Bell, W. (1982). Personal communication.
2. Cleaver, J. E. (1970). DNA damage and repair in light-sensitive human skin disease. *J. invest. Derm.* **54**, 181.
3. Jung, E. G. (1970). Investigations on dark repair in various light sensitive inherited disorders. *Humangenetik* **9**, 191.
4. Epstein, W. L., Fukuyama, K. and Epstein, J. H. (1971). Ultraviolet light, DNA repair and skin carcinogenesis in man. *Fedn. Proc.* **30**, 1766.
5. Rosenberg, L. E. and Scriver, C. H. (1980). Disorders of Amino Acid Metabolism. *In* 'Metabolic Control and Diseases', 8th ed. (Eds, Bondy, P. K. and Rosenberg, L. E.), p. 583. W. B. Saunders Company, Philadelphia.
6. Baron, D. N., Dent, C. E., Harris, H., Hart, E. W. and Jepson, J. B. (1956). Hereditary Pellagra-like Skin Rash with Temporary Cerebellar Ataxia, Constant Renal Amino-aciduria, and other Bizarre Biochemical Features. *Lancet* **ii**, 421.
7. Halvorsen, K. and Halvorsen, S. (1963). Hartnup disease. *Pediatrics* **31**, 29.

The clinical picture in Hartnup's disease is very variable and shows poikilodermatous changes.[1] Other patients with lesions resembling hydroa vacciniforme have been shown to have a Hartnup pattern of amino aciduria.[2, 3] Thus, the skin changes seen in Hartnup's disease may not be typically pellagrinous but they do appear to be precipitated by exposure to sunlight. One clinical case of Hartnup's disease did not have the typical amino acid excretion pattern.[4]

1. Clodi, P. H., Deutsch, E. and Niebauer, G. (1964a). Krankheitsbild mit poikilodermieartigen Hautveranderungen, Aminoacidurie und Indolaceturie. Beitrag zur Kenntnis des Hartnup-Syndrome. *Arch. klin. exp. Derm.* **218**, 165.
2. Clodi, P. H., Deutsch, E. and Niesbauer, G. (1964b). Hyperaminoacidurie bei Lichtdermatosen. *Wien. klin. Wschr.* **76**, 623.
3. Ashurst, P. J. (1969). Hydroa vacciniforme occurring in association with Hartnup's disease. *Br. J. Derm.* **81**, 486.
4. Borrie, P. F. and Lewis, C. A. (1962). Hartnup disease. *Proc. R. Soc. Med.* **55**, 231.

82 | Light Sensitivity Associated with Drugs and Chemicals

B. E. JOHNSON

Department of Dermatology, University of Dundee, Ninewells Hospital, Dundee, Scotland

PHYSIOL. PATHOPHYSIOL. OF SKIN Vol. 8
ISBN 0 12 380608 9

I. MOLECULAR MECHANISMS OF PHOTOSENSITIZATION[1,2,3,4]

Photochemistry (see page 2393) may be logically extended to introduce the concept of photosensitization at the molecular level which, in turn, serves as a basis for discussions of the applied aspects of chemical, drug and metabolite induced photosensitivity.

Photosensitization is a process in which abnormal reactions to normal solar radiation are produced in a system by the introduction of a specific radiation absorbing substance. A general definition may be given as "the action of one component (the photosensitizer) which causes another component in the system to react to radiation".[5] Within the context of skin photobiology, the process is usually considered in relation to supposedly normally harmless radiation such as UV-A or the visible spectrum. This radiation is absorbed by the "foreign" molecule and skin reactions result from the involvement of cell and tissue constituents during the dissipation of the absorbed energy. The pathways available for this energy dissipation vary according to the molecular structure of the photosensitizer, the nature of the biomolecule with which it is associated and whether or not molecular oxygen is involved.

Just as the molecular mechanisms of photosensitization vary, so do the mechanisms involved at the biological level. In micro-organisms and more complex cells in culture, photosensitization may be shown to be mediated primarily through changes in lipid, protein and nucleic acid constituents, causing membrane damage, inhibition of macro-molecular synthesis, mutation and cell death. In the skin, immediate or delayed responses of varying severity result directly from such cellular reactions and are included in a broad category of "phototoxicity". When immunologic mechanisms appear to be involved, the term "photo-

1. Blum, H. F. (1964). 'Photodynamic Action and Diseases Caused by Light'. Hafner Publishing Company, New York.
2. Pathak, M. A. (1969). Basic aspects of cutaneous photosensitization. *In* 'The Biologic Effects of Ultraviolet Radiation (with emphasis on the skin)' (Ed. Urbach, F.), pp. 489–511. Pergamon Press, Oxford.
3. Gallo, U. and Santamaria, L. (1972). 'Research Progress in Organic, Biological and Medicinal Chemistry', Vol. III, parts 1 and 2. North Holland, Amsterdam.
4. Spikes, J. D. (1977). Photosensitization. *In* 'The Science of Photobiology' (Ed. Smith, K. C.), pp. 87–110. Plenum Press, New York.
5. Lamola, A. A. (1974). Fundamental aspects of the spectroscopy and photochemistry of organic compounds; electronic energy transfer in biologic systems; and photosensitization. *In* 'Sunlight and Man' (Ed. Fitzpatrick, T. B.), pp. 17–55. University of Tokyo Press, Tokyo.

allergy" is usually used.[1,2,3] These aspects of photosensitization will be discussed in greater detail in the sections dealing with specific skin reaction.

The lifetime of the excited singlet state (designated ^1P) of photosensitizer molecules is very short, between 10^{-9} and 10^{-6} s. Fluorescence may be detected during its decay back to the ground state (P_0), but the possibility of interaction with neighbouring molecules to produce a photosensitized reaction is remote. Such an interaction requires a longer period excitation such as occurs in the triplet state which has a duration of 10^{-3} to 10, or even 100 s, and it is a general rule that photosensitized reactions proceed via the triplet state (^3P).

$$P_0 \rightarrow {}^1P \rightarrow {}^3P \rightarrow \text{Photosensitization}$$
$$\downarrow \quad \downarrow$$
$$P_0 \quad P_0$$

Although photosensitizing chemicals generally exhibit fluorescence on appropriate excitation, there is no direct correlation between the intensity of the fluorescence and the photosensitizing potential. In fact, many fluorescent compounds do not act as photosensitizers. The ability to form the triplet state is more relevant with regard to photosensitizing potential, as illustrated by Spikes in respect to the photosensitized inactivation of trypsin by compounds of the fluorescein series (Table 1).[4]

There are various pathways by which a triplet state photosensitizer can bring about change in the target, or substrate molecules. Type I reactions[5] are those in which electron or hydrogen atom transfer gives rise to reactive free radical forms of both the substrate and sensitizer. Subsequent reactions vary, but often from their interactions with molecular oxygen ($^3O_2$) result in a fully oxidized substrate and a regenerated photosensitizer.

1. Epstein, S. (1962). Photoallergy versus phototoxicity. *In* 'Dermatoses due to Environmental and Physical Factors' (Ed., Rees, R. B.), pp. 119–135. Charles C. Thomas, Springfield, Illinois.
2. Harber, L. C. and Baer, R. L. (1972). Pathogenic mechanisms of drug-induced photosensitivity. *J. Invest. Derm.* **58**, 327.
3. Herman, P. S. and Sams, W. M. Jr (1972). 'Soap Dermatitis'. Charles C. Thomas, Springfield, Illinois.
4. Spikes, J. D. (1977). Photosensitization. *In* 'The Science of Photobiology' (Ed., Smith, K. C.), pp. 87–110. Plenum Press, New York.
5. Foote, C. S. (1974). Photoreactions with molecular oxygen. *In* 'Progress in Photobiology'. Proc. of the VI International Congress on Photobiology (Ed., Schenck, G. O.). Deutsche Gesellschaft für Lichtforschung e.V., Frankfurt, 005.

1. $^3P + S \rightarrow P^+ + S^+$
2. $S^+ + {}^3O_2 \rightarrow Sox$
3. $P^+ + {}^3O_2 \rightarrow Po$

where ^3P is photosensitizer in its triplet state and S is substrate molecule.

Alternatively, the substrate may be oxidized directly by the oxygen superoxide generated when the free radical photosensitizer reacts with molecular oxygen. In some instances, normally unreactive substrate may

Table 1

Quantum yields for fluorescence, triplet state production and photosensitization by compounds of the fluorescein series

Photosensitizer	Fluorescence	Quantum field triplet state	Photosensitization
Fluorescein	0·92	0·05	0·00017
Tetrabromo-fluorescein (oesin Y)	0·19	0·71	0·0021
Tetraiodo-fluorescein	0·02	1·07	0·003

become susceptible to oxidation as a result of a light induced photosensitizer/substrate complex formation. The relative importance of these various Type I pathways remain unclear.

During the last 15 years, attention has been directed more to the Type II energy transfer reactions in which the excitation energy of the triplet state photosensitizer is transferred to ground state oxygen. The normal ground state of oxygen is itself a triplet; energy transfer results in the formation of the highly reactive, excited singlet state $^1O_2$, which may directly oxidize a variety of biologically important substrate molecules.[1, 2]

1. $^3P + {}^3O_2 \rightarrow P_o + {}^1O_2$
2. $^1O_2 + S \rightarrow S_{ox}$

Whether or not a specific photosensitization involves excited singlet

1. Wilson, T. and Hastings, J. W. (1970). Chemical and biological aspects of singlet excited molecular oxygen. In 'Photophysiology' (Ed. Giese, A. C.), Vol. V, pp. 50–95. Academic Press, London, Orlando and New York.
2. Foote, C. S. (1976). Photosensitized oxidation and singlet oxygen: consequences in biological systems. In 'Free Radicals in Biology' (Ed. Pryor, W. A.), Vol. II, pp. 85–133. Academic Press, London, Orlando and New York.

oxygen may be inferred from the results of *in vitro* studies. Sodium azide efficiently quenches excited singlet oxygen. If its addition to the reaction mixture results in inhibition of the photosensitization, then a Type II mechanism is probably involved. Similarly, the lifetime of $^1O_2$ in water (H_2O) is some 2 μs, but in deuterated or heavy water (D_2O) it is extended to around 20 μs. An increased reaction in D_2O would, again, indicate the involvement of a Type II mechanism.[1, 2]

Histidine or the cyclic tertiary diamine, DABCO, which interact with $^1O_2$, may also help to determine the involvement of the Type II mechanism in a given photosensitizer reaction.[3, 4] In addition, studies of O_2 uptake in an irradiated solution of photosensitizer, with or without furan, an $^1O_2$ acceptor, may give a purely photochemical indication of the preferred pathway for that photosensitizer.[5] Quantitative studies of the contribution of Type II reactions to photosensitized cellular damage may be pursued using 1,3-diphenylisobenzofuran as an intracellular singlet oxygen acceptor,[6] but careful controls are required.[7] Lamola[8] has suggested that differentiation between Type I and Type II reactions in complex biological systems might be made by the fact that 5- and 7-hydroperoxides of cholesterol result from free radical oxidation while with $^1O_2$ only the 5-hydroperoxide is produced.

In general, photosensitizers with π-π^* triplet transition, such as anthraquinones and benzophenones, react through the Type I mechanism. Acridines, xanthenes such as eosin Y and rose bengal, thiophenes such as methylene blue, flavins and porphyrins, with n-π^* triplets, produce $^1O_2$. The nature of the substrate may also play a role in determining the preferred pathway for photosensitized oxidations.

1. Nilsson, R., Merkel, P. B. and Kearns, D. R. (1972). Unambiguous evidence for the participation of singlet oxygen ($^1\Delta$) in photodynamic oxidation of amino acids. *Photochem. Photobiol.* **16**, 117–125.

2. Nilsson, R. and Kearns, D. R. (1973). A remarkable deuterium effect on the rate of photosensitized oxidation of alcohol dehydrogenase and trypsin. *Photochem. Photobiol.* **17**, 65–68.

3. Mathews-Roth, M. M. (1977). Photosensitization in Sarcina lutea: different mechanisms of exogenous and endogenous photosensitizers. *Photochem. Photobiol.* **25**, 599–600.

4. Anderson, S. M., Krinsky, N. I., Stone, M. J. and Clagett, D. C. (1974). Effect of singlet oxygen quenchers on oxidative damage to liposomes initiated by photosensitization or by radiofrequency discharge. *Photochem. Photobiol.* **20**, 65–69.

5. Davies, A. K., Hamblett, I., McKellar, J. F. and Phillips, G. O. (1975). Mechanism of photocontact dermatitis due to an anthraquinone disperse dye. *J. appl. Chem. Biotechnol.* **25**, 195–204.

6. Weishaupt, K. R., Gomer, C. J. and Dougherty, T. J. (1976). Identification of singlet oxygen as the cytotoxic agent in photodestruction of a murine tumour. *Cancer Res.* **36**, 2326–2329.

7. Rosenthal, I. (1976). Recent developments in singlet molecular oxygen chemistry. *Photochem. Photobiol.* **24**, 641–645.

8. Lamola, A. A. (1977). Photodegradation of biomembranes. *In* 'Research in Photobiology' (Ed. Castellani, A.), pp. 53–63. Plenum Press, New York.

Differentiation between Type I and Type II mechanisms simplifies a complex situation, but both may operate in the same photosensitized reaction. The pathway may change depending on pH, concentration of photosensitizer, or the nature of the solvent. However, differentiation may be useful for the understanding of the photosensitized reactions, and also possibly in practical terms for the protection against damage at cell and tissue level.

So far this discussion has emphasized the role of oxygen in photo-sensitization. This is appropriate because the majority of photosensitized reactions studied at molecular level are oxygen dependent. Although used for a variety of reactions, the term "Photodynamic Action", originally coined to separate the biologic effects from purely chemical effects,[1] should be restricted to oxygen-requiring reactions.[2,3] A close spatial relationship between photosensitizer and substrate molecules is required for the reaction to proceed, even when excited singlet oxygen is involved. In some cases, this may involve an obligate binding of photosensitizer to substrate, but in others such binding inhibits the reaction. Whether or not binding occurs, photodynamic action usually results in the regeneration of the photosensitizer ground state, and the behaviour here resembles that of a chemical catalyst. This can still occur even when binding to the substrate is a prerequisite for the reaction.

Apart from these "photodynamic", oxygen-dependent mechanisms, there are photosensitization processes of varying importance in which oxygen is not required. Moreover, the photosensitizers are consumed in the process, except for reactions like the acetophenone sensitized formation of thymine dimers in DNA.[4] The most familiar of these is the UV-A induced covalent binding of the furano-coumarin compounds known as psoralens (Fig. 1) to the pyrimidine bases, thymines in particular, of DNA.[5,6,7] The significance of close

1. Tappeiner, H. V. and Jodlbauer, A. (1904). Die sensibilizierende Wirkung fluorescierender Substanzen. *Dt. Arch. klin. Med.* **80**, 427.
2. Blum, H. F. (1964). 'Photodynamic Action and Diseases Caused by Light'. Hafner Publishing Company, New York.
3. Spikes, J. D. (1968). Photodynamic action. *In* 'Photophysiology' (Ed. Giese, A. C.), Vol. III, pp. 33–64. Academic Press, London, Orlando and New York.
4. Lamola, A. A. (1970). Triplet photosensitization and the photobiology of thymine dimers in DNA. *Pure appl. Chem.* **24**, 599–610.
5. Musajo, L. and Rodighiero, G. (1972). Mode of photosensitizing action of furocoumarins. *In* 'Photophysiology' (Ed. Giese, A. C.), Vol. VII, pp. 115–147. Academic Press, London, Orlando and New York.
6. Scott, B. R., Pathak, M. A. and Mohn, G. R. (1976). Molecular and genetic basis of furocoumarin reactions. *Mut. Res.* **39**, 29–74.
7. Song, P. S. and Tapley, K. J. Jr (1979). Photochemistry and Photobiology of Psoralens. *Photochem. Photobiol.* **29**, 1177–1197.

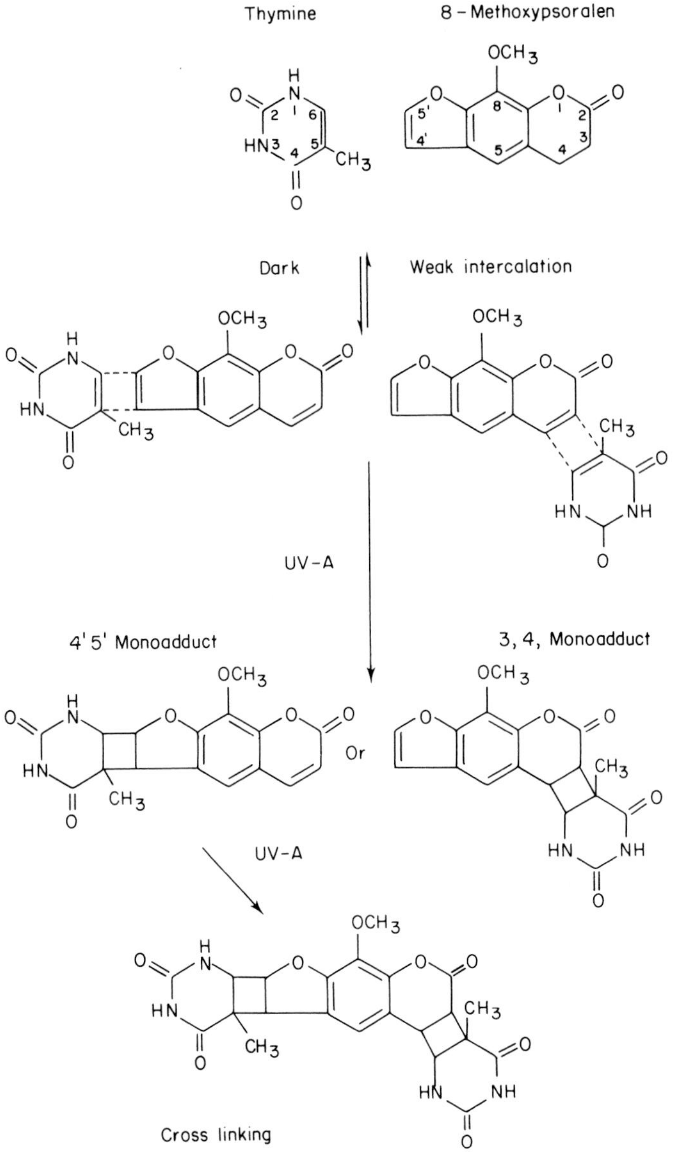

Fig. 1. Interactions between 8-methoxypsoralen and Thymine in DNA. In the dark, a weak, reversible intercalated binding occurs. Exposure to UV-A results in preferred binding at the 8-MOP 3,4 position but monovalent adducts are also formed at the 4′5′ position. Where the free end of the 4′5′ monoadduct is apposed to a Thymine on the other side of the DNA helix, further exposure to UV-A results in a cross link.

photosensitizer/substrate relationships is illustrated in this reaction by the possibility of alternative pathways for psoralen photoreactions with biological materials in solution. The UV-A induced triplet 8-MOP[1, 2] may interact with oxygen to produce $^1O_2$ with the potential for oxidation of biological substrates, as already discussed, and also in relation to enzyme inactivation.[3] Unusually, the 8-MOP itself may be oxidized with subsequent binding to protein.[4] In addition photobinding, independent of oxygen and the formation of biologically active 8-methoxypsoralen dimers may occur. However, the yields from these alternative reactions are relatively low. When psoralens are taken into cells, there appears to be a preferential association with DNA. The psoralen is held within the DNA double helix by weak binding forces so that an intercalated complex is formed. Unless the system is saturated with psoralen, this dark reaction is transient, and the psoralen diffuses out of the cell quite rapidly. However, if the system is exposed to UV-A, cyclo-addition photoproducts are formed between the psoralens and thymines with which they are associated. This covalent binding involves the 5,6 double bond of the thymine. With linear psoralens such as trimethylpsoralen (TMP), 8-methoxypsoralen, 5-methoxypsoralen, and psoralen itself, the reaction may involve either the 3,4 double bond of the coumarin moiety or the 4'5' double bond of the furan ring. The 3,4 bonding occurs more readily but the mono-adduct so formed does not absorb UV-A. The 4'5' monoadduct is fluorescent and when associated with DNA further exposure to UV-A leads to additional linkage across the DNA helix at the 3,4 double bond. In this manner, bifunctional psoralens may give rise to cross linked DNA. When angular compounds such as angelicin are used, the spatial arrangement is such that only mono-adducts are formed and therefore cross links cannot be formed. Similarly, only mono-adducts are possible if the 3,4 double bond of the psoralen is substituted as in 3-dimethyl-allyl-psoralen[5, 6] or 3-carbethoxypsoralen[7] (Fig. 2).

1. Pathak, M. A., Allen, B., Ingram, D. J. E. and Fellman, J. H. (1961). Photosensitization and effect of ultraviolet radiation on the production of unpaired electrons in the presence of furocoumarins. *Biochim. biophys. Acta* **54**, 506–515.

2. Yeargers, E. and Augenstein, L. (1965). Absorption and emission spectrum of psoralen and emission spectrum of psoralen and 8-methoxypsoralen in powders and in solution. *J. invest. Derm.* **44**, 181–187.

3. Poppe, W. and Grossweiner, L. I. (1975). Photodynamic sensitization by 8-methoxypsoralen via the singlet oxygen mechanism. *Photochem. Photobiol.* **22**, 217–219.

4. Yoshikawa, K., Mori, N., Sakakibara, S., Mizuno, N. and Song, P. S. (1979). Photoconjugation of 8-methoxypsoralen with proteins. *Photochem. Photobiol.* **29**, 1127–1133.

5. Rodighiero, G. and Dall'Acqua, F. (1976). Biochemical and Medical aspects of psoralens. *Photochem. Photobiol.* **24**, 647.

6. Vedaldi, D., Dall'Acqua, F., Cafieri and Rodighiero, G. (1979). 3-(**F**,-Dimethylallyl)-psoralen: A linear furocoumarin forming mainly 4', 5'-Monofunctional adducts with DNA. *Photochem. Photobiol.* **29**, 277.

7. Dubertret, L., Averbeck, D., Zajdela, F., Bisagni, E., Moustacchi, E., Touraine, H. and Latarjet, R. (1978). Photochemotherapy (PUVA) of psoriasis using 3-carbethoxypsoralen, a non-carcinogenic compound in mice. *Br. J. Derm.* **101**, 379.

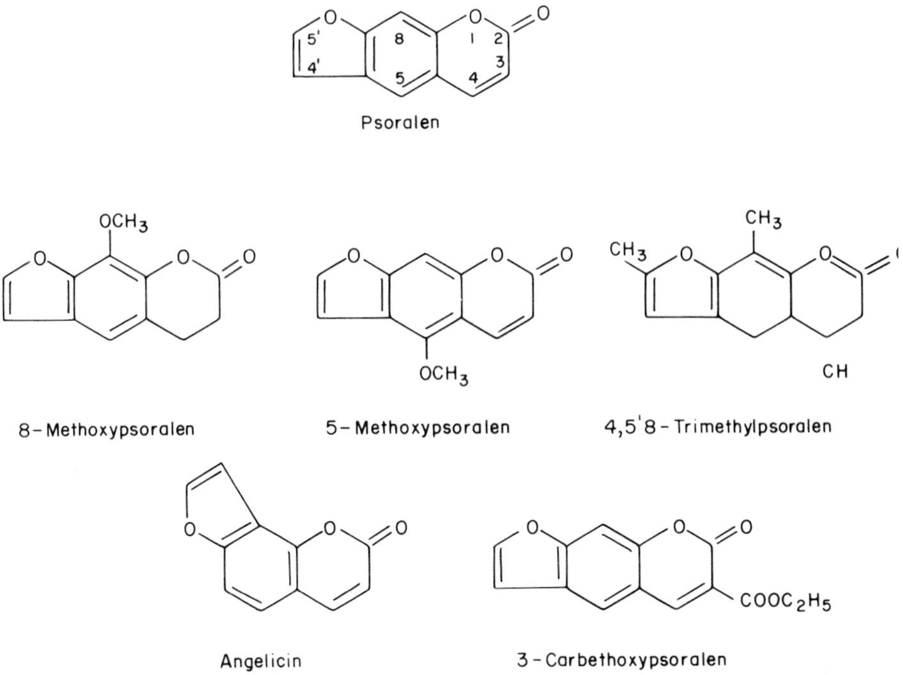

Psoralen

8-Methoxypsoralen

5-Methoxypsoralen

4,5'8-Trimethylpsoralen

Angelicin

3-Carbethoxypsoralen

Fig. 2. Molecular structures of Psoralen, 8-MOP, 5-MOP, Trimethylpsoralen, all of which are linear psoralens and form cross links, and of Angelicin, an angular furocoumarin, and 3-carbethoxypsoralen, which form monoadducts only.

Substitution in positions other than those directly involved in photo-addition may also change the photoreactivity of the psoralens. Thus, 5-methoxypsoralen and 8-methoxypsoralen are quite active, but the substitution of hydroxyl groups in the 5 or 8 positions inactivates the molecules. The anionic form produced by hydroxyl substitution has low triplet state yield on irradiation, and the triplet state energy available is dispersed throughout the whole molecule rather than being localized at the active sites of the 3,4 or 4'5' double bonds.[1] Conversely, substitution with methyl groups, other than at the 3 position, leads to an enhancement of photoreactivity.[2] The relative photosensitizing potential of various common psoralens has been summarized by Pathak, Kramer and Fitzpatrick.[3] Certain polycyclic aromatic hydrocarbons, such as benz-

1. Song, P. S. and Tapley, K. J. Jr (1979). Photochemistry and Photobiology of Psoralens. *Photochem. Photobiol.* **29**, 1177.

2. Pathak, M. A. (1969). Basic Aspects of Cutaneous Photosensitization. *In* 'The Biologic Effects of Ultraviolet Radiation with emphasis on the skin' (Ed. Urbach, F.), p. 489. Pergamon Press, Oxford.

3. Pathak, M. A., Kramer, D. M. and Fitzpatrick, T. B. (1974). Photobiology and Photochemistry of Furocoumarins (psoralens). *In* 'Sunlight and Man' (Ed. Fitzpatrick, T. B.), p. 335. University of Tokyo Press, Tokyo.

pyrene, have flat planar molecules which may also become intercalated between the DNA bases, and subsequent UV-irradiation may also lead to covalent binding of these chemicals into DNA.[1]

Although this type of photo-addition to DNA is not common and is usually associated with the psoralens, one other compound has also been shown to react in a similar manner. This is alpha-terthienyl, a thiophene derivative present in plants of the Compositae family[2] (Fig. 3). The importance of its photo-binding to DNA is not clear, however, since only mono-adducts are formed, and in the presence of oxygen in biological systems it nevertheless appears to photosensitize efficiently through the Type II photo-oxidation pathway.

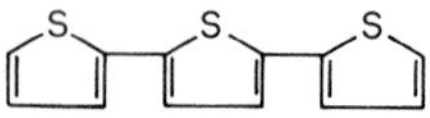

Alpha – terthienyl

Fig. 3. Molecular structure of α-terthienyl.

An oxygen independent photochemical reaction which gives rise to photosensitization in biological systems occurs with chlorpromazine. In solution, the photochemistry of this compound is complex,[3, 4, 5] but in neutral aqueous solution one or more of its photoproducts is cytotoxic to a greater extent than the original chlorpromazine.[6, 7] This is a simple chemical change that causes the apparent photosensitization and it may be relatively unimportant in the general problem of photosensitivity diseases. But a similar situation occurs with protriptyline[7] and the

1. Musajo, L. and Rodighiero, G. (1972). Photo-C_4-cyclo-addition reactions to the nucleic acids. *In* 'Research Progress in Organic, Biological, and Medicinal Chemistry', p. 155. North-Holland Publishing Co., Amsterdam.

2. Kagan, J., Gabriel, R. and Reed, S. (1980). Alpha-terthienyl, a non-photodynamic phototoxic compound. *Photochem. Photobiol.* **31**, 465.

3. Huang, C. L. and Sands, F. L. (1967). Effect of ultraviolet irradiation on chlorpromazine II. *J. pharmaceut. Sci.* **56**, 259.

4. Grant, F. W. and Greene, J. (1972). Phototoxicity and photonucleophilic aromatic substitution in chlorpromazine. *Toxicol. appl. Pharmac.* **23**, 71.

5. Davies, A. K., Navaratnam, S. and Phillips, G. O. (1976). Photochemistry of chlorpromazine (2-chloro-N-(3-dimethyl-aminopropyl)phenothiazine) in propan-2-ol solution. *J. chem. Soc., Perkin Trans II* **25**.

6. Johnson, B. E. (1974). Cellular mechanisms of chlorpromazine photosensitivity. *Proc. R. Soc. Med.* **67**, 871.

7. Kochevar, I. E. and Lamola, A. A. (1979). Chlorpromazine and protriptyline phototoxicity: photosensitized, oxygen independent red cell hemolysis. *Photochem. Photobiol.* **29**, 791.

reaction type may also be involved in the so-called photoallergic reactions that occur with chlorpromazine and sulphonamides.[1, 2, 3] With these compounds, irradiation leads to the formation of substances which act as contact allergens. A similar mechanism may be involved in the photosensitization obtained with the halogenated salicylanilides and related substances. Tetrachlorsalicylanilide (TCSA) in particular has induced the type of photosensitization leading to a sequential loss of chlorine atoms.[4, 5, 6] However, it appears that the photoproducts of TCSA alone do not function as complete antigens and that a UV-induced covalent binding to protein is an obligatory step in the process.[7] Cross reactions with other halogenated salicylanilides may be explained in terms of photoproduct formed. The UV-induced binding of photo-sensitizers to protein may not be the major feature of photosensitization leading to cellular damage, but the demonstration of such photobinding implies that the complex so formed has the potential to photosensitize and involve the immune system. In this context the protein binding occurring with 8-methoxypsoralen may well be the molecular mechanism which underlies the photoallergic reactions reported with psoralens.[8, 9, 10]

1. Rothstein, J., Schwarz, K., Schwarz-Speck, M. and Storck, H. (1966). Role of *in vivo* and *in vitro*-formed decomposition products of sulfanilamides and phenothiazines in photoallergy: Relationship of spectrophometric findings to *in vivo* reaction. *Int. Archs Allergy appl. Immun.* **29**, 1.

2. Ippen, H. (1969). Mechanisms of Photopathological Reactions. *In* 'The Biologic Effects of Ultraviolet Radiation with emphasis on the skin' (Ed. F. Urbach), p. 513. Pergamon Press, Oxford.

3. Aoki, K. and Saito, T. (1974). Studies on the mechanism of photosensitivity caused by sulfa drugs. *In* 'Sunlight and Man' (Ed. Fitzpatrick, T. B.), p. 431. University of Tokyo Press, Tokyo.

4. Coxon, J. A., Jenkins, F. P. and Welti, D. (1965). The effect of light on halogenated salicylanilide ions. *Photochem. Photobiol.* **4**, 713.

5. Davies, A. K., Hilal, N. W., McKellar, J. F. and Phillips, G. O. (1975). Photochemistry of tetrachlorsalicylanilide and its relation to the persistent light reactor. *Br. J. Derm.* **92**, 143.

6. Morikawa, F., Nakayama, Y., Fukuda, M., Hamona, M., Yokoyama, Y., Nagura, T., Ishihara, M. and Toda, K. (1974). Techniques for evaluation of phototoxicity and photoallergy in laboratory animals and man. *In* 'Sunlight and Man' (Ed. Fitzpatrick, T. B.), p. 529. University of Tokyo Press, Tokyo.

7. Kochevar, I. E. and Harber, L. C. (1977). Photoreactions of 3,3′, 4′,5-tetrachlorsalicylanilide with proteins. *J. invest. Derm.* **68**, 151.

8. Fulton, J. E. Jr and Willis, I. (1968). Photoallergy to Methoxsalen. *Archs Derm.* **98**, 445.

9. Llungren, B. (1977). Psoralen photoallergy caused by plant contact. *Contact Dermatitis* **3**, 85.

10. Plewig, G., Hofmann, Cornelia and Braun-Falco, O. (1978). Photoallergic Dermatitis from 8-methoxypsoralen. *Archs derm. Res.* **261**, 201.

II. PHOTOCONTACT AND DRUG-INDUCED PHOTOSENSITIVITY REACTIONS[1, 2, 3, 4]

A. Introduction

The various molecular mechanisms of photosensitization have already been discussed. Absorption of visible or UV radiation by different photosensitizing chemicals, by the transfer of energy or electrons, with or without the involvement of free radicals and oxygen, produce changes in various important biomolecules and thereby cause a variety of disturbances in biological systems. In skin, these may result from direct contact with the photosensitizing chemicals, as for example in cosmetics and toiletries, plants or their products, and as an occupational hazard. They may also be due to drugs which have photosensitizing properties circulating through, or accumulating in, the skin. Therefore, except for the special case of the porphyrias in which the photosensitization is due to a metabolic abnormality, the cutaneous manifestations are seen as photocontact of drug induced photosensitivity reactions.

B. Types of Photoreactions

The type of reaction developing may differ with different photosensitizers. In addition, a given photosensitizer may produce more than one type of reaction, depending on the manner in which it is introduced to the skin. It is proposed that these variations in photosensitized skin reactions may be classified under two main headings, depending on whether or not immunologic mechanisms are involved. Such a classification was introduced by Stephen Epstein in 1939 based on the observation that experimental sulphanilamide photosensitization can cause two distinct types of reaction.[5] The first, resembling sunburn, was obtained in all subjects tested, and occurred soon after the intradermal injection of the drug and exposure to sunlight. This type of reaction was familiar as part of the spectrum of "photodynamic action" first described

1. Blum, H. F. (1964). 'Photodynamic action and diseases caused by light'. Hafner Publishing Company, New York.
2. Harber, L. C. and Baer, R. L. (1972). Pathogenic mechanisms of drug-induced photosensitivity. *J. invest. Derm.* **58**, 327.
3. Herman, P. S. and Sams, W. M., Jr (1972). 'Soap Photodermatitis'. Charles C. Thomas, Springfield, Illinois.
4   Fitzpatrick, T. B. (Ed.) (1974). Phototoxicity and Photoallergy: Action of light on skin in presence of exogenous photosensitising agents including drugs. Section III of 'Sunlight and Man', p. 317. University of Tokyo Press, Tokyo.
5. Epstein, S. (1939). Photoallergy and primary photosensitivity to sulfanilamide. *J. invest. Derm.* **2**, 43.

at the beginning of this century and represents the direct result of cellular damage: this was called "phototoxicity".[1] The second, obtained in fewer subjects appeared 10 days later following a second exposure of sunlight. It was more severe, and of an eczematous nature; because it resembled the delayed hypersensitivity reactions of contact dermatitis, it was thought also to have an immunological basis and was called "photoallergy". Similar experimental results were obtained by Burckhardt, who emphasized the increased intensity of the second reaction and the characteristic histologic picture of eczema which was not present in the phototoxic reaction.[2, 3]

These early studies illustrated some of the basic features of photosensitized skin reactions. A single compound may produce different reactions in the skin through quite different cellular mechanisms. Where the concentration of photosensitizer in the skin is sufficiently high, and an appropriate radiation wavelength and exposure dose used, a phototoxic reaction is usually obtained in all test subjects although the ease with which it can be elicited varies. Moreover, this occurs on the first exposure of the subject to the procedure. On the other hand subjects taking the drug orally may not become photosensitive because the required skin concentration is not attained. In some cases, however, a reaction may be obtained at lower concentrations because of repeated exposures to both drug and sunlight.

A number of authors have presented tables to illustrate the differences between these two major classes of photosensitization.[4, 5, 6] A typical example is shown in Table 2, but it should be stressed that the differentiation is indicative rather than definitive, especially with regard to the details of photoallergy.[7]

The various complex pathways involved in both phototoxicity and photoallergy may be conveniently simplified in diagrammatic form, as shown in Fig. 4, which is derived and expanded from that of Harber, Baer

1. Blum, H. F. (1964). 'Photodynamic action and diseases caused by light'. Hafner Publishing Company, New York.
2. Burckhardt, W. (1941). Untersuchungen über die Photoaktivitat einiger Sulfonilamide. Dermatologica **83**, 63.
3. Burckhardt, W. (1948). Photoallergische Ekzeme durch Sulfonilamidsalben. Dermatologica **96**, 280.
4. Rothenstein, J., Schwarz, K., Schwarz-Speck, M. and Storck, H. (1966). Role of in vivo and in vitro formed decomposition products of sulfanilamides and phenothiazines in photoallergy: relationship of spectrophotometric findings to in vivo reactions. Int. Archs Allergy **29**, 1.
5. Jillson, O. F. (1969). Testing for phototoxicity and photoallergy. In 'The biologic effects of ultraviolet radiation with emphasis on the skin' (Ed. Urbach, F.), p. 533. Pergamon Press, Oxford.
6. Harber, L. C. and Baer, R. L. (1972). Pathogenic mechanisms of drug-induced photosensitivity. J. invest. Derm. **58**, 327.
7. Magnus, I. A. (1976). 'Dermatological Photobiology'. Blackwell, Oxford.

Table 2

Phototoxicity	Photoallergy
Positive photopatch test in all subjects	Positive photopatch test in only a few subjects
No previous exposure required	Previous exposure essential
Relatively high concentration of substance required	Relatively low concentration of substance required
Wavelength dependence matches absorption spectrum	Wavelength dependence not obviously restricted by absorption spectrum
Sunburn-like dusky erythema reaction or smarting with immediate erythema and wealing. May be delayed	Eczematous reaction or wealing May be delayed to 96 h
Pigmentation probable	Pigmentation not usual
No reaction at unexposed sites	Distal flares may occur on exposed sites and at sites previously producing a positive patch test reaction
In vitro test evidence of cytotoxicity	*In vitro* tests evidence of lymphocyte transformation and macrophage inhibition possible
No evidence of cellular immune involvement on *in vitro* testing	
No passive transfer	Passive transfer possible
Possible cross reactions with similar compounds not relevant. Does not lead to persistent light reaction	Possible cross reactions with similar chemical compounds. Can be associated with contact allergic reactions and with the state of persistent light reaction

and Bickers.[1] The contents of both the table and the diagram are discussed in the following sections which deal in more detail with the cellular mechanisms of phototoxicity and photoallergy.

III. PHOTOTOXICITY

A. Cellular Effects

The cellular effects of phototoxicity were first recognized in 1900 when Raab reported that Paramecia were killed when exposed to a

1. Harber, L. C., Baer, R. L. and Bickers, D. R. (1974). Techniques of evaluation of phototoxicity and photoallergy in biologic systems, including man with particular emphasis on immunologic aspects. *In* 'Sunlight and Man' (Ed. Fitzpatrick, T. B.), p. 515. University of Tokyo Press, Tokyo.

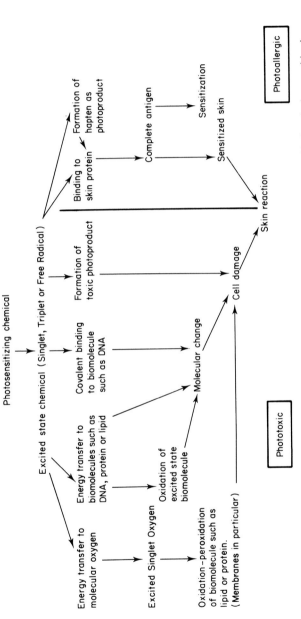

Visible or ultraviolet radiation

+

Photosensitizing chemical

Excited state chemical (Singlet, Triplet or Free Radical)

Energy transfer to molecular oxygen

Energy transfer to biomolecules such as DNA, protein or lipid

Covalent binding to biomolecule such as DNA

Formation of toxic photoproduct

Binding to skin protein

Formation of hapten as photoproduct

Excited Singlet Oxygen

Oxidation of excited state biomolecule

Complete antigen

Sensitization

Oxidation-peroxidation of biomolecule such as lipid or protein. (Membranes in particular)

Molecular change

Sensitized skin

Sensitized skin

Cell damage

Skin reaction

Phototoxic

Photoallergic

Fig. 4. Diagrammatic representation of the various pathways for drug or environmental chemical-induced photosensitization including mechanisms for both Phototoxicity and Photoallergy.

combination of acridine and sunlight.[1] This lethal effect varied directly with the light intensity but it did not occur in the absence of acridine. It was also abolished when a solution of acridine was used as an optical filter to the incident sunlight, a result which clearly and simply illustrated the fundamental principle that photosensitization depends specifically on the absorption of radiation by the photosensitizer. The radiation not absorbed by the acridine molecule was without effect.

This original work was rapidly expanded, especially by Tappeiner and Jodlbauer[2] to study the effects of various chemicals such as eosin and fluorescein on a variety of organisms, and this work was well reviewed by Blum.[3] A survey of the literature up to 1940 showed the importance of oxygen in these reactions in that it was required for photosensitization in enzymes, other proteins, toxins, viruses, bacteria, protozoa, mammalian erythrocytes, isolated muscle, and whole frog and human skin. The compounds investigated included Rose Bengal, Methylene Blue, Eosin, Erythrosin, Haematoporphyrin, Hypericin, neutral red, and methyl-cholanthrene. However, more recent studies of photosensitized reactions involving substances such as the psoralens have shown that oxygen independent processes also have an important place in the overall picture of phototoxicity.

The extension of the concept of phototoxicity from unicellular organisms to human skin was rapid. An abnormal urinary pigment, thought to be haematoporphyrin, was detected in patients with sunlight-induced bullous eruptions as early as 1898,[4] but it was 10 years later when this compound was recognized to be a photodynamic agent.[5] Porphyrin photosensitization as the basis for some light sensitive dermatoses was postulated in 1909.[6] Although haematoporphyrin itself is not a natural porphyrin and therefore does not play a part in the photosensitivity of the porphyrias, its action is typical of a number of photosensitizers. Its effect in human skin was dramatically illustrated by Meyer-Betz as a persistent urticarial reaction in himself after intravenous injection of this substance

1. Raab, O. (1900). Über die Wirkung fluorescierender Stoffe auf Infusorien. *Z. Biol.* **39**, 524.
2. Tappeiner, H. V. and Jodlbauer, A. (1907). Die sensibilizierende Wirkung fluorescierender Substanzen. Leipzig. F. C. W. Vogel. This is a series of papers reprinted from *D. Arch. klin. Med.* 1904–1906.
3. Blum, H. F. (1964). 'Photodynamic action and diseases caused by light'. Hafner Publishing Company, New York.
4. Anderson, T. M. (1898). Hydroa aestivale in two brothers complicated with the presence of haematoporphyrin in the urine. *Br. J. Derm.* **10**, 1.
5. Hausmann, W. (1908). Über die sensibilisierende Wirkung tierischer Farbstoffe und ihre physiologische Bedentung, *Biochem. Z.* **14**, 247.
6. Ehrmann, S. (1909). Weitare Untersuchungen über Lichtwirkung bei Hydron aestivalis (Bazin). Summer eruption (nach Hutchinson). *Archs Derm. Syph.* **97**, 75.

and exposure to sunlight.[1] Phototoxicity of the acridines to human skin was clearly demonstrated in 1925 when trypaflavine treatment produced a severe photosensitivity.[2] The use of Rose Bengal in liver function tests also gave rise to light-induced erythema and oedema,[3] and the introduction of the sulphonamides with their photosensitizing action was another major example of this type of cutaneous phototoxicity in man. Also, similar reactions had been observed in association with exposure to coal tar products as early as 1913,[4] and hyperpigmentation resulting from contact with cologne followed by exposure to sunlight was described in 1916.[5] The association of the typical phytophotodermatitis reactions of erythema, blistering and intense hyperpigmentation and exposure to sunlight was first suggested in the 1930s. In 1938, Kuske presented evidence that the plant substances responsible for this type of photosensitization were furocoumarins, an entirely new group of chemicals as far as the known photosensitizers were concerned.[6]

There are various useful lists of photosensitizing compounds,[7] the most comprehensive being that of Santamaria and Prino.[8] Epstein and his colleagues tabulated the photosensitizing polycyclic hydrocarbons along with their carcinogenic potential,[9] and others with greater relevance for dermatological photobiology have been prepared by Pathak[10] with special reference to psoralens.[11] Magnus has prepared a list of photo-

1. Meyer-Betz, F. (1913). Untersuchungen über die biologische (photodynamische) Wirkung der Haemato porphyrins und anderer Derivate des Blute und Gallenfarbstoffes. *Dt. Arch. klin. Med.* **112**, 476.
2. Jausion, H. and Marceron, L. (1925). Le 'coup de lumière' acridinique; son traitement preventif par la resorcine. *Bull. Soc. fr Derm. Syph.* **32**, 358.
3. Fiessinger, N., Ableaux-Fernet, M. and Aussannaire, M. (1937). Les reactions de photosensibilisation dans l'épreuve du rose bengal. *Bull. Soc. fr. Derm.* **44**, 1768.
4. Lewin, J. (1913). Über photodynamische Wirkungen von Inhaltsstoffen des Steinkohlenteerpechs am Menschen. *Munch. Med. Wochschr.* **60**, 1529.
5. Freund, E. (1916). Über bisher noch nicht beschriebene kunstliche Hautverfärbungen. *Derm. Wochschr.* **63**, 931.
6. Kuske, H. (1938). Experimentelle Untersuchungen zur Photosensibilisierung der Haut durch pflanzliche Wirkstoffe. I. Lichtensibilisierung der Furocoumarine als Ursache verschiedener phytogener Dermatosen. *Archs Derm. Syph.* **187**, 112.
7. Fowlks, W. L. (1959). The mechanism of the photodynamic effect. *J. invest. Derm.* **32**, 233.
8. Santamaria, L. and Prino, G. (1972). List of the photodynamic substances. In 'Research Progress in Organic, Biological and Medicinal Chemistry', Vol. 3, part 1 (Eds Gallo, U. and Santamaria, L.), p. XI. North Holland or American Elsevier.
9. Epstein, S. S., Small, M., Falk, H. L. and Mantel, N. (1964). On the association between photodynamic and carcinogenic activities in polycyclic compounds. *Cancer Res.* **24**, 855.
10. Pathak, M. A. (1969). Basic aspects of cutaneous photosensitization. In 'The biologic effects of ultraviolet radiation with emphasis on the skin' (Ed. Urbach, F.), p. 489. Pergamon Press, Oxford.
11. Pathak, M. A. and Fitzpatrick, T. B. (1959). Relationship of molecular configuration to the activity of furocoumarins which increase the cutaneous responses following long wave ultraviolet radiation. *J. invest. Derm.* **32**, 255.

sensitizing drugs commonly prescribed in the UK.[1] Others have presented the more common photosensitizing substances,[2,3,4] and Table 3 is representative of these.

B. Intracellular Reactions with Porphyrins

Cellular responses to photosensitization are mediated through a number of pathways, but the majority of oxygen-dependent reactions involve

Table 3

Phototoxic compounds

Dyestuffs	Thiazines:	Methylene blue, Toluidine blue.
	Xanthenes:	Fluorescein, halogenated fluoresceins such as Eosin, Erythrosin, Rose Bengal.
	Anthraquinones:	Anthraquinone, Benzanthrone, Disperse Blue 35.
Polycylic hydrocarbons in pitch and coal tar		Anthracene, Acridine, 1,2-Benzanthracene and other derivatives.
Plant extracts *Perfumes*	Psoralens.	8-methoxypsoralen (Xanthotoxin, Methoxsalen), 5-methoxypsoralen (Bergapten), Trimethylpsoralen (Tripsoralen). Other derivatives.
	Polyacetylenes and alphaterthienyl.	
Drugs	Tranquilizers:	Chlorpromazine and other phenothiazines, Protriptyline.
	Antibiotics:	Tetracyclines (Demethylchlortetracycline), Sulphonamides, Nalidix acid, Griseofulvin.
	Diuretics:	Chlorthiazides, Frusemide.
	Bacteriostatics:	Halogenated Salicylanilides.
Miscellaneous	Sunscreens:	Amyl o-dimethylaminobenzoic acid.
	Oral contraceptives.	
	Cyclamate sweetener.	

A number of these substances also appear in the table of photoallergic compounds (see page 2593).

1. Magnus, I. A. (1976). 'Dermatological Photobiology'. Blackwell, Oxford.
2. Harber, L. C., Baer, R. L. and Bickers, D. R. (1974). Techniques of evaluation of phototoxicity and photoallergy in biologic systems, including man, with particular emphasis on immunologic aspects. *In* 'Sunlight and Man' (Ed. Fitzpatrick, T. B.), p. 515. University of Tokyo Press, Tokyo.
3. Parrish, J. A., Anderson, R. R., Urbach, F. and Pitts, D. (1978). 'UV-A. Biologic effects of ultraviolet radiation with emphasis on human responses to longwave ultraviolet.' Plenum Press, New York.
4. Emmet, E. A. (1979). Phototoxicity from exogenous agents. *Photochem. Photobiol.* **30**, 429.

damage to some part of the complex lipo-protein membrane system of the cell. This is well illustrated by the *in vitro* studies of photosensitized red blood cell haemolysis.[1, 2] The original studies of photohaemolysis with fluorescein and its derivatives, rose bengal, and erythrosin established that it had the characteristics of colloid osmotic haemolysis, potassium leakage preceding the actual haemolysis (Fig. 5). Moreover, the reaction could be abolished by excluding oxygen from the system. This model has been used, not only to investigate the mechanisms of phototoxicity,[3, 4, 5]

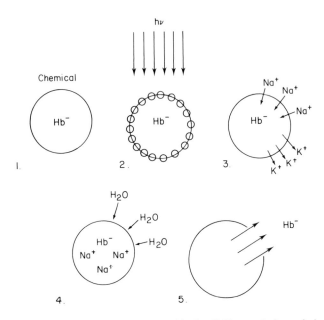

Fig. 5. Diagrammatic representation of photosensitized colloid osmotic haemolysis, one of the commonest model systems for studying phototoxicity. 1. Chemical is added to a suspension of red blood cells. 2. The mixture of RBCs and photosensitizer is exposed to appropriate radiation. 3. Photosensitized damage to the RBC membrane results in potassium leak and sodium entry to the cell. 4. Inside of the cell becomes hypertonic and water is taken in with resultant swelling of the cell. 5. The cell membrane ruptures releasing the contained haemoglobin.

1. Davson, H. and Ponder, E. (1940). Photodynamically induced cation permeability and its relation to haemolysis. *J. cell. comp. Physiol.* **15**, 67.

2. Blum, H. F. (1964). 'Photodynamic action and diseases caused by light'. Hafner Publishing Company, New York.

3. Cook, J. S. and Blum, H. F. (1959). Dose relationships and oxygen dependence in ultraviolet and photodynamic hemolysis. *J. cell. comp. Physiol.* **53**, 41.

4. Nilsson, R., Swanbeck, G. and Wennersten, G. (1975). Primary mechanisms of erythrocyte photolysis induced by biological sensitizers and phototoxic drugs. *Photochem. Photobiol.* **22**, 183.

5. Schothorst, A. A. and Suurmond, D. (1977). The role of oxygen in the photodamaging effect on erythrocytes of some photoallergic and phototoxic compounds. *Acta derm-venereol.* **57**, 127.

but also to serve as a screening test for suspected phototoxic compounds.[1,2] Its use is, of course, restricted by the fact that the red cell does not contain DNA, RNA or any cytoplasmic organelles; phototoxic compounds which react with these cell constituents cannot therefore be identified. None the less, where cell membrane mediated photosensitivity reactions are thought to be present, this test is extremely useful.

Porphyrin photosensitization has been used in recent studies of the phototoxic membrane damage in cells. In particular, the protoporphyrin containing erythrocytes of patients with erythropoietic protoporphyria were shown to haemolyse on exposure to 400 nm radiation[3] with the characteristics of colloid osmotic haemolysis typical of the photo-haemolysis obtained with photodynamic substances.[4,5] This reaction is oxygen dependent[5,6] and with minor variations due to differences in cellular binding sites[7] it can be reproduced in normal red blood cells by pre-incubation with protoporphyrin.[5,8,9] The importance of the lipid solubility characteristics of the photosensitizer in this system is illustrated by the inability to induce a similar photohaemolysis with either uroporphyrin or coproporphyrin, both of which are relatively hydrophilic.[8]

The mechanisms involved in this oxygen-dependent membrane damage are still not clear, but protection may be obtained with anti-oxidants such as alpha-tocopherol[3] and beta-carotene.[9,10,11] Like the

1. Kahn, G. and Fleischaker, B. (1971). Red blood cell hemolysis by photosensitizing compounds. *J. invest. Derm.* **56**, 85.

2. Freeman, R. G. (1970). Interaction of phototoxic compounds with cells in tissue culture. *Archs Derm.* **102**, 521.

3. Harber, L. C., Fleischer, A. S. and Baer, R. L. (1964). Erythropoietic protoporphyria and photohaemolysis. *J. Am. med. Ass.* **189**, 191.

4. Fleischer, A. S., Harber, L. C., Cook, J. S. and Baer, R. L. (1966). Mechanism of *in vitro* photohaemolysis in erythropoietic protoporphyria. *J. invest. Derm.* **46**, 505.

5. Schothorst, A. A., van Steveninck, J., Went, L. N. and Suurmond, D. (1970). Protoporphyrin-induced photohaemolysis in protoporphyria and in normal red blood cells. *Clinica chim. Acta* **28**, 241.

6. Hsu, J., Goldstein, B. D. and Harber, L. C. (1971). Photoreactions associated with *in vitro* hemolysis in erythropoietic protoporphyria. *Photochem. Photobiol.* **13**, 67.

7. Lamola, A. A. (1977). Photodegradation of Biomembranes. *In* 'Research in Photobiology' (Ed. Castellani, A.), p. 53. Plenum Press, New York.

8. Haining, R. G., Hulse, T. E. and Labbe, R. F. (1969). Photohemolysis: the comparative behaviour of erythrocytes from patients with different types of porphyria. *Proc. Soc. exp. Biol. Med.* **132**, 625.

9. Goldstein, B. D. and Harber, L. C. (1972). Erythropoietic protoporphyria: lipid peroxidation and red cell membrane damage associated with photohemolysis. *J. clin. Invest.* **51**, 892.

10. Swanbeck, G. and Wennersten, G. (1973). Effect of beta-carotene on photohemolysis. *Acta derm-venereol. (Stockholm)* **53**, 283.

11. Moshell, A. and Bjornson, L. (1977). Photoprotection in erythropoietic protoporphyria: mechanism of photoprotection by beta-carotene. *J. invest. Derm.* **68**, 157.

photohaemolysis with haematoporphyrin,[1] the relative contributions of singlet oxygen quenching and free radical scavenging to this protection are not certain. The importance of -SH groups to the maintenance of biomembrane integrity is illustrated by the inhibition of photohaemolysis by dithiothreitol[2] and by cysteine and various mercapto-compounds.[3] Although the mechanisms are not clear, membrane-SH is decreased in photosensitized red blood cells, as is acetylcholinesterase activity,[4] although ATP and glutathione producing enzymes are not affected.[5] A reduction in unsaturated fatty acid content is thought to follow the photosensitized formation of lipid peroxides[4] which, by free radical (Type I) or singlet oxygen (Type II) mechanism, may be the major initial step in photosensitized damage to biomembranes generally. However, the photo-oxidation of amino acid membrane constituents may be equally or more important.[6] Cross linking of membrane-bound protein can occur,[7, 8] and the formation of cholesterol 5-alpha-hydroperoxide, which induces membrane instability, has been detected in protoporphyrin sensitized membrane.[9]

Such detailed investigations of phototoxicity at the cellular level with other photosensitizers are uncommon. Kynurenic acid, a tryptophan derivative which may act as an endogenous photosensitizer in human skin, induces a photohaemolysis which can be inhibited by beta-carotene.[10] There is good evidence that this is mediated through excited singlet

1. Nilsson, R., Swanbeck, G. and Wennersten, G. (1975). Primary mechanisms of erythrocyte photolysis induced by biological sensitizers and phototoxic drugs. *Photochem. Photobiol.* **22**, 183.
2. Harber, L. C., Hsu, J., Hsu, H. and Goldstein, B. D. (1972). Studies of photoprotection against porphyrin photosensitization using dithiothreitol and glycerol. *J. invest. Derm.* **58**, 383.
3. Suurmond, D., van Steveninck, J. and Went, L. N. (1970). Some clinical and fundamental aspects of erythropoietic protoporphyria. *Br. J. Derm.* **82**, 323.
4. Goldstein, B. D. and Harber, L. C. (1972). Erythropoietic protoporphyria: lipid peroxidation and red cell membrane damage associated with photohemolysis. *J. clin. Invest.* **51**, 892.
5. Schothorst, A. A., van Steveninck, J., Went, L. N. and Suurmond, D. (1970). Protoporphyrin-induced photohemolysis in protoporphyria and in normal red blood cells. *Clin. chim. Acta* **28**, 41.
6. Schothorst, A. A., van Steveninck, J., Went, L. N. and Suurmond, D. (1972). Photodynamic damage of the erythrocyte membrane caused by protoporphyrin in protoporphyria and in normal red blood cells. *Clinica. chim. Acta* **39**, 161.
7. Girotti, A. (1976). Photodynamic action of protoporphyrin IX on human erythrocytes: cross linking of membrane proteins. *Biochem. biophys. Res. Commun.* **72**, 1367.
8. DeGoeij, A., Ververgaert, P. and van Steveninck, J. (1975). Photodynamic effects of protoporphyrin on the architecture of erythrocyte membranes in protoporphyria and in normal red blood cells. *Clinica chim. Acta* **62**, 287.
9. Lamola, A. A., Yamane, T. and Trozzolo, A. M. (1973). Cholesterol hydroperoxide formation in red cell membranes and photohemolysis in erythropoietic protoporphyria. *Science* **179**, 1131.
10. Swanbeck, G. and Wennersten, G. (1974). Photohemolytic activity of tryptophan and phenylalanine metabolites. *Acta derm-venereol.* **54**, 99.

oxygen,[1,2] but here again it is not clear whether unsaturated fatty acids, amino acids, or cholesterol are the principle membrane constituents involved. The photodynamic lysis of liposomes and model membrane systems consisting of unsaturated fatty acid containing phospholipid[3] or of phospholipid and cholesterol,[4,5,6] resemble the lysis of the red cell membrane, but nevertheless oxidation of amino acids of the protein within the membranes is still probably important. It seems that any chemical or drug which produces an oxygen dependent photohaemolysis probably acts at the cellular level in much the same way as protoporphyrin or haematoporphyrin.

C. Intracellular Reactions with Other Agents

Using potassium loss as an indication of photosensitized damage to erythrocytes, oxygen dependence has been clearly demonstrated for anthracene as well as protoporphyrin.[7] There is some suggestion that a similar effect is obtained with bithionol, tribromosalicylanilide, promethazine, demethylchlortetracycline, sulphanilamide and chlorpromazine.

These studies of photohaemolysis provide good evidence for the plasma membrane as the primary target for phototoxic damage to the cell. However, Slater and Riley[8] found that the lysosome membrane, especially in epidermal cells, is specifically damaged by photosensitization with phylloerythrin, the porphyrin derived from chlorophyll, which is responsible for photosensitivity reactions in cattle and sheep with liver damage.[9]

While accepting that other cell constituents might be directly

1. Swanbeck, G., Wennersten, G. and Nilsson, R. (1974). Participation of singlet state excited oxygen in photohaemolysis induced by kynurenic acid. *Acta derm-venereol.* **54**, 433.
2. Nilsson, R., Swanbeck, G. and Wennersten, G. (1975). Primary mechanisms of erythrocyte photolysis induced by biological sensitizers and phototoxic drugs. *Photochem. Photobiol.* **22**, 183.
3. Felmeister, A. and Tolat, S. V. (1970). Phospholipid spherules as a model to assess photosensitizing properties of drugs. *J. pharm. Sci.* **59**, 856.
4. Anderson, S. M. and Krinsky, N. I. (1973). Protective action of carotenoid pigments against photodynamic damage to liposomes. *Photochem. Photobiol.* **18**, 403.
5. Anderson, S. M., Krinsky, N. I. and Stone, M. J. (1974). Effect of singlet oxygen quenchers on oxidative damage to liposomes initiated by photosensitization or by radiofrequency discharge. *Photochem. Photobiol.* **20**, 65.
6. Copeland, E. S., Alving, C. R. and Grenan, M. M. (1976). Light-induced leakage of spin label marker from liposomes in the presence of phototoxic phenothiazines. *Photochem. Photobiol.* **24**, 41.
7. Schothorst, A. A. and Suurmond, D. (1977). The role of oxygen in the photodamaging effect on erythrocytes of some photoallergic and phototoxic compounds. *Acta derm-venereol.* **57**, 127.
8. Slater, T. F. and Riley, P. A. (1966). Photosensitization and lysosomal damage. *Nature* **209**, 151.
9. Clare, N. T. (1956). Photodynamic action and its pathological effects. *In* 'Radiation Biology (Ed. Hollaender, A.), Vol. III, p. 693. McGraw-Hill, New York.

damaged, they emphasized the possibility of widespread cellular damage resulting from the release of hydrolytic enzymes following photo-sensitization restricted to lysosome membranes. There appear to be two major pathways for the involvement of membrane damage in the photosensitized killing of nucleated mammalian cells (Fig. 6). Rose bengal and eosin do not penetrate living cells and only produce damage

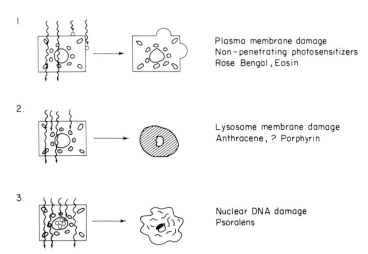

Fig. 6. Diagrammatic representation of the three major cellular mechanisms postulated for phototoxicity. 1. Plasma membrane damage when photosensitizer is adsorbed onto the membrane and does not penetrate the cell. This type of damage may also occur with penetrating chemicals if sufficient remains in the membrane. 2. Lysosome membrane damage when photosensitizer is concentrated within lysosomes and the photosensitization leads to the release of hydrolytic enzymes. 3. DNA damage when the photosensitizer has a specific interaction with DNA. It should be emphasized that other cellular targets may exist and also that for some photosensitizers, more than one target may be affected.

to the plasma membrane: cell death occurs from characteristic cytoplas-mic extrusions in the form of surface blebbing. Anthracene, uropor-phyria, neutral red and acridine, however, enter the cell and are concentrated within lysosomes. Where plasma membrane damage is prevented by removal of excess chemical, photosensitization then causes cytoplasmic vacuolation, nuclear pyknosis and a rounding up of the cell body: reactions that are ascribed to the intracellular release of lysosomal enzymes.[1] Photosensitized release of acid hydrolases by acridine orange

1. Allison, A. C., Magnus, I. A. and Young, M. R. (1966). Role of lysosomes and of cell membranes in photosensitization. *Nature* **209**, 874.

without profound ultrastructural damage to lysosome membranes can occur, and then observed changes in other cell structures appear to depend on the action of these enzymes.[1] Both plasma membrane and cytoplasmic photosensitization occur in fibroblasts treated with haematoporphyrin, but the site of the cytoplasmic effect is not defined.[2] Damage confined to the plasma membrane occurs in kynurenic acid photosensitization.[3, 4]

Further investigations of fibroblast photosensitization by porphyrins has shown that a water soluble protoporphyrin is taken into the cell and concentrated in the lysosome.[5] However, there is no evidence that lysosomal enzymes are responsible for fibroblast death,[6] and it is concluded that the mechanism for protoporphyrin photosensitization of nucleated cells is probably similar to that occurring in photohaemolysis of red blood cells in erythropoietic protoporphyria.

The anthraquinone dye, disperse blue 35, also photosensitizes by damage to membranes, probably through the excited singlet oxygen pathway.[7]

The importance of protein and lipid for the maintenance of membrane integrity and the facility with which they may be shown to undergo photooxidation has led to the neglect of nucleic acids as a possible target for photodynamic action. However, it is evident that methylene blue and related compounds may sensitize the photodynamic destruction of guanine residues in nucleic acids.[8] The mechanisms involved have not been established, but for the less lipophilic porphyrins[9] and other water

1. Hawkins, H. K., Ericsson, J. L. E., Biberfield, P. and Trump, B. F. (1972). Lysosomes and phagosome stability in lethal cell injury. *Am. J. Pathol.* **68**, 255.
2. Fritsch, P., Gschnait, F., Honigsmann, H. and Wolff, K. (1976). Protective action of beta-carotene against lethal photosensitization of fibroblasts *in vitro*. *Br. J. Derm.* **94**, 263.
3. Wennersten, G. and Brunk, U. (1977). Cellular aspects of phototoxic reactions induced by kynurenic acid. I. Establishment of an experimental model utilising *in vitro* cultivated cells. *Acta derm-venereol.* **57**, 201.
4. Wennersten, G. and Brunk, U. (1978). Cellular aspects of phototoxic reactions induced by kynurenic acid. II. Fine structural analysis and cytochemistry on cultivated cells. *Acta derm-venereol. (Stockholm)* **58**, 297.
5. Schothorst, A. A., Suurmond, D. and Ploem, J. (1977). *In vitro* studies on the protoporphyrin uptake and photosensitivity of normal skin fibroblasts and fibroblasts from patients with erythropoietic protoporphyria. *J. invest. Derm.* **69**, 551.
6. Wakulchik, S. D., Schiltz, J. R. and Bickers, D. R. (1980). Photolysis of protoporphyrin-treated human fibroblasts *in vitro*: studies on the mechanism. *J. Lab. clin. Med.* **96**, 158.
7. Davies, A. K., Hamblett, I., McKellar, J. F. and Phillips, G. O. (1975). Mechanism of photocontact dermatitis due to an anthraquinone disperse dye. *J. appl. Chem. Biotechnol.* **25**, 195.
8. Spikes, J. D. (1977). Photosensitization. In 'The Science of Photobiology' (Ed. Smith, K. C.), p. 87. Plenum Press, New York.
9. West, J., Breitbart, R. and Pathak, M. A. (1980). Photosensitization of DNA by Uro-, Copro- and Protoporphyrins. Abstr. 8th Intern'l. Photobiol. Congress, Strasbourg.

soluble photosensitizers, this action may produce cellular change similar to that brought about by other DNA damaging agents.

D. Intracellular Reactions with Psoralens

Although the photosensitized reactions obtained with psoralens are obviously phototoxic the mechanisms involved differ from those previously discussed because oxygen was not required.[1,2] This was well illustrated in a comparative study between 8-methoxypsoralen and toluidine blue photosensitized in the killing of the bacterium, *Sarcina lutea*.[3] Evidence for the photosensitized interaction of psoralens with DNA was first reported in 1965,[4] and the details of these interactions are discussed in the section on molecular mechanisms in photosensitization. It is clear that monofunctional adducts, especially to thymine, and cross links between pyrimidines in the DNA double helix, give rise to the inhibition of DNA synthesis and cellular proliferation, chromosome damage, mutation, and cell death.[5,6,7] Because this form of photosensitization has been used successfully in the treatment of psoriasis and other conditions, the cellular events involved are discussed in detail in the section on photochemotherapy (see page 2651). Discussion here is restricted to the aspects of psoralen phototoxicity as it appears in phytophotodermatitis, and to the changes resulting from exposure to bergamot oil in perfume preparations. The *Candida albicans* test developed by Daniels[8] has proved useful in studies with psoralens, even though it may fail to detect phototoxicity with sulphanilamides and demethylchlortetracycline[8] and may give different results from those obtained on the skin with

1. Musajo, L., Rodighiero, G. and Santamaria, L. (1957). Le sostanze fotodinamiche con particolare riguado alle furocoumarine. *Atti. Soc. ital. Patol.* **5**, 1.
2. Oginsky, E. L., Green, G. S., Griffith, D. G. and Fowlks, W. L. (1959). Lethal photosensitization of bacteria with 8-methoxypsoralen to long wavelength ultraviolet radiation. *J. Bacteriol.* **78**, 821.
3. Matthews, M. M. (1963). Comparative studies of lethal photosensitization of Sarcina lutea by 8-methoxypsoralen and by toluidine blue. *J. Bacteriol.* **85**, 322.
4. Musajo, L., Rodighiero, G. and dall'Acqua, F. (1965). Evidences of a photoreaction of the photosensitizing furocoumarins with DNA and with pyrimidine nucleosides and nucleotides. *Experientia* **21**, 24.
5. Pathak, M. A., Kramer, D. M. and Fitzpatrick, T. B. (1974). Photobiology and photochemistry of furocoumarins (psoralens). *In* 'Sunlight and Man' (Ed. Fitzpatrick, T. B.), p. 335. University of Tokyo Press, Tokyo.
6. Musajo, L., Rodighiero, G., Caporale, G., dall'Acqua, F., Marciani, S., Bordin, F., Baccichetti, F. and Bevilacqua, R. (1974). Photoreaction between skin-photosensitizing furocoumarins and nucleic acids. *In* 'Sunlight and Man' (Ed. Fitzpatrick, T. B.), p. 369. University of Tokyo Press, Tokyo.
7. Song, P.-S. and Tapley, K. J., Jr. (1978). Photochemistry and photobiology of psoralens. *Photochem. Photobiol.* **29**, 1177.
8. Daniels, F., Jr. (1965). A simple microbiological method for demonstrating phototoxic compounds. *J. invest Derm.* **44**, 259.

quinoline methanols[1] and tetramethylthiurammonosulphate.[2] Microgram quantities of administered 8-MOP found in animal tissues can be detected by this method,[3] although the more sensitive *Staphylococcus aureus* model is required for the lesser amounts present in human plasma during photochemotherapy.[4] Apart from screening for phototoxicity in various plants, the method has been used to assess the 8-MOP and 5-MOP content of both *Dictamnus alba*, the gas plant,[5] and *Heracleum mantegazzianum*, the giant hogweed,[6] both well recognized agents in producing phytophotodermatitis.

This method was also used in a survey of the 5-MOP content of bergamot oil[7] and other perfume materials[8] to give quantitative estimates of the photosensitizer.

The photosensitizing potential of various plants of the *Compositae* family was first recognized by the use of the *C. albicans* test.[9, 10] This led to the isolation of a new group of phototoxic compounds, namely the polyacetylenes and thiophene derivatives such as alpha-terthienyl.[11] An oxygen independent covalent binding to DNA, similar to that of the psoralens but restricted to mono-adducts, has been suggested as the phototoxic mechanism for alphaterthienyl.[12] However, the cellular mechanisms are more complex than those of the psoralens in that alpha-terthienyl photohaemolysis is much more marked.[13] The author has found that

1. Ison, A. E. and Davis, C. M. (1969). Phototoxicity of quinoline methanols and other drugs in mice and yeast. *J. invest. Derm.* **52**, 193.
2. Muller, R. and Mitchell, J. C. (1971). Psoralen-type phototoxicity of tetramethylthiurammonosulphide for *Candida albicans*; not for mouse or man. *J. invest Derm.* **56**, 340.
3. Becker, S. W. and West, B. (1965). Detection of photosensitizers in tissue. *Archs Derm.* **92**, 457.
4. Glew, W. B., Roberts, W. P., Malinin, G. I. and Nigra, T. P. (1980). Quantitative determination by bioassay of photoactive 8-methoxypsoralen in serum. *J. invest. Derm.* **75**, 230.
5. Moller, H. (1978). Phototoxicity of *Dictamnus alba*. *Contact Dermatitis* **4**, 264.
6. Gumar, A. W. S. (1976). 'A quantitative study of phytophotodermatitis'. Thesis, University of Dundee, Scotland.
7. Zaynoun, S. T., Johnson, B. E. and Frain-Bell, W. (1977). A study of oil of bergamot and its importance as a phototoxic agent. I. Characterisation and quantitation of the photoactive component. *Br. J. Derm.* **96**, 475.
8. Zaynoun, S. T. (1978). The quantitative analysis of bergapten in perfumes. *J. Soc. cosmet Chem.* **29**, 247.
9. Camm, E. L., Towers, G. H. N. and Mitchell, J. C. (1975). UV-mediated antibiotic activity of some Compositae species. *Phytochem* **14**, 2007.
10. Towers, G. H. N., Wat, C. K., Graham, E. A., Bandoni, R. J., Chan, G. F. Q., Mitchell, J. C. and Lam, J. (1977). Ultraviolet-mediated antibiotic activity of species of Compositae caused by polyacetylenic compounds. *Lloydia* **40**, 487.
11. Towers, G. H. N. (1979). Contact hypersensitivity and photodermatitis evoked by compositae. *In* 'Toxic Plants' (Ed. Kinghorn, A. D.), p. 171. Columbia University Press, New York.
12. Kagan, J., Gabriel, R. and Reed, S. A. (1980). Alpha-terthienyl, a non-photodynamic phototoxic compound. *Photochem. Photobiol.* **31**, 465.
13. Wat, C. K., MacRae, W. D., Yamamoto, E., Towers, G. H. N. and Lam, J. (1980). Phototoxic effects of naturally occurring polyacetylenes and alphaterthienyl on human erythrocytes. *Photochem. Photobiol.* **32**, 167.

ethanol extracts of various *Compositae* have a considerable phototoxic potential in terms of membrane damage,[1, 2] but do not have lethal effects against *C. albicans*.

E. Phototoxicity due to Chlorpromazine and Other Compounds

It seems that at the cellular level the phototoxic effects of a number of compounds may be produced through more than one pathway. This complex situation is well illustrated by chlorpromazine (CPZ) phototoxicity which shows lethal effects against viruses,[3, 4] bacteria,[5, 6] and cultured mammalian cells:[6, 7, 8] it also exhibits photohaemolysis[7, 9, 10, 11] and cytogenetic changes.[12] Photosensitized binding of CPZ to protein,[13] RNA, and DNA[14, 15] occurs, and the photosensitized oxidation of

1. Frain-Bell, W., Hetherington, A. and Johnson, B. E. (1979). Contact allergic sensitivity to chrysanthemum and the photosensitivity dermatitis and actinic reticuloid syndrome. *Br. J. Derm.* **101**, 491.

2. Addo, H. A., Johnson, B. E. and Frain-Bell. W. (1980). Abstract. A study of the relationship between contact allergic sensitivity and persistent light reaction. *Brit. J. Derm.* **103**, 20.

3. Matsuo, I., Ohkido, M., Fujita, H. and Suzuki, K. (1980). Chlorpromazine photosensitization. I. Effect of near-UV irradiation on bacteriophages sensitized with chlorpromazine. *Photochem. Photobiol.* **31**, 169.

4. Day, R. S. and Dimattina, M. (1977). Photodynamic action of chlorpromazine in adeovirus 5: repairable damage and single strand breaks. *Chem.–biol. Interactions* **17**, 89.

5. Matsuo, I., Ohkido, M., Fujita, H. and Suzuki, K. (1980). Chlorpromazine photosensitization. II. Failure to detect any evidence for involvement of DNA damage in the photodynamic killing of *Escherichia coli* in the presence of chlorpromazine. *Photochem. Photobiol.* **31**, 175.

6. Garraz, G., Dugois, P. and Dugois, J. (1962). Photosensibilisants et radiosensibilisants. 1er memoire: definitions et techniques d'étude. *Thérapie* **17**, 189.

7. Johnson, B. E. (1974). Cellular mechanisms of chlorpromazine photosensitivity. *Proc. R. Soc. Med.* **67**, 871.

8. Ljunggren, B., Cohen, S. R., Carter, D. M. and Wayne, S. I. (1980). Chlorpromazine phototoxicity: growth inhibition and DNA-interaction in normal human fibroblasts. *J. Invest. Derm.* **75**, 253.

9. Kahn, G. and Fleischaker, B. (1971). Red blood cell haemolysis by photosensitising compounds. *J. invest. Derm.* **56**, 85.

10. Freeman, R. G. (1970). Interaction of phototoxic compounds with cells in tissue culture. *Archs Derm.* **102**, 521.

11. Kochevar, I. E. and Lamola, A. A. (1979). Chlorpromazine and protriptyline phototoxicity: photosensitized, oxygen independent red cell haemolysis. *Photochem. Photobiol.* **29**, 791.

12. Kelly-Gaevert, F. and Legator, M. S. (1973). Photoactivation of chlorpromazine cytogenetic and mutagenic effect. *Mut. Res.* **21**, 101.

13. Alani, M. D. and Dunne, J. H. (1973). Effects of longwave ultraviolet radiation on photosensitizing and related compounds. II. *In vitro* binding to soluble epidermal proteins. *Br. J. Derm.* **89**, 367.

14. Rosenthal, I., Ben-Hur, E., Prager, A. and Riklis, E. (1978). Photochemical reactions of chlorpromazine; chemical and biochemical implications. *Photochem. Photobiol.* **28**, 591.

15. Kahn, G. and Davis, B. P. (1970). *In vitro* studies on longwave ultraviolet light-dependent reactions of the skin photosensitizer chlorpromazine with nucleic acids, purines and pyrimidines. *J. invest. Derm.* **55**, 47.

liposomes has been reported.[1] However, photohaemolysis with CPZ is independent of oxygen and appears to be due to the membrane damaging effects of a cytotoxic photoproduct.[2, 3] Non-dividing cells are also killed, probably due to damage to the plasma membrane.[2] This photomimetic effect of the CPZ photoproduct was first observed in the killing of Ehrlich tumour cells.[3] Similarly, the binding of CPZ to DNA occurs as the result of the formation of a stable photoproduct.[4] Conversely, CPZ photosensitized damage to DNA in viruses[5] and normal human fibroblasts,[6] as well as inhibition of fibroblast proliferation,[6] appears to be due to a genuine photosensitization reaction rather than to a toxic photoproduct.

It has been suggested that the action of a toxic photoproduct, "photofluorescein", was responsible for the photohaemolysis with fluorescein,[7] but the more conventional photodynamic mechanisms would seem more likely. Nonetheless, photohaemolysis obtained with protriptyline, a tranquillizer with many reported instances of photosensitivity reactions,[8] is due mainly to the lytic effect of a photoproduct[9, 10] and some part of tetrachlorsalicylanilide phototoxicity may also depend on this mechanism.[11]

The problem of chlorpromazine phototoxicity is further complicated by the possibility that the reactions observed are due to drug metabolites rather than to the parent compound. Even topically applied compounds may be changed by epidermal metabolic processes. In an excellent series

1. Copeland, E. S., Alving, C. R. and Grenan, M. M. (1976). Light-induced leakage of spin label marker from liposomes in the presence of phototoxic phenothiazines. *Photochem. Photobiol.* **24**, 41.
2. Johnson, B. E. (1974). Cellular mechanisms of chlorpromazine photosensitivity. *Proc. R. Soc. Med.* **67**, 871.
3. Garraz, G. and Beriel, H. (1962). Photosensibilisants et radiosensibilisants. 2e memoire: les photomimetiques. *Thérapie* **17**, 195.
4. Chung, F.-L. and Kochevar, I. E. (1979). Photoreactions of chlorpromazine with DNA, American Chemical Society, 10th Northeast Annual Meeting, Syracuse, Abstract.
5. Day, R. S. and Dimattina, M. (1977). Photodynamic action of chlorpromazine on adenovirus 5: repairable damage and single strand breaks. *Chem.–biol. Interactions* **17**, 89.
6. Ljunggren, B., Cohen, S. R., Carter, D. M. and Wayne, S. I. (1980). Chlorpromazine phototoxicity: growth inhibition and DNA-interaction in normal human fibroblasts. *J. invest. Derm.* **75**, 258.
7. Menke, J. F. (1935). The hemolytic action of photofluorescein. *Biol. Bull.* **68**, 360.
8. Magnus, I. A. (1976). 'Dermatological Photobiology'. Blackwell Scientific Publications, Oxford.
9. Kochevar, I. E. and Lamola, A. A. (1979). Chlorpromazine and Protriptyline phototoxicity: photosensitized, oxygen independent red cell hemolysis. *Photochem. Photobiol.* **29**, 791.
10. Kochevar, I. E. (1980). Possible mechanisms of toxicity due to photochemical products of protriptyline. *Toxicol. appl. Pharmacol.* **54**, 258.
11. Kahn, G. and Fleischaker, B. (1971). Evaluation of phototoxicity of salicylanilides and similar compounds by photohemolysis. *J. invest. Derm.* **56**, 91.

of investigations, Ljunggren and Moller, using the increase in weight of irradiated mouse tail as a quantitative measure of phototoxicity, showed the major metabolites of CPZ, two demethylated compounds, the sulphoxide, 7-hydroxyl-CPZ and 2-chlorphenothiazine were all photo-toxic: the demethyl compounds having a greater phototoxicity than the parent compound.[1] They also found that 7-hydroxymethyl nalidixic acid, the major metabolite of nalidixic acid, was equally effective as the parent compound.[2]

Other studies of phototoxicity in animals have mainly been concerned with the development of screening techniques. Mice,[3, 4, 5, 6, 7] rats,[6] guinea-pigs,[6, 8, 9] rabbits,[6] and pigs[6, 7, 10] have all been used in these studies: the phototoxicity being determined as erythema or oedema in flank skin, or as an increase in ear thickness in mice and guinea-pigs. Although there is some inter-species difference,[6] a general picture of chemical and drug phototoxicity is obtained by topical, intradermal or systemic administration, followed by exposure to the appropriate radiation. Some difficulty has been encountered in experimentally demonstrating the phototoxicity of some substances which clearly had phototoxic properties in humans. For example, reactions were not elicited with either demethylchlortetracycline or chlorthiazide in guinea-pigs using artificial sources of UVR,[9] but positive results were obtained when natural sunlight was used.[11] Intradermal injections of nalidixic acid

1. Ljunggren, B. and Moller, H. (1977). Phenothiazine phototoxicity: an experimental study on chlorpromazine and its metabolites. *J. invest Derm.* **68**, 313.
2. Ljunggren, B. and Moller, H. (1978). Drug phototoxicity in mice. *Acta derm-venereol. (Stockholm)* **78**, 1.
3. Ison, A. E. and Blank, H. (1967). Testing phototoxicity in mice. *J. invest. Derm.* **49**, 508.
4. Rothe, W. E. and Jacobus, D. P. (1968). Laboratory evaluation of the phototoxicity potency of quinoline methanols. *J. med. Chem.* **11**, 366.
5. Gloxuber, C. (1970). Prüfung von Kosmetik-Grundstoffen auf fototoxische Wirkung. *J. Soc. cosmet. Chem.* **21**, 825.
6. Morikawa, F., Nakayama, Y., Fukuda, M., Hamano, M., Yokoyama, Y., Nagura, T., Ishihara, M. and Toda, K. (1974). Techniques for evaluation of phototoxicity and photoallergy in laboratory animals and man. In 'Sunlight and Man' (Ed. Fitzpatrick, T. B.), p. 529. University of Tokyo Press, Tokyo.
7. Forbes, P. D., Urbach, F. and Davies, R. E. (1977). Phototoxicity testing of fragrance raw materials. *Food Cosmetic Toxicol.* **15**, 55.
8. Stott, C. W., Stasse, J., Bonomo, R. and Campbell, A. H. (1970). Evaluation of the phototoxic potential of topically applied agents using long-wave ultraviolet light. *J. invest. Derm.* **55**, 335.
9. Sams, W. M. (1966). The experimental production of drug phototoxicity in guinea pigs: II Using artificial light sources. *Archs Derm.* **94**, 773.
10. Bay, W. W., Gleiser, C. A., Dukes, T. W. and Brown, R. S. (1970). The experimental production and evaluation of drug-induced phototoxicity in swine. *Toxicol. appl. Pharmacol.* **17**, 538.
11. Sams, W. M. Jr and Epstein, J. H. (1967). The experimental production of drug phototoxicity in guinea pigs. I Using sunlight. *J. invest. Derm.* **48**, 89.

failed to elicit a phototoxic reaction in mouse flank skin,[1] and repeated attempts to induce sulphanilamide phototoxicity in mouse skin[2] were unsuccessful. However, both drugs could be shown to be phototoxic in the mouse tail test,[3] and sulphanilamide phototoxicity has been demonstrated in mouse flank skin using monochromatic radiation around 390 nm: shorter wavelengths around 300 nm produced doubtful reactions.[4] This result is surprising in view of the fact that sulphanilamide does not absorb at these longer wavelengths. Other drugs, such as griseofulvin, may induce a porphyria type of photosensitivity in mice through effects on the liver,[5,6] but there is no evidence of such a mechanism with sulphanilamide.

The characteristics of the skin reactions and the wavelengths for the phototoxic responses to CPZ have also been determined in mice. The vascular reaction varied with increasing exposure dose from a mild oedema, as detected with a plasma bound blue dye, through a marked erythema and stasis to ulceration: maximum oedema occurred within 4–6 h. Although neither histamine nor kinins appeared to be involved, some suppression of the reaction was obtained with ε-amino-caproic acid and soya bean trypsin inhibitor, as indication that plasmin or some protease system was involved. The action spectrum showed a broad peak around 330 nm with activity up to about 380 nm.[7] This wavelength dependency matched the studies using window glass, filtered sunlight, or "blacklight" in mice,[8] and similar sources with guinea-pigs.[9,10] The use of animals in studies of 8-MOP photosensitization is reviewed in the section on photochemotherapy (see page 2621).

Although CPZ may directly activate mammalian tyrosinase,[11] it is

1. Ramsay, C. A. and Obreshkova, E. (1974). Photosensitivity from nalidixic acid. *Br. J. Derm.* **91**, 523.
2. Blum, H. F. (1941). Studies of photosensitivity due to sulfanilamide. *J. invest. Derm.* **4**, 159.
3. Ljunggren, B. and Moller, H. (1978). Drug phototoxicity in mice. *Acta derm-venereol. (Stockholm)* **78**, 1.
4. Stratigos, J. D. and Magnus, I. A. (1968). Photosensitivity of demethylchlortetracycline and sulphanilamide. *Br. J. Derm.* **80**, 391.
5. DeMatteis, F. and Rimington, C. (1963). Disturbance of porphyrin metabolism caused by grizeofulvin in mice. *Br. J. Derm.* **75**, 91.
6. Konrad, K., Honigsmann, H., Gschnait, F. and Wolff, K. (1975). Mouse model for protoporphyria. II Cellular and subcellular events in the photosensitivity flare of the skin. *J. invest. Derm.* **65**, 300.
7. Hunter, J. A. A., Bhutani, L. K. and Magnus, I. A. (1970). Chlorpromazine photosensitivity in mice: its action spectrum and the effect of anti-inflammatory agents. *Br. J. Derm.* **82**, 157.
8. Ison, A. and Blank, H. (1967). Testing drug phototoxicity in mice. *J. invest. Derm.* **49**, 508.
9. Sams, W. M. Jr. (1966). Experimental production of drug phototoxicity in guinea pigs, using artificial light sources. *Archs Derm.* **94**, 773.
10. Sams, W. M. Jr. and Epstein, J. H. (1967). Experimental production of drug phototoxicity in guinea pigs, using sunlight. *J. invest Derm.* **48**, 89.
11. van Woert, M. H. (1972). Activation of tyrosinase by chlorpromazine. *In* 'Pigmentation: Its genesis and biologic control' (Ed. Riley, V.), p. 503. Apleton-Century-Crofts, New York.

doubtful whether this action is involved in the phototoxicity reactions. Melanin may bind CPZ,[1] and when the drug is present in tissues in high concentration, this binding occurs *in vivo*.[2,3] The abnormal pigmentation observed in exposed skin areas of patients treated with high doses of CPZ, 1 g or more per day, over a period of months, is probably related to this phenomenon rather than to increased melanogenesis alone.[4,5,6] However, there does appear to be an increase in melanin deposition in dermal macrophages in the skin of these patients[6] and the blue–purple colouration probably depends mainly on this dermal CPZ–melanin deposit. As with phototoxicity due to other agents, further studies are required to establish the cellular and tissue interactions involved in CPZ and other phenothiazine induced phototoxicity.

F. Nature of the Phototoxic Reactions

The phototoxic reactions of human skin vary depending on the drug or chemical involved. The all-embracing term "exaggerated sunburn" is therefore incorrect, and should only be used where there is a clear similarity of the type of reaction and its time course.

The reactions obtained with coal tar, pitch and associated compounds after contact with the skin and exposure to sunlight or UV-A have a distinct pathophysiology.[7,8] Either natural or experimental exposure leads to a burning sensation of the skin during exposure. If the exposure is limited, there may be no physical sign of photosensitization, but if it is continued the intensity of the burning (pitch smarts) increases and becomes painful. Erythema of the exposed area occurs and may be associated with a surrounding flare. With higher doses, a weal may be produced which subsides after an hour or so, the flare fading to leave an erythema restricted to the exposed site. With these higher exposure doses, the immediate erythema may fade slightly but then becomes more

1. Forest, I. S., Gutmann, F. and Keyser, H. (1966). *In vitro* interaction of chlorpromazine and melanin. *Agressologie* **7**, 147.
2. Greiner, A. C. and Berry, K. (1964). Skin pigmentation and corneal and lens opacities with prolonged chlorpromazine therapy. *Can. med. Ass. J.* **90**, 663.
3. Satanove, A. (1965). Pigmentation due to phenothiazines in high and prolonged dosage. *J. Am. med. Ass.* **191**, 263.
4. Zelickson, A. S. and Zeller, H. C. (1964). A new and unusual reaction to chlorpromazine. *J. Am. med. Ass.* **188**, 394.
5. Zelickson, A. S. (1966). Skin changes in chlorpromazine treatment. *J. Am. med. Ass.* **198**, 341.
6. Lever, W. F. and Schaumberg-Lever, G. (1975). *In* 'Histopathology of the Skin', 5th Ed., p. 241. J. B. Lippincott, Philadelphia.
7. Crow, K. D., Alexander, E., Buck, W. H. L., Johnson, B. E., Magnus, I. A. and Porter, A. D. (1961). Photosensitivity due to pitch. *Br. J. Derm.* **73**, 220.
8. Kaidbey, K. H. and Kligman, A. M. (1977). Clinical and histological study of coal tar phototoxicity in humans. *Archs Derm.* **113**, 592.

intense again, reaching a maximum at between 24 and 48 h. This delayed erythema then fades gradually to be replaced by hyperpigmentation which can be marked in individuals having a high level of natural pigmentation. With lower exposure or in dark complexioned individuals, the reactions are often restricted to an immediate erythema and delayed hyperpigmentation phases.

The oxygen dependent membrane damaging photosensitization effects of coal tar and its constituents, such as anthracene, which can be demonstrated *in vitro* at the cellular level, may be related to these phototoxic reactions in skin.[1] However, locating the cellular or sub-cellular sites of phototoxicity is much more difficult in the *in vivo* situations. The immediate erythema, flare, and wealing reactions can be abolished by restricting the circulation and thereby lowering the oxygen tension in the skin at the time of irradiation. These early reactions appear to be due to damage to plasma membranes rather than to cytoplasmic organelles. The immediate erythema and urticarial reactions might arise from mast cell damage and resulting histamine release,[2] and in some cases skin histamine depletion or antihistamine administration results in a decreased reaction.[3] However, in the majority of cases these procedures have no effect[4] and they never diminished the induced pain. It may be that there is involvement of the epidermal nerve endings in this immediate response along with direct damage to the vascular en-dothelium. The delayed phase of coal tar phototoxicity is also diminished by lowering the oxygen tension in the skin.[3] The histopathology of the reaction (Fig. 7) shows epidermal changes after 24 h ranging from intercellular oedema to degeneration of basal cells in the more severe reactions. By 48 h the architecture of the whole epidermis is disturbed but, although the majority of keratinocytes appear vacuolated, those in the more superficial layers become swollen and lose their characteristic staining properties.[3,5] The dermal changes consist of slight oedema with vasodilatation and a sparse infiltrate of mononuclear cells which decrease with time. The epidermal changes may reflect phototoxic damage to

1. Ito, T. (1978). Cellular and subcellular mechanisms of photodynamic action: the $^1O_2$ hypothesis as a driving force in recent research. *Photochem. Photobiol.* **28**, 493.

2. Allison, A. C., Magnus, I. A. and Young, M. R. (1966). Role of lysosomes and of cell membranes in photosensitization. *Nature* **209**, 874.

3. Kaidbey, K. H. and Kligman, A. M. (1977). Clinical and histological study of coal tar phototoxicity in humans. *Archs Derm.* **113**, 592.

4. Crow, K. D., Alexander, E., Buck, W. H. L., Johnson, B. E., Magnus, I. A. and Porter, A. D. (1961). Photosensitivity due to pitch. *Br. J. Derm.* **73**, 220.

5. Burckhardt, W. (1969). Photoallergy and phototoxicity due to drugs. *In* 'The Biologic Effects of Ultraviolet Radiation with emphasis on the skin' (Ed. Urbach, F.), p. 527. Pergamon Press, Oxford.

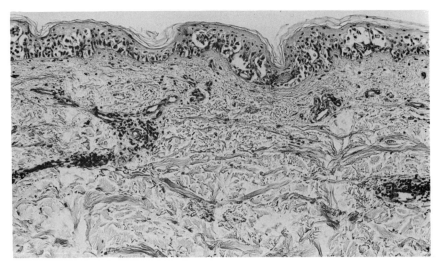

Fig. 7. Histopathology of a severe phototoxic reaction of the type produced by coal tar 24 h after exposure. Vacuolar degeneration of the basal and suprabasal layer cells in the epidermis gives rise to microvesicles but there is no evidence of apoptosis. The perivascular infiltrate is unremarkable. Compare with Fig. 10, the histopathology of typical photoallergic reaction.

keratinocyte lysosomes,[1] and the delayed erythema may result from the release of vaso-active agents from the damaged epidermis. Whether or not the hyperpigmentation is suppressed by arterial occlusion is not stated. This pigmentation, which is similar to that induced by psoralens, is a major complaint of the affected subjects.[2]

As well as the oxygen-dependent photosensitized damage to membranes, coal tar[3] and anthracene[4, 5] may form UV-A-induced covalent cross links in DNA. This covalent binding is considered to be responsible for the photosensitized inhibition of DNA synthesis demonstrated in mouse epidermis.[6] However, there is no evidence of inhibition of DNA

1. Allison, A. C., Magnus, I. A. and Young, M. R. (1966). Role of lysosomes and of cell membranes in photosensitization. *Nature* **203**, 874.
2. Foerster, H. R. and Schwartz, L. (1939). Industrial dermatitis and melanosis due to photosensitization. *Archs Derm. Syph.* **39**, 55.
3. Pathak, M. A. and Biswas, R. K. (1977). Skin photosensitization and DNA cross-linking ability of photochemotherapeutic agents. *J. invest. Derm.* **68**, 236.
4. Blackburn, G. M., Buckingham, J., Fenwick, R. G. *et al.* (1973). Photochemical binding of anthracene and other aromatic hydrocarbons to deoxyribonucleic acid with attendant loss of tritium. *J. chem. Soc. (Perkin I)* **1**, 2809.
5. Blackburn, G. M. and Taussig, P. E. (1975). The photocarcinogenicity of anthracene: photochemical binding to DNA in tissue culture. *Biochem. J.* **149**, 289.
6. Walter, J. F. and DeQuoy, P. R. (1978). Anthracene with near ultraviolet light inhibiting epidermal proliferation. *Archs Derm.* **114**, 1463.

synthesis in human skin photosensitized with either coal tar or anthracene, and it may require an exposure dose in excess of that which would be tolerated to show such an effect.[1]

The photo-reactions due to contact with the anthraquinone, disperse blue[2,3] and with the dyestuffs intermediate, benzanthrone,[4,5,6] appear to be identical with those induced by coal tar and its constituents.

A similar reaction pattern is observed in the photosensitivity associated with the manufacture of "UV-cured" inks where the phototoxic agent has been identified as a mixture of amyl-dimethylaminobenzoate isomers.[7] Although photosensitization does not occur following the topical application of methylene blue, eosin, or rose bengal on intact skin, a typical coal tar phototoxicity can be induced by these compounds if the skin is scarified before their application.[3] The same reactions can be induced by rose bengal after intradermal injection.[8,9] However, with rose bengal the delayed erythema response is not clearly defined and the resulting pigmentation, though present, may be less well marked. Since neither eosin nor rose bengal penetrate living cells, the phototoxic action of these dyes should be directed against the plasma membranes of the exposed cells.

A comparison of the cutaneous phototoxicity reactions obtained using these two dyes with those obtained with antiracene which is taken up into cells, might help to determine the relative importance of damage to various cellular compartments to the overall picture of this type of phototoxicity. A comparison between the effects of intravenous and intradermal administration of this type of photosensitizer may also be helpful in this respect.[10]

1. Parrish, J. A., Morison, W. L., Gonzalez, E., Krop, T., White, H. A. D. and Rosario, R. (1978). Therapy of psoriasis by tar photosensitization. *J. invest. Derm.* **70**, 111.
2. Gardiner, J. S., Dickson, A., MacLeod, T. M. and Frain-Bell, W. (1971). The investigation of photocontact dermatitis in a dye manufacturing process. *Br. J. Derm.* **85**, 264.
3. Kaidbey, K. H. and Kligman, A. M. (1978). Identification of topical photosensitizing agents in humans. *J. invest. Derm.* **70**, 149.
4. Trivedi, D. H. and Niyogi, A. K. (1968). Benzanthrone hazard in dye-factory. *Indian J. indust. Med.* **14**, 13.
5. Singh, G. B. (1970). Toxicity of dyes with special reference to benzanthrone. *Indian J. indust. Med.* **16**, 122.
6. Authors' personal observation.
7. Emmett, E. A., Taphorn, B. R. and Kominsky, J. R. (1977). Phototoxicity occurring during the manufacture of ultraviolet-cured ink. *Archs Derm.* **113**, 770.
8. Blum, H. F. (1964). 'Photodynamic action and diseases caused by light'. Hafner Publishing Co., New York.
9. Zaynoun, S. T., McVittie, E. and Hunter, J. A. A. (1977). Melanosomal pattern in phototoxic pigmentary responses induced by topical psoralens and other photosensitizers. *Clin. exp. Derm.* **2**, 243.
10. Allison, A. C., Magnus, I. A. and Young, M. R. (1966). Role of lysosomes and of cell membranes in photosensitization. *Nature* **209**, 874.

This type of phototoxic reaction appears to be the main manifestation of "photodynamic action" in the skin. The first descriptions, however, confused it with natural sunburn in addition to the phototoxic reaction.[1] The majority of more recent studies have avoided this confusion.

Drug induced phototoxicity reactions may be elicited in human skin by intradermal injections of the drug followed by exposure of the injection sites to the appropriate radiation,[2] and for screening purposes this method is more reliable than patch test procedures.[3]

IV. CLINICAL ASPECTS OF PHOTOTOXICITY

A. Furocoumarins

Phototoxicity caused by furocoumarins (psoralens)[4] is seen as a phyto-photodermatitis.[5] Klaber suggested this term for these reactions produced in skin by external contact with plants or plant materials followed by exposure to sunlight.[6]

Plants identified as producing phytophotodermatitis due to their content of photosensitizing psoralens are restricted to four families, the Umbelliferae, Rutaceae, Moraceae, and Leguminosae[7] (see Table 4). There are also some plants which are reported to evoke phytophotoder-matitis, but not through psoralen photosensitization, and these are shown in Table 5. The importance of UV-A in the production of the skin reactions was demonstrated in early investigations.[8, 9] Typically, the reactions are initiated by contact with the plant and exposure to sunlight. The response is seen first some 24 h later as erythema which may be

1. Blum, H. F. (1964). 'Photodynamic action and diseases caused by light'. Hafner Publishing Co., New York.
2. Kaidbey, K. H. and Kligman, A. M. (1978). Identification of systemic phototoxic drugs by human intradermal assay. *J. invest. Derm.* **70**, 272.
3. Kligman, A. M. and Breit, R. (1968). The identification of phototoxic drugs by human assay. *J. invest. Derm.* **51**, 90.
4. Musajo, L. and Rodighiero, G. (1962). The skin-photosensitizing furocoumarins. *Experentia* **18**, 153.
5. Pathak, M. A. (1974). Phytophotodermatitis. *In* 'Sunlight and Man' (Ed. Fitzpatrick, T. B.), p. 495. University of Tokyo Press, Tokyo.
6. Klaber, R. (1942). Phyto-photodermatitis. *Br. J. Derm.* **54**, 194.
7. Pathak, M. A., Daniels, F., Jr and Fitzpatrick, T. B. (1962). Presently known distribution of Furocoumarins (Psoralens) in plants. *J. invest. Derm.* **39**, 225.
8. Behcet, H., Ottenstein, B., Lion, K. and Dessauer, F. (1939). Les dermatiques des figues recherchés des influences chimiques, physiques et allergiques pouvant provoquer la dermatite des figues. *Ann. Dermatol. Syph* **10**, 32.
9. Jensen, T. and Hansen, K. J. (1939). Active spectral range for phytogenic photodermatitis produced by Pastinaca sativa (dermatitis bullosa striata pratensis, Oppenheim). *Archs Derm.* **40**, 566.

Table 4

Drug and chemical induced photosensitivity—phytophotodermatitis

Plants commonly reported to elicit phytophotodermatitis containing photoactive psoralens[1,2]

Order	Botanical name	Common name
Moraceae	*Ficus carica*	Fig
Umbelliferae	*Ammi majus*	Atrillal
	Angelica archangelica	Angelica
	Anethum graveolene	Dill
	Apium graveolens	Celery
	Daucus carota	Wilt carot
	Daucus sativa	Garden carrot
	Foeniculum vulgare	Fennel
	Heracleum gigantum	Garden parsnip
	Heracleum mantegazzianum	Giant hogweed
	Heracleum sphondylium	Cow parsnip
	Pastinaca sativa	Wild parsnip
	Peucedanum oreoselium	Parsley
	Peucedanum ostruthium	Masterwort
Rutaceae	*Citrus aurantifolia*	Lime
	Citrus aurantium	Lime
	Citrus bergamia	Bergamot lime
	Dictamnus alba	Gas plant
	Phebalium argenteum	Blister bush
	Ruta graveolens	Common rue
Leguminosae	*Psoralea coryfolia*	Bavachi

Table 5

Drug and chemical induced photosensitivity—phytophotodermatitis

Plants reported to evoke phytophotodermatitus but not through psoralen photosensitization[1,2]

Order	Botanical name	Common name
Compositae	*Achilles millefolium*	Yarrow
Ranunculaceae	*Ranunculas* species	Buttercup
Cruciferae	*Brassica* species	Mustard
Convolvulaceae	*Convolvulus arvensis*	Bind weed
Rosaceae	*Agrimony eupatoria*	Agrimony
Chenopediaceae	*Chenopedium* species	Goose foot
Hypericaceae	*Hypericum perforatum*	Saint John's wort

1. Based on table in Pathak, M. A., Fitzpatrick, T. B. and Daniels, F., Jr. (1962). Presently known distribution of furocoumarins (Psoralens) in plants. *J. invest. Derm.* **39**, 225.
2. The reader is advised to consult the text, 'Botanical Dermatology' by Mitchell, J. and Rook, A., Greengrass Ltd, Vancouver, B.C., 1979.

painful, distributed in a pattern clearly related to the contact with the plant. Bullae develop during the next 24 h and then may coalesce to produce a bizarre pattern (Fig. 8). These subside quite quickly and where there is minimal residual damage the reaction develops as an intense hyperpigmentation which may persist for months. When there is more severe damage, a single phototoxic episode may give rise to pigmentary changes which persist for a long time.[1] The intensity of the erythema and the extent of the blistering depend on the intensity of solar exposure. When this is minimal, only erythema occurs and this may take 72 h or more to develop followed by hyperpigmentation. However, pigmentation may develop without any preceding erythema.

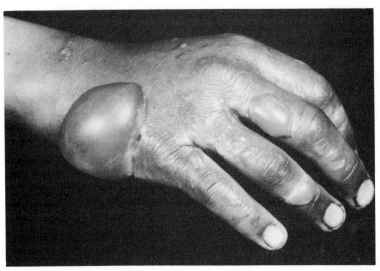

Fig. 8. A severe example of phytophotodermatitis. This is not the typical "Dermatitis bullosa striata pratensis" of Oppenheim but it is a common presentation after contact with *Heracleum mantegazzianum*, the Giant Hogweed, as a plaything.

Another form of psoralen phototoxicity is known as berlock dermatitis,[2] first described by Freund in 1916 as a transient erythema rapidly followed by hyperpigmentation on skin sites to which eau de cologne had been applied prior to sun exposure 24 h or more earlier.[3]

1. Jain, S. R. (1969). Investigations on the essential oil of heracleum mantegazzianum. *Planta Med.* **17**, 230.
2. Harber, L. C., Harris, H., Leider, M. and Baer, R. L. (1964). Berloque dermatitis. A technique for its deliberate reproduction. *Archs Derm.* **90**, 572.
3. Freund, E. (1976). Über bischer noch nicht beschriebene kunstliche Hautverfarbungen. *Derm. Wschr.* **63**, 931.

This is now a recognized photosensitivity reaction associated with perfumed materials containing bergamot oil.[1, 2, 3] This extract from the Bergamot Lime (*Citrus bergamia*) contains an active ingredient, bergapten, which is 5-methoxypsoralen. When the perfume has a high bergamot oil content and the skin exposed to intense sunlight, the skin reactions may be equally severe as those seen in phytophotodermatitis.[4] Usually, however, the reaction is a mild erythema followed by an intense hyperpigmentation in a distribution depending on the sites of application of the perfumed material.[3]

Studies of both 8-methoxypsoralen and bergamot oil phototoxicity have shown that a number of factors may influence the reactions obtained. Hydration of the skin may result in an increased intensity,[5, 6, 7] as it does in the case of UV-erythema.[8] The interval between applying the photosensitizer and exposure of the skin to radiation is important and maximal photosensitization with bergamot oil or 8-methoxypsoralen is obtained when this interval is between 1 and 2 h.[9, 10] The nature of the vehicle has an effect on this interval; for example, when ethanol is used as the vehicle phototoxicity may be elicited after longer periods than with paraffin molle flavin.[10]

The cellular mechanisms involved in these forms of psoralen phototoxicity are mediated through covalent binding to DNA. The major effect is on the epidermis and with moderate reactions the histological picture is similar to that of ordinary sunburn but with a slight delay in the appearance of the "sunburn cells". Increases in exposure result in increased numbers of these cells and in disintegration of the

1. Marzulli, F. N. and Maibach. H. I. (1970). Perfume phototoxicity. *J. Soc. cosmet. Chem.* **21**, 695.
2. Zaynoun, S. T., Johnson, B. E. and Frain-Bell, W. (1977). A study of oil of bergamot and its importance as a phototoxic agent. I. Characterisation and quantification of the photoactive component. *Br. J. Derm.* **96**, 475.
3. Zaynoun, S. T. (1978). The quantitative analysis of bergapten in perfumes. *J. Soc. cosmet. Chem.* **29**, 247.
4. Burdick, K. H. (1966). Phototoxicity of Shalimar perfume. *Archs Derm.* **93**, 425.
5. Harber, L. C. and Baer, R. L. (1965). Effect of humidity on the photosensitive response to 8-methoxypsoralen. *J. invest. Derm.* **44**, 61.
6. Levine, G. M. and Harber, L. C. (1969). The effect of humidity on the phototoxic response to 8-MOP in guinea pigs. *Acta derm-venereol. (Stockholm).* **49**, 82.
7. Zaynoun, S. T., Johnson, B. E. and Frain-Bell, W. (1977). A study of oil of bergamot and its importance as a phototoxic agent. II. Factors which affect the phototoxic reaction induced by bergamot oil and psoralen derivatives. *Contact Dermatol.* **3**, 225.
8. Cattano, A. N. (1970). Photosensitivity following treatment with occlusive dressings. *Archs Derm.* **102**, 276.
9. Arora, S. K. and Willis, I. (1976). Factors influencing methoxsalen phototoxicity in vitiliginous skin. *Archs Derm.* **112**, 327.
10. Zaynoun, S. T., Johnson, B. E. and Frain-Bell, W. (1977). A study of oil of bergamot and its importance as a phototoxic agent. II. Factors which affect the phototoxic reaction induced by bergamot oil and psoralen derivatives. *Contact Dermatol.* **3**, 276.

prickle cells. The bullae are therefore intraepidermal, but in severe cases the basal layer may also be involved and the blisters are subepidermal.

The increase in pigmentation observed in these reactions appears to depend not only on the activation of melanogenesis but also on an increase in the size of the melanosomes transferred to the keratinocytes.[1] Although the complete change from the small, multiple melanosome pattern of caucasoids to the large single melanosome pattern of negroids, as was originally postulated,[2] does not occur: there is an increase in numbers of these large melanosomes in the keratinocytes.[3, 4] Whether there is an increase in melanocyte population due to psoralen photo-toxicity is not clearly established.[5] However, earlier investigations with psoralens and sunlight for the treatment of vitiligo indicated that, although there was not a numerical increase of melanocytes, nevertheless their DOPA reactivity did increase.[6]

Phototoxic reactions have been induced experimentally in skin with α-terthienyl, but the role of this thiophene and polacetylenes contained in plants of the Compositae family[7] in human phototoxic reactions is uncertain. Where such reactions have been reported they appear to be similar to those with coal tar.

The erythema produced in sun-exposed areas of patients with solar keratoses treated with topical 5-fluorouracil appears to be a form of phototoxicity, but the mechanisms involved remain obscure.[8]

B. Tetracyclines

Photosensitivity reactions obtained with the tetracycline group of drugs were mainly due to demethylchlortetracycline (DMCT) and were

1. Pathak, M. A., Jimbow, K., Parrish, J. A. Kaidbey, K. M., Kligman, A. M. and Fitzpatrick, T. B. (1976). Effect of UV-A, UV-B and psoralen on *in vivo* human melanin pigmentation. *In* 'Pigment Cell' (Ed. Riley, V.), Vol. 3, p. 291. S. Karger, Basel.
2. Toda, K., Pathak, M. A., Parrish, J. A., Fitzpatrick, T. B. and Quevedo, W. C., Jr. (1972). Alterations of racial differences in melanosomes distribution in human epidermis after exposure to ultraviolet light. *Nature New Biol.* **236**, 143.
3. Konrad, K. and Wolff, K. (1973). Hyperpigmentation, melanosome size and distribution patterns of melanosomes. *Archs Derm.* **107**, 853.
4. Zaynoun, S. T., McVittie, E. and Hunter, J. A. A. (1977). Melanosomal pattern in phototoxic pigmentary responses induced by topical psoralens and other photosensitizers. *Clin. exp. Derm.* **2**, 243.
5. Rosdahl, I. K. and Swanbeck, G. (1980). Effects of PUVA on the epidermal melanocyte population in psoriatic patients. *Acta derm-venereol. (Stockholm)* **60**, 21.
6. Jarrett, A. and Szabo, G. (1956). The pathological varieties of vitiligo and their response to treatment with melidinine. *Br. J. Derm.* **68**, 313.
7. Towers, G. H. N. (1980). Photosensitizers from plants and their photodynamic action. *Prog. Phytochem.* **6**, 183.
8. Dillaha, C. J., Jansen, G. T., Honeycutt, W. M. and Bradford, A. C. (1963). Selective cytotoxic effect of topical 5-fluorouracil. *Archs Derm.* **88**, 247.

generally described as exaggerated sunburn.[1, 2, 3] This was clearly demonstrated in normal subjects receiving oral DMCT (600 mg per day) and exposed to natural sunlight[4, 5] or the emission from a carbon arc source.[4] An erythema with oedema developed more rapidly than a normal sunburn, was of greater intensity, and persisted longer. Tetracycline itself did not produce these reactions.

Although the majority of phototoxic reactions associated with the tetracycline group is due to DMCT, similar reactions are observed with other members, in particular chlortetracycline (CT)[5] and doxycycline.[6, 7] A survey of tetracycline phototoxicity in Japan and other countries indicates that they were mainly reactions due to DMCT, and rarely to CT and doxycycline. Also reactions to metacycline, minocycline and oxytetracycline were very rarely seen.[8] Apart from the exaggerated sunburn and photoonycholysis, phototoxicity induced by DMCT may present as a lichenoid reaction, developing 10–20 days after the exposure and persisting for about 2 months.[9, 10] In addition, with high doses of tetracycline itself, followed by exposure to strong sunlight, reactions are observed which resemble those of porphyria cutanea tarda.[11]

The histological picture of DMCT induced phototoxicity in human skin shows mild oedema, vasodilatation and a minimal cellular infiltrate in the dermis. While changes in the architecture of the epidermis are present with vacuolation and homogenization of the suprabasal layers, the damage is mild compared to that obtained with topical applications of photosensitizers.[12]

1. Morris, W. E. (1960). Photosensitivity due to tetracycline derivative. *J. Am. med. Ass.* **172**, 121.
2. Falk, M. (1960). Light sensitivity due to demethylchlortetracycline. *J. Am. med. Ass.* **172**, 122.
3. Fuhrman, D. L. and Brown, B. W. (1960). Demethylchlortetracycline, American Medical Association. *Arch. Derm.* **82**, 244.
4. Harber, L. C., Tromovitch, T. A. and Baer, R. L. (1961). Studies on photosensitivity due to demethylchlortetracycline. *J. Invest. Derm.* **37**, 189.
5. Blank, H., Cullen, S. I. and Catalano, P. M. (1968). Photosensitivity studies with de-methylchlortetracycline and doxycycline. *Archs Derm.* **97**, 1.
6. Verhagen, H. (1965). Photosensitivity due to chlortetracycline. *Dermatologica* **130**, 439.
7. Frost, P., Weinstein, G. D. and Gomez, E. C. (1972). Phototoxic potential of minocycline and doxycycline. *Archs Derm.* **105**, 681.
8. Tanioku, K. and Ono, K. (1974). Phototoxic and photoallergic problems in Japan. In 'Sunlight and Man' (Ed. Fitzpatrick, T. B.), p. 483. University of Tokyo Press, Tokyo.
9. Jones, H. E. *et al.* (1972). Photosensitive lichenoid eruption with demeclocycline. *Archs Derm.* **106**, 58.
10. Maibach, H. I., Epstein, J. H. and Sams, W. M., Jr. (1974). Letter: Photosensitive lichenoid eruption associated with demeclocycline. *Archs Derm.* **109**, 97.
11. Epstein, J. H. *et al.* (1978). Porphyria-like cutaneous changes induced by tetracycline hydrochloride photosensitization. *Archs Derm.* **112**, 661.
12. Epstein, J. H. (1974). Phototoxicity and photoallergy: clinical syndromes. In 'Sunlight and Man' (Ed. Fitzpatrick, T. B.), p. 459. University of Tokyo Press, Tokyo.

The wavelength responsible for the reaction to DMCT appears somewhat confused. One early study suggested that the sunburning wavelengths were responsible because a window glass filter abolished the response.[1] However, it also reported that in some subjects the response could still be obtained with this filter. Using a mylar filter to cut off the sunburning wavelengths below 310 nm, it is possible to clearly differentiate the phototoxic reaction induced by DMCT from normal sunburn.[2] Artificial sources of UV-B failed to produce the reaction, and it would seem that the results obtained by Stratigos and Magnus[3] for mouse DMCT phototoxicity also apply to humans.[4] Onocholysis, a relatively common finding with photosensitivity to DMCT,[1, 5, 6] is observed some 3–6 weeks after the phototoxic reaction. It is unlikely that wavelengths below 320 nm would penetrate the nail, but the longer wavelength UV-A may well act directly on the nail bed.[3]

The mechanisms involved in DMCT phototoxicity in the skin have not been defined. Cells in culture are killed[7, 8] and, although there is no evidence of phototoxicity with the *Candida* test,[9] membrane damage through an oxygen dependent, free radical mechanism is indicated by photohaemolysis studies.[10, 11] The sunburn type of reaction may result from this kind of damage but the lichenoid reaction is not easily explained: it may be on a special type of skin reactivity in certain persons.

1. Orentreich, N., Harber, L. C. and Tromovitch, T. A. (1961). Photosensitivity and photo-onycholysis due to demethylchlortetracycline. *Am. med. Ass. Archs Derm.* **83**, 730.

2. Maibach, H. I., Sams, W. M. and Epstein, J. H. (1967). Screening for drug toxicity by wavelengths greater than 3100 Å. *Archs Derm.* **95**, 12.

3. Stratigos, J. D. and Magnus, I. A. (1968). Photosensitivity by demethylchlortetracycline and sulphanilamide. *Br. J. Derm.* **80**, 391.

4. Ramsay, C. A. (1977). Longwave ultraviolet radiation sensitivity induced by oxytetracycline: a case report. *Clin. exp. Derm.* **2**, 255.

5. Segal, B. M. (1963). Photosensitivity, nail discolouration, and onycholysis. *Archs intern. Med.* **112**, 165.

6. Frank, S. B., Cohen, H. J. and Minkin, W. (1971). Photo-onycholysis due to tetracycline hydrochloride and doxycycline. *Archs Derm.* **103**, 520.

7. Freeman, R. G., Murtishaw, W. and Knox, J. M. (1970). Tissue culture techniques in the study of cell photobiology and phototoxicity. *J. invest. Derm.* **54**, 164.

8. Chang, T. W. and Weinstein, L. (1964). Photosensitization of human cell cultures by demethylchlortetracycline. *Proc. Soc. exp. Biol. Med.* **116**, 509.

9. Daniels, F. (1965). A simple microbiological method for demonstrating phototoxic compounds. *J. invest. Derm.* **44**, 259.

10. Schothorst, A. A. and Suurmond, D. (1977). The role of oxygen in the photodamaging effect of erythrocytes of some photoallergic and phototoxic compounds. *Acta derm-venereol. (Stockholm)* **57**, 127.

11. Nilsson, R., Swanbeck, G. and Wennersten, G. (1975). Primary mechanisms of erythrocyte photolysis induced by biological sensitizers and phototoxic drugs. *Photochem. Photobiol.* **22**, 183.

C. Phenothiazines

Phototoxicity is part of the complex pattern of skin reactions to the phenothiazines in general and to chlorpromazine in particular.[1, 2, 3] Phototoxic reactions in human skin due to phenothiazine itself were described in 1940 as sunburn, chemical burning or "dermatitis".[4] Regular reports followed in the veterinary literature of photosensitivity reactions of the eyes and skin of stock animals, and even pheasants treated with phenothiazine as a pesticide.[5]

Chlorpromazine-induced phototoxicity in human skin was first clearly defined by Schulz, Wiskemann and Wulf in 1956, using photopatch test techniques and xenon arc irradiation.[6] The reaction obtained in this and other studies appears to qualify it as of the "exaggerated sunburn" type, but an intense erythema with oedema and itching may develop during exposure to strong sunlight.[7, 8, 9] An early reaction may be obtained with experimental phototesting. With patch test procedures, an early discolouration of the skin is produced in the exposed area, erythema appearing in 30 min.[9] With intradermal injections of high concentrations of the drug, an immediate phototoxic weal is produced,[10] but the burning sensation associated with dyes and coal tar does not appear to play a part in this reaction.

Although Schulz and his colleagues demonstrated the effectiveness of long wavelength UVR in the phototoxicity due to CPZ,[6] other investigators suggested that only the "sunburn wavelengths" were

1. Mullins, J. F., Cohen, I. M. and Farrington, E. S. (1956). Cutaneous sensitivity reactions to chlorpromazine. *J. Am. med. Ass.* **162**, 946.
2. Calnan, C. D. (1958). Studies in contact dermatitis: V Photosensitivity from chlorpromazine. *Trans. St John's Hosp. dermatol. Soc.* **48**, 26.
3. Calnan, C. D., Frain-Bell, W. and Cuthbert, J. W. (1961). Occupational dermatitis from chlorpromazine. *Trans. St John's Hosp. dermatol. Soc.* **46**, 48.
4. DeEds, F., Wilson, R. H. and Thomas, J. O. (1940). Photosensitization by phenothiazine. *J. Am. med. Ass.* **114**, 2095.
5. Enzie, F. D. and Whitmore, G. E. (1953). Photosensitization keratitis in young goats following treatment with phenothiazine. *J. Am. vet. Ass. Sept. 1953*, p. 237.
6. Schulz, K. H., Wiskemann, A. and Wulf, K. (1956). Klinische und experimentelle Untersuchungen über die photodynamische Wirksamkeit von Phenothiazinderivaten, insbesondere von Megaphen. *Arch. klin. exp. Derm.* **202**, 285.
7. Epstein, J. H., Brunsting, L. A., Petersen, M. C. and Schwarz, B. E. (1957). A study of photosensitivity occurring with chlorpromazine therapy. *J. invest. Derm.* **28**, 329.
8. Cahn, M. M. and Levy, E. J. (1957). Ultraviolet light factor in chlorpromazine dermatitis. *Archs Derm.* **75**, 38.
9. Epstein, S. (1968). Chlorpromazine photosensitivity. *Archs Derm.* **98**, 354.
10. Horio, M. (1975). Chlorpromazine photoallergy: co-existence of immediate and delayed type. *Archs Derm.* **111**, 1469.

involved. More recent investigations have confirmed the major part played by UV-A in this reaction in man.[1, 2] There is little reason to suppose that the action spectrum varies greatly from that obtained in mice, which extends from 320–380 nm with a broad peak of activity centred around 330. There is no evidence that CPZ produces an intensification of the normal sunburn reaction with wavelengths below 320 nm.[3]

The acute phototoxic reactions obtained in patients on high dose CPZ or other phenothiazines are probably due to the photosensitizing properties of metabolites rather than to those of the parent compounds.[4, 5] However, the cellular reactions involved probably differ little from those obtained with CPZ *in vitro*. If the photosensitized interactions between CPZ and DNA are relevant to cutaneous phototoxicity, it should be possible to demonstrate an inhibition of epidermal DNA synthesis as in the case of psoralens. However, in one comparative study of these reactions in mouse skin, CPZ was without effect.[6] Moreover, the photosensitized killing of *E. coli* involves neither DNA damage[7] nor excited singlet oxygen.[8] Although further investigations are necessary, it would appear that the phototoxic effects of CPZ are directed against cell membranes: probably the plasma membrane rather than those of the intracellular organelles.[8] An oxygen dependent photosensitized damage to liposome membranes appeared in one study to parallel the photo-toxicity of the various phenothiazines in mouse skin.[9] Other workers,

1. Kligman, A. M. and Breit, R. (1968). The identification of phototoxic drugs by human assay. *J. invest. Derm.* **51**, 90.
2. Kaidbey, K. H. and Kligman, A. M. (1978). Identification of topical photosensitizing agents in humans. *J. invest. Derm.* **70**, 149.
3. Hunter, J. A. A., Bhutani, L. K. and Magnus, I. A. (1970). Chlorpromazine photosensitivity in mice: its action spectrum and the effect of anti-inflammatory agents. *Br. J. Derm.* **82**, 157.
4. Ljunggren, B. and Moller, H. (1977). Phenothiazine phototoxicity: an experimental study on chlorpromazine and its metabolites. *J. invest. Derm.* **68**, 313.
5. Ljunggren, B. and Moller, H. (1977). Phenothiazine phototoxicity: an experimental study on chlorpromazine and related tricyclic drugs. *Acta derm-venereol. (Stockholm)* **57**, 325.
6. Walter, J. F. and DeQuoy, P. R. (1978). Anthracene with near ultraviolet light inhibiting epidermal proliferation. *Archs Derm.* **114**, 1463.
7. Matsuo, I., Ohkido, M., Fujita, H. and Suzuki, K. (1980). Chlorpromazine photosensitization II. Failure to detect any evidence for involvement of DNA damage in the photodynamic killing of *Escherichia coli* in the presence of chlorpromazine. *Photochem. Photobiol.* **31**, 175.
8. Rosenthal, I., Ben-Hur, E., Prager, A. and Riklis, E. (1978). Photochemical reactions of chlorpromazine; chemical and biochemical implications. *Photochem. Photobiol.* **28**, 591.
9. Copeland, E. S., Alving, C. R. and Grenan, M. M. (1976). Light-induced leakage of spin label marker from liposomes in the presence of phototoxic phenothiazines. *Photochem. Photobiol.* **24**, 41.

however, found different relative phototoxic potentials of phenothiazine compounds.[1,2]

It is not known whether CPZ phototoxicity in human or animal skin is oxygen dependent. If it is not, the toxic photoproduct demonstrated by UV-irradiation of CPZ *in vitro* may be an important factor in the clinical phototoxicity. In support of this, the intradermal injection of irradiated CPZ in mice[3] and in guinea-pigs[4] produced reactions similar to those obtained with more conventional phototesting procedures. The membrane damaging effect obtained in these experiments would be through a detergent-like action rather than the primary structural alteration that occurs with oxygen dependent photosensitization.[5] The photoproduct has not been identified, but it is probably a CPZ dimer rather than promazine, 2,hydroxypromazine, or CPZ sulphoxide, which are the identified photoproducts of CPZ.[5]

The CPZ photosensitized release of histamine from rat peritoneal mast cells[6] and guinea-pig skin[7] *in vitro* indicates possible mast cell damage with histamine release. However, there is no histamine involvement in mouse skin CPZ phototoxicity,[8] neither is there any evidence for such an action in human skin.

D. Nalidixic Acid Photosensitivity

Cutaneous photosensitivity reactions associated with nalidixic acid, an antibacterial agent used in the treatment of urinary tract infection, take the form of bullae, varying in size from a millimetre to several centimetres in diameter. The blisters are usually tense and have a sharply demarcated erythema at their base. They may be painful or pruritic but usually heal without scarring, leaving varying degrees of post-inflammatory hyper-

1. Schulz, K. H., Wiskemann, A. and Wulf, K. (1956). Klinische und experimentelle Untersuchungen über die photodynamische Wirksamkeit von Phenothiazinderivaten, insbesondere von Megaphen. *Arch. klin. exp. Derm.* **202**, 285.
2. Ljunggren, B. and Moller, H. (1977). Phenothiazine phototoxicity: an experimental study on chlorpromazine and related tricyclic drugs. *Acta derm-venereol. (Stockholm)* **57**, 325.
3. Johnson, B. E. (1974). Cellular mechanisms of chlorpromazine photosensitivity. *Proc. R. Soc. Med.* **67**, 871.
4. Ljunggren, B. (1977). Phenothiazine phototoxicity: toxic chlorpromazine photoproducts. *J. invest. Derm.* **69**, 383.
5. Kochevar, I. E. and Lamola, A. A. (1979). Chlorpromazine and protriptyline phototoxicity: photosensitized, oxygen independent red cell hemolysis. *Photochem. Photobiol.* **29**, 791.
6. Frisk-Holmberg, M. (1971). On the mechanism of chlorpromazine-induced histamine release from rat mast cells. *Acta physiol. scand.* **83**, 412.
7. Lanb, S. K. and Tomlinson, D. R. (1976). Chlorpromazine-induced histamine release from guinea pig skin *in vitro* and photosensitive reaction. *Archs derm. Res.* **225**, 219.
8. Hunter, J. A. A., Bhutani, L. K. and Magnus, I. A. (1970). Chlorpromazine photosensitivity in mice: its action spectrum and the effect of anti-inflammatory agents. *Br. J. Derm.* **82**, 15.

pigmentation. They develop in exposed areas, favouring the dorsal surfaces of hands and feet but also occurring on the lower legs and face after periods of treatment which may vary from a few days up to a year or more, and follow an exposure to intense sunlight. A preponderance of females in the reported cases is probably due to the prescribing pattern of the drug rather than any sex difference in response. The variation in time for the development of lesions depends on the chance of exposure to the required intensity of sunlight. The photosensitivity appears to persist in that new lesions may develop on exposure 2 or 3 months after the drug has been withdrawn. Also, as with porphyria cutanea tarda, it has been suggested that trauma may give rise to some of these lesions.[1, 2, 3, 4, 5, 6] The reaction on facial skin may be limited to an erythema.[5]

Histological examination shows separation at the dermo–epidermal junction. Early damage to the epidermis is minimal, but there may be some basophilic degeneration of the collagen in the superficial dermis and a mild perivascular lymphohistiocytic infiltrate.[5] There is no evidence of perivascular deposits of PAS-positive material, as is found in the porphyrias.

The results of phototesting in patients have been variable. In some all reactions were negative.[3] In others there was an increased sensitivity to the sunburn wavelengths,[5, 7] and abnormal responses to UV-A and even visible radiation have been reported.[8, 9] Bullae have been elicited by phototesting with both UV-B and UV-A,[5] but the majority of positive reactions were limited to an erythema. Monochromator testing was difficult to interpret, but there was evidence of abnormal sensitivity to 320 and 340 nm radiation.[4] Photopatch tests have been consistently negative in both patients and normal controls. However, phototoxic reactions to UV-A are consistently induced in the mouse tail test after oral administration of both nalidixic acid and its main metabolite, 7-

1. Zelickson, A. S. (1964). Phototoxic reaction with nalidixic acid. *J. Am. med. Ass.* **190**, 556.
2. Burry, J. N. and Crosby, R. W. L. (1966). A case of phototoxicity due to nalidixic acid. *Med. J. Aust.* **2**, 698.
3. Baes, H. (1968). Photosensitivity caused by nalidixic acid. *Dermatologica* **136**, 61.
4. Ramsay, C. A. and Obreshkova, E. (1974). Photosensitivity from nalidixic acid. *Br. J. Derm.* **91**, 523.
5. Brauner, G. J. (1975). Bullous photoreaction to nalidixic acid. *Am. J. Med.* **58**, 576.
6. Burry, J. N. (1974). Persistent phototoxicity due to nalidixic acid. *Archs Derm.* **109**, 263.
7. Birkett, D. A., Garretts, M. and Stevenson, C. J. (1968). Phototoxic bullous eruptions due to nalidixic acid. *Br. J. Derm.* **81**, 342.
8. Haven, E. and Eerts, J. (1967). Lichtovergewoenlichend Verodtzaakt de Halidixin Zuur. *Arch. Belg. Derm. Syth.* **23**, 421.
9. Brehm, G. and Korting, G. W. (1970). Bullöse Hautreaktion auf Nalidixinsäurer. *Med. Welt.* **11**, 423.

hydroxynalidixic acid.[1] Also intradermal injections of nalidixic acid in humans gave consistently positive reactions to UV-A.[2] The absorption spectrum of nalidixic acid shows a broad absorption between 320 and 340 nm, and it is this absorption which is related to the phototoxicity reactions (Fig. 9).

The mechanisms involved in this type of drug-induced photosensitivity are not known. Before the unequivocal demonstration of phototoxicity by intradermal injections, the failure to obtain a reaction in normal subjects,

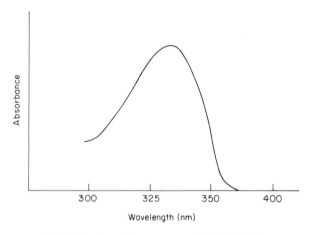

Fig. 9. The absorption spectrum of Nalidixic Acid.

the long period of drug taking before the development of reactions, and the continuation of skin reactivity after cessation of drug administration were taken to be indications of a photoallergic mechanism. However, because the drug is patently phototoxic and also because there is no evidence of immunologic involvement, the reactions are now considered to be phototoxic. Also attempts to demonstrate an associated lymphocyte transformation for this drug have failed.[3]

The formation of bullae and increased skin fragility in nalidixic acid phototoxicity are similar to those seen in porphyria cutanea tarda, but

1. Ljunggren, B. and Moller, H. (1978). Drug phototoxicity in mice. *Acta derm-venereol. (Stockholm)* **58**, 1.
2. Kaidbey, K. H. and Kligman, A. M. (1978). Identification of systemic phototoxic drugs by human intradermal assay. *J. invest. Derm.* **70**, 272.
3. Alexander, S. and Forman, L. (1971). Which of the drugs cause the rash? Or the value of the lymphocyte transformation test in eruptions caused by nalidixic acid. *Br. J. Derm.* **84**, 429.

there is no evidence of abnormal porphyrin metabolism in these patients.[1, 2] Phototoxicity has been demonstrated at the cellular level with *C. albicans*,[3] but the present author has found only minimal photo-haemolysis with both nalidixic acid and hydroxynalidixic acid. The cellular mechanisms here may, therefore, be similar to those due to the more water soluble porphyrins, and this is reflected in the similar appearance of the resulting reactions

E. Frusemide

Blisters similar to those with nalidixic acid may develop in the exposed skin of patients on high doses of the diuretic, frusemide.[4] It is thought that these are also phototoxic blisters.[5, 6] These reactions have been associated with haemodialysis, but in the cases reported there always appears to be a high dose frusemide.[6, 7] Phototests in some patients failed to produce evidence of abnormal photosensitivity, but the phototesting procedure may not have used appropriate exposures or wavelengths. Sunlight does appear to be involved and the cases are mainly patients with renal failure or other conditions which could lead to high blood concentrations of the drug.[8] Positive phototest reactions are obtained after intradermal injections but the quantity of drug required (1 mg to produce 100% positive reactions) is very high.[9] The causative wavelengths were demonstrated to be in the UV-A ranges.

In most patients on dialysis with these lesions, no porphyric abnormality is present and the skin changes are attributed to frusemide induced phototoxicity.[5, 6, 7, 8] Rarely, renal failure causes increased plasma por-

1. Birkett, D. A., Garretts, M. and Stevenson, C. J. (1968). Phototoxic bullous eruptions due to nalidixic acid. *Br. J. Derm.* **81**, 342.
2. Ramsay, C. A. and Obreshkova, E. (1974). Photosensitivity from nalidixic acid. *Br. J. Derm.* **91**, 523.
3. Louis, P., Wiskemann, A. and Schulz, K. H. (1973). Bullose Photodermatitis durch Nalidixin-saure. *Haitarzt* **24**, 445.
4. Ebringer, A., Adam, W. R. and Parkin, J. D. (1969). Bullous haemorrhagic eruption associated with frusemide. *Med. J. Aust.* **1**, 763.
5. Burry, J. B. and Lawrence, J. R. (1976). Phototoxic blisters from high frusemide dosage. *Br. J. Derm.* **94**, 495.
6. Kennedy, A. C. and Lyell, A. (1976). Acquired epidermolysis bullosa due to high dose frusemide. *Br. Med. J.* **1**(6024), 1509.
7. Keczkes, K. and Karr, M. J. (1976). Bullous dermatosis of chronic renal failure. *Br. J. Derm.* **95**, 541.
8. Rotstein, H. (1978). Photosensitive bullous eruption associated with chronic renal failure. *Aust. J. Derm.* **19**, 58.
9. Kaidbey, K. H. and Kligman, A. M. (1978). Identification of systemic phototoxic drugs by human intradermal assay. *J. invest Derm.* **70**, 272.

phyrin levels,[1] and in these cases the bullae may represent lesions associated with this form of porphyria cutanea tarda acquisita.

F. Other Drugs Causing Phototoxic Reactions

Phototoxic skin reactions to other drugs such as chlorthiazide, griseofulvin, chlordiazepoxide and quinidine may be induced experimentally.[2,3,4,5] Reactions similar to those attributed to phototoxicity with CPZ and DMCT have been observed in patients treated with chlorthiazide,[6,7] griseofulvin,[8] chlordiazepoxide[9] and possibly quinidine[10] as part of the pattern of their side-effects.[11] Photosensitivity due to the cyclamate artificial sweeteners may also be phototoxic.[12,13]

Similar phototoxic reactions have been reported following the use of oral contraceptives,[14,15,16] but the major problem here appears to be an increased response of the melanocyte system to sunlight due to the

1. Poh-Fitzpatrick, M. P., Bellet, N., DeLeo, V. B., Grossman, M. E. and Harber, L. C. (1978). Porphyria Cutanea Tarda in two patients treated with hemodialysis for chronic renal failure. *New Engl. J. Med.* **299**, 292.
2. Kligman, A. M. and Breit, R. (1968). The identification of phototoxic drugs by human assay. *J. invest. Derm.* **51**, 90.
3. Ison, A. E. and Davis, C. M. (1969). Phototoxicity of quinoline methanols and other drugs in mice and yeast. *J. invest. Derm.* **52**, 193.
4. Ljunggren, B. and Moller, H. (1978). Drug phototoxicity in mice. *Acta derma-venereol. (Stockholm)* **58**, 1.
5. Kaidbey, K. H. and Kligman, A. M. (1978). Identification of systemic phototoxic drugs by human intradermal assay. *J. invest. derm.* **70**, 272.
6. Norins, A. L. (1959). Chlorothiazide drug eruption involving photosensitization. *Archs Derm.* **79**, 592.
7. Harber, L. C., Lashinsky, A. M. and Baer, R. L. (1959). Photosensitivity due to chlorothiazide and hydrochlorothiazide. *New Engl. J. Med.* **261**, 1378.
8. Chang, T. W. (1965). Cold urticaria and photosensitivity due to griesofulvin. *J. Am. med. Ass.* **193**, 848.
9. Luton, F. E. and Finchum, R. N. (1965). Photosensitivity reaction to chlordiazepoxide. *Archs Derm.* **86**, 58.
10. Widmer, O., Zurcher, K. and Krebs, A. (1976). Hautnebenwirkungen interner Arzneimittel. IV. C. Medikamentose Lichtempfindlichkeit (Photosensibilitat). *Dermatologica* **152**, 216.
11. Parrish, J. A., White, H. A. D. and Pathak, M. A. (1979). Photomedicine. *In* 'Dermatology in General Medicine', 2nd edition (Eds Fitzpatrick, T. B., Eisen, A. Z., Wolff, K., Freedberg, I. M. and Austen, K. F.), p. 942. McGraw-Hill, New York.
12. Lamberg, S. I. (1967). A new photosensitizer: the artificial sweetener cyclamate. *J. Am. med Ass.* **201**, 747.
13. Yong, J. M. and Sanderson, K. V. (1969). Photosensitivity dermatitis and renal tubular acidosis after ingestion of calcium cyclamate. *Lancet* **ii**, 1273.
14. Erickson, L. R. and Peterka, E. S. (1968). Sunlight sensitivity from oral contraceptives. *J. Am. med Ass.* **203**, 980.
15. Oosterhuis, W. W. (1968). Photosensitization by oral contraceptives. *Nederl. T. Geneesk.* **112**, 2154.
16. Elgart, M. L. and Higdon, R. S. (1971). Photosensitivity caused by oral contraceptives. *Med. Ann. D.C.* **40**, 501.

hormones, which results in melasma.[1, 2] Oestrogens alone may also induce photosensitivity reactions.[3]

Studies with photohaemolysis have shown that the halogenated salicylanilides and related compounds possess a phototoxic potential.[4, 5] Phototoxic skin reactions have been elicited with TCSA, bithional, and also with jadit (4-chloro-2-hydroxybenzoic acid-N-n-butylamide).[6, 7]

A final example of this exaggerated sunburn type of phototoxic skin reaction is seen in the erythema and oedema which can develop in the yellow or red areas of tattoos and is due to cadmium sulphide.[8, 9] This photoaction has been demonstrated to be mediated through excited singlet oxygen and directed against cell membranes, in particular, the plasma membrane.[10]

It seems that there are four main types of drug and chemical induced phototoxicity in skin which may be clearly defined at least in clinical terms. A single "typical" phototoxic reaction does not exist.

First, there is the immediate burning and wealing reaction, followed by a delayed erythema and hyperpigmentation. These reactions are almost certainly mediated through cell membrane damage. Secondly, there is what might truly be termed the "exaggerated sunburn response", and is possibly due to membrane damage in which oxygen may not be involved. Third is the unusual blistering response in an abnormally fragile skin induced by prolonged treatment with nalidixic acid or frusemide, which resembles the skin reactions in porphyria cutanea tarda and probably results from photosensitization of a biological target other than membranes. Finally, there is the characteristic delayed erythema, intense hyperpigmentation and blistering reactions associated with the

1. Mathison, I. W. and Haas, K. L. (1970). Drug photosensitivity I. Light and photosensitivities observed during oral contraceptive therapy: a review. *Obs. Gynaecol. Survey* **25**, 389.
2. Horkay, I., Tamasi, P., Krekooa, A. and Dalmy, L. (1975). Photodermatoses induced by oral contraceptives. *Archs derm. Res.* **253**, 53.
3. Young, J. W. (1964). A list of photosensitizing agents of interest to the Dermatologist. *Bull. Ass. Mil. Derm.* **13**, 33.
4. Oleniacz, W. S., Singer, E. J., Doyle, A. B. and Vinson, L. J. (1968). Induction of photohaemolysis by tetrachlorsalicylanilide. *J. pharm. Sci.* **57**, 2136.
5. Khan, G. and Fleischaker, B. (1971). II. Evaluation of phototoxicity of salicylanilides and similar compounds by photohemolysis. *J. invest. Derm.* **56**, 91.
6. Kobayashi, F., Wada, Y. and Mizuno, N. (1974). Comparative studies on phototoxicity of chemicals. *J. Derm.* **1**, 93.
7. Kaidbey, K. H. and Kligman, A. M. (1978). Identification of topical photosensitizing agents in humans. *J. invest. Derm.* **70**, 149.
8. Bjornberg, A. (1963). Reactions to light in yellow tattoos from cadmium sulfide. *Archs Derm.* **88**, 267.
9. Goldstein, N. (1967). Mercury-cadmium sensitivity in tattoos. A photoallergic reaction in red pigment. *Ann. intern. Med.* **67**, 948.
10. Wennersten, G. (1977). Photodynamic aspects of some metal complexes. *Acta derm-venereol. (Stockholm)* **57**, 519.

Table 6

Drug induced phototoxicity obtained by intradermal injection[1]

Drug name	Effective wavelengths	Amount of drug (μg)
Sulphanilamide*	UV-B	500
Sulphapyridine	UV-B	500
Demethlychlortetracycline	UV-A	200
Tetracycline	UV-A	200
Chlorthiazide	UV-B and UV-A	250
Chlorpromazine	UV-A	100
Prochlorperazine	UV-A	250
Griseofulvin	UV-A	250
Nalidixic acid	UV-A	150
Frusemide	UV-A	500
Quinidine	UV-A	250
Vinblastin	UV-B	0·2

* Other studies have shown reactions to be produced by UV-B alone,[2] UV-A,[3] and UV-A and visible radiation.[4]

1. Kaidbey, K. H. and Kligman, A. M. (1978). Identification of topical photosensitizing agents in humans. *J. invest. Derm.* **70**, 149.
2. Blum, H. F. (1941). Studies of photosensitivity due to sulfanilamide. *J. invest. Derm.* **4**, 159.
3. Kligman, A. M. and Breit, R. (1968). The identification of phototoxic drugs by human assay. *J. invest. Derm.* **51**, 90.
4. Burckhardt, W. (1941). Untersuchungen über die Photoaktivitat einiger Sulfanilamide. *Dermatologica* **83**, 63.

psoralens, brought about by damage to DNA and presenting an entirely distinct form of phototoxicity.

V. PHOTOALLERGY[1, 2, 3, 4]

The photosensitivity reactions occurring in some subjects 10 days after an initial phototoxic response to intradermal sulphanilamide and exposure to sunlight were clinically quite distinct from the initial response. These more closely resembled eczematous reactions seen in the allergic-type

1. Harber, L. C. and Baer, R. L. (1972). Pathogenic mechanisms of drug induced photosensitivity. *J. invest. Derm.* **58**, 327.
2. Epstein, J. H. (1972). Photo-allergy: A review. *Archs Derm.* **106**, 741.
3. Amos, H. E. (1973). Photoallergy: A critical survey. *Trans St John's Hosp. derm. Soc.* **59**, 147.
4. Emmet, E. A. (1978). Drug photoallergy. *Int J. Derm.* **17**, 370.

contact reaction.[1] Burckhardt[2] confirmed the photosensitive nature of the reaction and that it occurred in limited numbers of subjects showing an initial phototoxic response. He also observed that an urticarial element might occur and that cross photosensitivity could be demonstrated with sulphonamide derivatives which had little or no photosensitizing potential on their own. The importance of sunlight in the skin reactions due to topical treatment with sulphanilamide was suggested by Peterkin.[3]

The reactions were restricted to sun-exposed areas of skin and could be reproduced by photopatch, but not by the conventional closed patch tests.[4] The histopathology showed the characteristic perivascular lymphocytic infiltrate and epidermal spongiosis of contact eczema.

It was suggested that the reactions observed were typical contact sensitivity reactions, the hapten involved being a photoproduct of the sulphonamide.[4] This explanation was shown to be true for photosensitivity reactions induced by Nadisan, a sulphonamide derivative (1-butyl-3-sulphanil): the patients gave positive closed patch tests with p-hydroxylaminobenzane sulphonamide (PHABSA), an oxidative photoproduct of the parent compound.[5,6] Experimental studies with guineapigs have shown that animals sensitized to sulphanilamide plus irradiation also react to PHABSA. Similarly, animals sensitized to PHABSA react to challenge with sulphanilamide plus irradiation. In both types of experiment, the procedures failed to produce reactions in non-sensitized controls.[7,8] However, only two out of 10 patients with sulphanilamide-induced photoallergy were shown to react to PHABSA.[9] It is possible

1. Epstein, S. (1939). Photoallergy and primary photosensitivity to sulfanilamide. *J. invest. Derm.* **2**, 43.
2. Burckhardt, W. (1941). Untersuchungen über die Photoaktivitat einiger Sulfanilamide. *Dermatologica* **83**, 63.
3. Peterkin, G. A. (1945). Sulphonamide rashes. An analysis of 500 cases seen in North Africa and Italy. *Br. med J.* **2**, 1.
4. Burckhardt, W. (1948). Photoallergische Ekzeme durch Sulfanilamidsalben. *Dermatologica* **96**, 280.
5. Burckhardt, W., Schwarz, K. and Schwarz-Speck, M. (1957). Photoallergische Ekzeme durch Nadisan. *Schweiz. med. Wschr.* **87**, 954.
6. Shinn, L., Main, E. R. and Mellon, R. R. (1939). Conversion of sulfanilamide into p-hydroxylamino-benzene-sulphonamide by ultraviolet irradiation. *Proc. Soc. exp. Biol.* **52**, 736.
7. Schwarz, K. and Speck, M. (1957). Experimentelle Untersuchungen zur Frage der Photoallergie der Sulfonamide. *Dermatologica* **114**, 232.
8. Aoki, K., Shimotoge, M. and Saito, T. (1974). Studies on photosensitivity caused by sulfa drugs. 6. Sensitization with p-hydroxylaminobenzene sulfonamide and histamine metabolism. *J. Derm.* **1**, 99.
9. Rothenstein, J., Schwarz, K., Schwarz-Speck, M. and Storck, H. (1966). Role of *in vivo* and *in vitro* formed decomposition products of sulfanilamides and phenothiazines in photoallergy; relationship of spectrophotometric findings to *in vivo* reactions. *Int. Archs Allergy* **29**, 1.

that in most cases the formation of a complete allergen is part of the photosensitization involving the UV-induced binding of the hapten to protein. However, photocoupling of sulphanilamide to protein failed to produce positive patch test reactions,[1] and it remains uncertain as to why PHABSA did not consistently produce reactions in these patients.

The clinical similarities between skin responses to photosensitization and delayed hypersensitivity reactions of contact dermatitis eruptions would appear to justify the concept of photoallergy. It is postulated that once the photosensitizer is in the skin absorption of the appropriate radiation results in the formation of allergen. This may be simply a photochemical reaction, the photoproduct then acts as hapten in the same way as a contact allergen. Alternatively, some photosensitized change involving skin protein may be required, either to produce an active carrier protein, or, by photoactivated binding to a protein, to produce a complete allergen which would not have otherwise been formed without the irradiation.[2] As the number of drugs and chemicals producing these suspected photoallergic reactions has increased (Table 7 and Fig. 10), opportunities to study their mechanisms have also increased.

Of the sulphonamides, sulphanilamide has shown the greatest photosensitizing potential, although others may induce similar reactions and exhibit cross-sensitization reactions. Other sulphonamide derivatives, such as the antidiabetic sulphonylureas, carbutamide (Nadisan®)[3] and chlorpropamide,[4,5] have been classed as photoallergic drugs. Cross reactions with sulphonamide have also been obtained with tolbutamide.[4] The photosensitivity reactions induced by the diuretic and antihypertensive thiazide derivatives, chlorthiazide (Diaril®) and hydrochlorthiazide (Hydrodiuril®) are also classed, in part, as photoallergy.[6,7] Some of the skin eruptions resemble lichen planus and are similar to reactions due to quinacrine, gold salts or arsenicals which are

1. Sulser, H. (1962). Photochemische Kuppling des Sulfanilamides und aromatischer Amine an Elweiss und andere hochmolekulare Verbindungen. *Arch. klin. exp. Derm.* **215**, 266.
2. Storck, H. (1965). Photoallergy and photosensitivity. *Archs Derm.* **91**, 469.
3. Burckhardt, W., Schwarz, K. and Schwarz-Speck, M. (1957). Photoallergische Ekzeme durch Nadisan. *Schweiz. med. Wschr.* **87**, 954.
4. Hitselberger, J. F. and Fosnaugh, R. P. (1962). Photosensitivity due to chlorpropamide. *J. Am. med. Ass.* **180**, 162.
5. Feuerman, E. and Frumkin, A. (1973). Photodermatitis induced by chlorpropamide. *Dermatologica* **146**, 25.
6. Norins, A. L. (1959). Chlorthiazide drug eruption involving photosensitization. *Archs Derm.* **79**, 592.
7. Harber, L. C., Lashinsky, A. M. and Baer, R. L. (1959). Skin manifestations of photosensitivity due to chlorthiazide and hydrochlorthiazide: preliminary report. *J. invest. Derm.* **33**, 83.

Table 7

Photoallergic compounds

Sulphonamides and sulphonylureas	Sulphanilamide
	Tolbutamide
	Carbutamide
	Chlorpropamide
Phenothiazines	Promethazine
	Chlorpromazine
Thiazides	Chlorthiazide
	Hydrochlorthiazide
Halogenated salicylanilides and	3,5,3′,4′Tetrachlorosalicylanilide (TCSA)
related substances	3,5,4′Tribromosalicylanilide (TBS)
	3,4,4′Trichlorocarbanilide (TCC)
	Hexachlorophene
	Bithionol
	Jadit®
	Fentichor
Triacetyldiphenolisatin	
Quinoxaline-n-dioxide	
Psoralens	8-methoxypsoralen
	5-methoxyangelicin (Isobergapten)
	6-methoxyangelicin (Spodin)
6-Methyl coumarin	
Musk ambrette	

This list is intended to be representative rather than comprehensive.

thought to be allergic.[1] The ability to reproduce these lesions by phototesting thiazide sensitive patients shows that they are photosensitivity reactions rather than true lichen planus. The flaring of previously damaged skin in sites remote from the phototesting site is taken as further evidence of the involvement of immunological mechanisms in photoallergy.[1]

Skin reactions obtained with sulphonamides, were usually of the photocontact eczema type; phototoxicity was rarely encountered, and contact sensitivity was very rare. The skin reactions with the phenothiazines, on the other hand, are complex.[2,3,4] Phototoxic reactions are

1. Harber, L. G., Lashinsky, A. M. and Baer, R. L. (1959). Photosensitivity due to chlorthiazide and hydrochlorthiazide. *New Engl. J. Med.* **261**, 1378.
2. Sidi, E., Hincky, M. and Gervais, A. (1955). Allergic sensitization and photosensitization to Phenergan cream. *J. invest. Derm.* **24**, 345.
3. Schulz, K. H., Wiskemann, A. and Wulf, K. (1956). Klinische und experimentelle Untersuchungen über die photodynamische Wirksamkeit von Phenothiazinderivaten, insbesondere von Megaphen. *Arch. klin. exp. Derm.* **202**, 285.
4. Epstein, S. and Rowe, R. (1957). Photoallergy and Photocross-sensitivity to Phenergan. *J. invest. Derm.* **29**, 319.

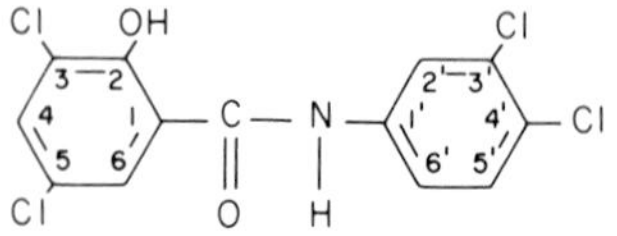

Cl OH Cl

3 2 2' 3'
4 1 1' 4' Cl
5 6 6' 5'

Cl C — N
‖ |
O H

3,3',4',5 Tetrachlorosalicylanilide

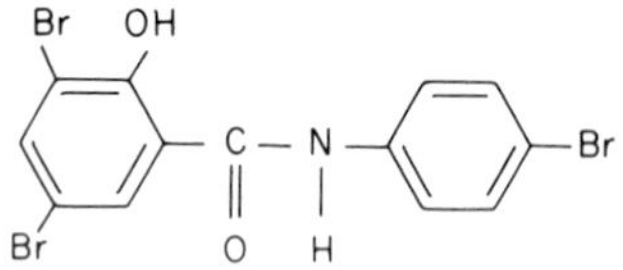

Br OH

C — N Br
‖ |
Br O H

3,4',5 Tribromosalicylanilide

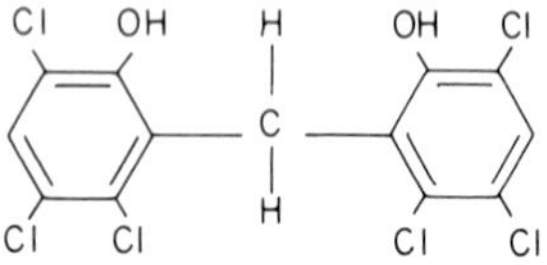

Cl OH H OH Cl

C

Cl Cl H Cl Cl

Hexachlorophene

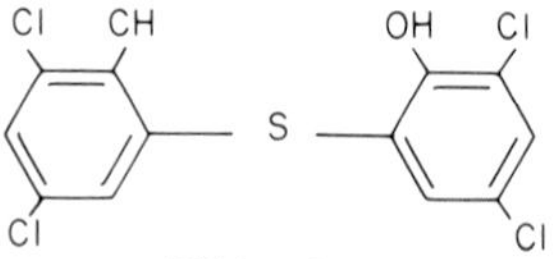

Cl CH OH Cl

S

Cl Cl

Bithionol

OH

Cl C — N — C₄H₉

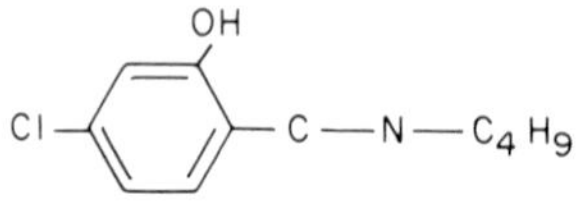

4 - Chloro - 2 - Hydroxybenzoic acid
N - n - Butylamide

Fig. 10. The molecular structures of the common photosensitizing halogenated salicylanilides and related chemicals.

relatively common in patients on high dosage chlorpromazine (CPZ). If an eczematous reaction is seen in these patients, there is usually some evidence of previous sensitization by contact.[1] This typical allergic contact eczema is more often seen in workers in manufacturing processes, nurses, and others handling the drug.[2] In some cases, this reaction is a straightforward contact eczema in which irradiation is not involved. In

1. Calnan, C. D. (1958). Studies in contact dermatitis. V. Photosensitivity from chlorpromazine. Trans. St John's Hosp. derm. Soc. **48**, 26.
2. Calnan, C. D., Frain-Bell, W. and Cuthbert, J. W. (1961–62). Occupational dermatitis from chlorpromazine. Trans. St John's Hosp. derm. Soc. **46**, 48.

some, the reaction is produced only when the skin is exposed to sunlight, while in others exposure increases the intensity of the skin reaction. Similar reactions are obtained with promethazine (Phenergan®) when used as the topical antihistamine.[1,2] Rarely is an immediate urticarial reaction obtained with CPZ photosensitization. This has the characteristics of an immediate hypersensitivity reaction being elicited in a sensitized individual with concentrations of CPZ which gave negative results in normal controls. However, these patients gave positive passive transfer tests.[3]

The histopathology of photocontact eczema reactions obtained with the phenothiazines, like that due to sulphanilamide, appears to be identical to that of contact allergic eczema.[4] Although the established reactions produced by phototoxic and photoallergic mechanisms may appear similar, both clinically and histologically, this is because secondary processes of damage and repair have become superimposed on the initial reactions. The majority of photoallergic reactions can be clearly differentiated from those of phototoxicity if the histopathology of the initial stages of the reactions are examined. This is done by biopsying the phototest sites during the first 48 h of their evolution. With such a procedure, the typical lymphocytic infiltrate and epidermal spongiosis and vesiculation are seen in photoallergic reactions (Fig. 11), but these are not in any of the earlier stages of the phototoxicity reactions.[5,6,7] An alternative to this eczematous picture is the photoallergic response with thiazides in which the histopathology is typical of the lichen planus.[8]

Interest in the concept of photoallergy was increased in the 1960s following reports of photosensitivity due to 3,4′5′5 tetrachlorosalicylanilide (TCSA) introduced into soaps as a bacteriostat.[9,10,11] The major

1. Sidi, E., Hincky, M. and Gervais, A. (1955). Allergic sensitization and photosensitization to Phenergan cream. *New Engl. J. Med.* **261**, 1378.
2. Epstein, S. (1960). Allergic photocontact dermatitis from promethazine (Phenergan). *A.M.A. Archs Derm.* **81**, 175.
3. Horio, T. (1975). Chlorpromazine photoallergy: co-existence of immediate and delayed type. *Archs Derm.* **111**, 1469.
4. Epstein, S. (1968). Chlorpromazine photosensitivity. *Archs Derm.* **98**, 354.
5. Miescher, G. (1957). Zur Histologie der lichtbedingten Reaktionen. *Dermatologica* **115**, 345.
6. Jung, E. G. and Hardmeier, T. (1967). Zur Histologie der photoallergischen Testreaction. *Dermatologica* **135**, 243.
7. Epstein, J. H. (1974). Phototoxicity and photoallergy: clinical syndromes. In 'Sunlight and Man' (Eds Fitzpatrick, T. B., Pathak, M. A., Harber, L. C., Seiji, M. and Kukita, A.), p. 459. University of Tokyo Press, Tokyo.
8. Harber, L. C., Lashinsky, A. M. and Baer, R. L. (1959). Photosensitivity due to chlorothiazide and hydrochlorothiazide. *New Engl. J. Med.* **261**, 1378.
9. Wilkinson, D. S. (1961). Photodermatitis due to tetrachlorosalicylanilide. *Br. J. Derm.* **73**, 213.
10. Calnan, C. D., Harman, R. R. M. and Wells, G. C. (1961). Photodermatitis from soaps. *Br. med. J.* **ii**, 1266.
11. Crow, K. D. (1961). Photodermatitis from soap. *Br. med. J.* **ii**, 1565.

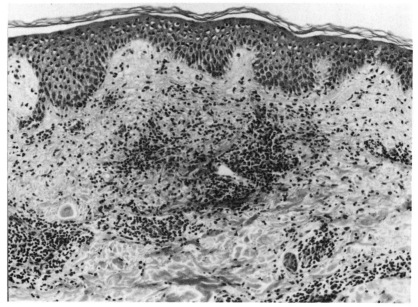

Fig. 11. Histopathology of an induced photoallergic response with chlorpromazine 40 h after exposure. Epidermal changes are relatively mild with some spongiosis but there is a heavy dermal infiltrate mainly of lymphocytes. (Courtesy of Dr H. A. Addo)

features of the reaction resembled those of a typical delayed hyper-sensitivity type of allergic contact dermatitis. Further studies in man revealed a complex pattern of photosensitivity, contact sensitivity and cross reactions to TCSA and related compounds such as 3,4′5 tri-bromosalicylanilide, hexachlorophene, bithionol, bromochlorosalicyla-nilide (Multifungin®), fenticlor and 4-chloro-2-hydroxybenzoic acid-N-n-butylamide (Jadit®).[1, 2, 3, 4, 5, 6, 7, 8, 9, 10] There is some similarity in the

1. Wilkinson, D. S. (1962). Further experiences with halogenated salicylanilides. *Br. J. Derm.* **74**, 295.
2. Wilkinson, D. S. (1962). Patch test reactions to certain halogenated salicylanilides. *Br. J. Derm.* **74**, 302.
3. Vinson, L. J. and Flatt, R. S. (1962). Photosensitization by tetrachlorosalicylanilide. *J. invest. Derm.* **38**, 327.
4. Jillson, O. F. and Baughman, R. D. (1963). Contact photodermatitis from bithionol. *Archs Derm.* **88**, 409.
5. Baughman, R. D. (1964). Contact photodermatitis from bithionol II. Cross sensitivities to hexachlorophene and salicylanilides. *Archs Derm.* **90**, 153.
6. Fregert, S. and Möller, H. (1964). Photo cross-sensitization among halogen–hydroxybenzoic acid derivatives. *J. invest. Derm.* **43**, 271.

molecular structure of these chemicals but the presence, and position, of the halogen atoms appears to be of greatest importance for producing the photosensitivity reactions.

The withdrawal of these halogenated phenolic compounds from the market resulted in a significant fall in the incidence of apparent photocontact dermatitis.[1] However, similar reactions have since been reported in association with exposure to quinoxaline-n-dioxide (Quindoxin®), an animal feedstuff additive[2] and to the fragrance materials 6-methylcoumarin[3, 4] and musk ambrette,[5, 6] and here again the possibility of an immune based reaction is raised.

Experimental studies using guinea-pigs confirmed that animals may be photosensitized to halogenated salicylanilides in the same way that sensitization to contact allergic agents such as dinitrochlorbenzene (DNCB) is achieved except that exposure to UVR is required for both induction and elicitation phases of the process.[7, 8, 9, 10, 11, 12] The photo-

1. Smith, S. Z. and Epstein, J. H. (1977). Photocontact dermatitis to halogenated salicylanilides and related compounds. *Archs Derm.* **113**, 1372.
2. Zaynoun, S., Johnson, B. E. and Frain-Bell, W. (1976). The investigation of quindoxin photosensitivity. *Contact Dermatitis* **2**, 343.
3. Kaidbey, K. H. and Kligman, A. M. (1978). Photocontact allergy to 6-methylcoumarin. *Contact Dermatitis* **4**, 277.
4. Jackson, R. T., Nesbitt, L. T. and Deleo, V. A. (1980). 6-Methylcoumarin photocontact dermatitis. *J. Am. Acad. Derm.* **2**, 124.
5. Raugi, G. J., Storrs, J. and Larsen, W. G. (1979). Photoallergic contact dermatitis to men's perfumes. *Contact Dermatitis* **5**, 251.
6. Giovizaao, V. J., Harber, L. C., Armstrong, R. B. and Kochevar, I. E. (1980). Photoallergic contact dermatitis to musk ambrette: clinical report of two patients with persistent light reactor patterns. *J. Am. Acad. Derm.* **3**, 384.
7. Vinson, L. J. and Borselli, V. F. (1966). A guinea pig assay of the photosensitizing potential of topical germicides. *J. Soc. cosmet. Chem.* **17**, 123.
8. Harber, L. C., Targovnik, S. E. and Baer, R. L. (1967). Contact photosensitivity to halogenated salicylanilides: In man and guinea pigs. *Archs Derm.* **96**, 646.
9. Harber, L. C., Targovnik, S. E. and Baer, R. L. (1968). Studies on contact photosensitivity to hexachlorophene and trichlorocarbanilide in guinea pigs and man. *J. invest. Derm.* **51**, 373.
10. Cripps, D. J. and Enta, T. (1970). Absorption and action spectra studies on bithionol and halogenated salicylanilide photosensitivity. *Br. J. Derm.* **82**, 230.
11. Morikawa, F., Nakayama, Y., Fukuda, M., Hamano, M., Yokoyama, Y., Nagura, T., Ishihara, M. and Toda, K. (1974). Techniques for evaluation of phototoxicity and photoallergy in laboratory animals and man. In 'Sunlight and Man' (Ed. Fitzpatrick, T. B.), p. 529. University of Tokyo Press, Tokyo.
12. Horio, T. (1976). The induction of photocontact sensitivity in guinea pigs without UVB radiation. *J. invest. Derm.* **67**, 591.

7. Harber, L. C., Harris, H. and Baer, R. L. (1966). Photoallergic contact dermatitis: due to halogenated salicylanilides and related compounds. *Archs Derm.* **94**, 255.
8. Harber, L. C., Harris, H. and Baer, R. L. (1966). Structural features of photoallergy to salicylanilides and related compounds. *J. invest. Derm.* **46**, 303.
9. Burry, J. N. (1967). Photo-allergic contact dermatitis from halogenated phenolic compounds. *Aust. J. Derm.* **9**, 142.
10. Herman, P. S. and Sams, W. M., Jr. (1972). 'Soap Photodermatitis. Photosensitivity to Halogenated Salicylanilides'. Charles C. Thomas, Springfield, Illinois.

sensitivity may be transferred passively with immune peritoneal cells[1] and the same kind of complex pattern of cross reactions as seen in man may be observed.[2] Photoallergic contact dermatitis to musk ambrette may also be easily induced in guinea-pigs if Freund's complete adjuvant is used in the induction phase.[3] Mice are easily photosensitized with TCSA, the photosensitivity being transferred passively with cells unequivocally identified as T lymphocytes. In mice, at least, the contact photosensitivity reactions obtained with TCSA are clearly examples of T-cell mediated delayed hypersensitivity.[4] Moreover, the induction of the photosensitivity depends on the Langerhans cell population of the mouse epidermis,[4] just as does the induction of plain contact sensitivity to 2,4-dinitro-1-fluorobenzene (DNFB) and other allergens.[5, 6, 7] Additional evidence that so-called photoallergic reactions generally might be cell mediated immune responses comes from the demonstration of photosensitized lymphoblast transformation with Jadit[8] and TCSA photosensitized macrophage migration inhibition[9] for which, it is of interest, a carrier protein was required during irradiation.

If it is accepted that these reactions are indeed cell mediated, the nature of the complete antigen becomes of particular interest. The photochemistry of the halogenated salicylanilides may proceed through successive losses of halogen atoms and stable photoproducts may be isolated.[10, 11, 12]

1. Harber, L. C. and Baer, R. L. (1969). Mechanisms of drug photosensitivity reactions. *Suppl. Toxicol. appl. Pharmacol.* **3**, 58.

2. Morikawa, F., Nakayama, Y., Fukuda, M., Hamano, M., Yokoyama, Y., Nagura, T., Ishihara, M. and Toda, K. (1974). Techniques for evaluation of phototoxicity and photoallergy in laboratory animals and man. *In* 'Sunlight and Man' (Ed. Fitzpatrick, T. B.), p. 529. University of Tokyo Press, Tokyo.

3. Ichikawa, H., Armstrong, R. B. and Harber, L. C. (1981). Photoallergic contact dermatitis in guinea pigs: improved induction technique using Freund's complete adjuvant. *J. invest. Derm.* **76**, 498.

4. Miyachi, Y. and Takigawa, M. (1982). Mechanisms of contact photosensitivity in mice: II. Langerhans cells are required for successful induction of contact photosensitivity to TCSA. *J. invest. Derm.* **78**, 363.

5 Silberberg, I. (1973). Apposition of mononuclear cells to Langerhans cells in contact allergic reactions. *Acta derm-venereol.* **53**, 1.

6. Silberberg, I., Baer, R. L. and Rosenthal, S. A. (1976). The role of Langerhans cells in allergic contact hypersensitivity. A review of findings in man and guinea pigs. *J. invest. Derm.* **66**, 210.

7. Toews, G. B., Bergstresser, P. R., Streilein, J. W. and Sullivan, S. (1980). Epidermal Langerhans cell density determines whether contact hypersensitivity or unresponsiveness follows skin painting with DNFB. *J. Immunol.* **124**, 445.

8. Jung, E. G., Hornke, J. and Hajdu, P. (1968). Photoallergie durch 4-Chlor-2-hydroxybenzoesaur-N-butylamid. *Arch. klin. exp. Derm.* **233**, 287.

9. Herman, P. S. and Sams, W. M., Jr. (1971). Requirement for carrier protein in salicylanilide sensitivity: the migration inhibition test in contact photoallergy. *J. Lab. clin. Med.* **77**, 572.

10. Jenkins, F. P., Welti, D. and Baines, D. (1964). Photochemical reactions of Tetrachlorosalicylanilide. *Nature* **201**, 827.

11. Coxon, J. A., Jenkins, F. P. and Welti, D. (1965). The effect of light on halogenated salicylanilide ions. *Photochem. Photobiol.* **4**, 713.

12. Davies, A. K., Hild, N. S., McKellar, J. F. and Phillips, G. O. (197). Photochemistry of Tetrachlorosalicylanilide and its relevance to the persistent light reactor. *Br. J. Derm.* **92**, 143.

It is possible that the apparent photosensitivity is due to plain contact sensitivity reactions to these stable photoproducts.[1] However, the highly reactive radical intermediate of irradiated TCSA binds readily with protein[2, 3, 4] and it is this reaction which is more likely involved in the formation of complete antigen.[5, 6, 7]

VI. PHOTOPROTECTIVE AGENTS

A. Topical Agents

The successful treatment of light sensitivity depends on a knowledge of the natural history of the specific photodermatoses, the determination of the responsible wavelengths, and where possible of any other aetiological factors. Damaged skin will usually not tolerate topically applied photoprotective chemicals unless the reaction is first suppressed, and this often justifies the initial short-term topical application of steroid preparations. Although these preparations might be expected to affect ultraviolet induced reactions as part of their general anti-inflammatory suppressive action,[8, 9] the mechanisms involved in such suppression remain obscure. Although the stabilization of lysosome membranes would help to minimize an inflammatory action, it is still not known whether lysosomal hydrolase release plays a part in the reaction to UV. It may well be therefore that the anti-inflammatory action of steroid preparations is related to the inhibition of fatty acid, prostaglandin precursor release, resulting from the induction of a phosopholipase inhibitor.[10] In subjects most severely affected the suppression of the

1. Willis, I. and Kligman, A. M. (1968). The mechanism of photoallergic contact dermatitis. *J. invest. Derm.* **51**, 378.
2. Jenkins, F. P., Welti, D. and Baines, D. (1964). Photochemical reactions of Tetrachlorosalicylanilide. *Nature* **201**, 827.
3. Kochevar, I. E. and Harber, L. C. (1977). Photoreactions of 3,3'4'5-Tetrachlorosalicylanilide with proteins. *J. invest. Derm.* **68**, 151.
4. Barratt, M. D. (1981). The photochemical binding of tetrachlorosalicylanilide to bovine insulin. *Photochem. Photobiophys.* **3**, 59.
5. Epstein, J. H. (1972). Photoallergy: a review. *Archs Derm.* **106**, 741.
6. Harber, L. C., Baer, R. L. and Bickers, D. R. (1974). Techniques of evaluation of phototoxicity and photoallergy in biologic systems, including man, with particular emphasis on immunologic aspects. *In* 'Sunlight and Man' (Ed. Fitzpatrick, T. B.), p. 518. University of Tokyo Press, Tokyo.
7. Kochevar, I. E. (1979). Photoallergic responses to chemicals. *Photochem. Photobiol.* **30**, 437.
8. Ljunggren, B. and Moller, H. (1973). Influence of corticosteroids on ultraviolet light erythema and pigmentation in man. *Arch Forsch.* **248**, 1.
9. Kaidbey, K. M. and Kurban, A. K. (1976). The influence of corticosteroids and topical indomethacin on sunburn erythema. *J. invest. Derm.* **66**, 153.
10. Flower, R. J. and Blackwell, G. J. (1979). Anti-inflammatory steroids induce biosynthesis of a phospholipase A_2 inhibitor which prevents prostaglandin generation. *Nature* **278**, 456.

reaction can only be achieved by a period of nursing behind special blinds whose materials screen off the responsible wavelengths of UV and visible radiation.[1, 2]

Some of the commonly used and effective photoprotective agents are listed in Table 8. They all protect against UV-B wavelengths although para-aminobenzoic acid and its esters are more effective than the others in protecting against shorter UV wavelengths. The advantage of the benzophenones is that they have the additional ability to protect against UV-A. A mixture of dihydroxyacetone and naphthoquinone is said to protect throughout the UV and visible spectrum, dihydroxyacetone

Table 8

Chemical	Approximate range of sunlight absorbance
Para aminobenzoic acid	290–320 nm
Para aminobenzoic acid esters	290–320 nm
glyceryl	
amyl dimethyl	
octyl dimethyl	
Cinnamates	290–320 nm
Salicylates	290–330 nm
Anthranilates	320–350 nm
Benzophenones	290–360 nm
Dihydroxyacetone/naphthoquinone mixture	approx. 290–450 nm
Titanium dioxide	Whole spectrum

See: Roelandts, R., Vanfree, J., Bonamie, A., Kerkhofs, L. and Degreef, H. (1983). A survey of UV-absorbers in commercially available sun products. *Int. J. Derm.* (in press).

protecting against UV-A and visible up to 500 nm peak, and the naphthoquinone protecting against the UV-B wavelengths. Such protection appears to result from a chemical reaction of dihydroxy-acetone with keratin.[3]

A selection of chemicals suitable for sunscreens is initially based on

1. Herd, Joyce, Sturrock, I. and Frain-Bell, W. (1973). The use of plastic material for the protection of patients with severe photodermatoses. *Br. J. Derm.* **88**, 283.
2. Frain-Bell, W. (1978). 'What is that thing called light?' Dowling Oration. *Br. J. Derm.* **84**, 266.
3. Fusaro, R. M. and Runge, W. J. (1962). Clinical experience with a topical light filter. *J. Am. med. Ass.* **182**, 1120.

spectrophometric studies.[1, 2, 3, 4] Their ultimate value, however, depends on the efficacy of the screening chemical to protect (protection factor) against natural sunlight or artificially produced solar simulator irradiation.[5, 6] Any photoprotective chemical which on account of its structure is able to absorb UV or visible may well have the capacity to produce a reaction within the skin following absorption of the incident radiation. All these chemical substances are to a variable degree capable of producing contact allergic sensitivity, phototoxicity, and presumably also photoallergy.

Both contact and photocontact reactions to sunscreen preparations have been reported. Difficulties arise, however, in the interpretation of the results of irradiation on a contact allergic reaction (the photopatch test). This makes the true incidence of photoallergic reactions due to these preparations difficult to assess. Phototoxic reactions may occur, and where these are associated with PABA and its esters, they appear to be restricted to the amyl dimethylaminobenzoate.[7] Also, the ortho isomer, amylodimethylaminobenzoic acid is strongly phototoxic and is responsible for the phototoxicity of UV-cured inks,[8] but the para form, amyl p-dimethylaminobenzoate has a very limited phototoxic potential. When phototoxic reactions occur with the PABA ester, Padimate A, used as a sunscreen, they may well be due to contamination of the para isomer with the ortho compound.[8, 9] However, allergic photocontact reactions have been confirmed with para aminobenzoic acid and its esters,[10] with cinnoxate (2-ethoxyethyl p-methoxycinnamate),[11, 12, 13] and with benzophenones such as oxybenzone and deoxybenzone.[14]

1. MacLeod, T. M. and Frain-Bell, W. (1971). The study of the efficacy of some agents used for the protection of the skin from exposure to light. *Br. J. Derm.* **84**, 266.
2. Robertson, D. F. and Groves, G. A. (1972). The selection and use of topical sunscreens. *Med. J. Aust.* **18**, 109.
3. Robertson, D. F. and Groves, G. A. (1977). Classification of sunscreen preparations. *Aust. J. Derm.* **18**, 109.
4. Sayre, R. M., Poh Agin, Patricia, Desrochers, Deborah L. and Marlow, E. (1980). Sunscreen testing methods: *in vitro* predictions of effectiveness. *J. Soc. cosmet. Chem.* **31**, 133.
5. Frain-Bell, W. (1978). 'What is that thing called light?' Dowling Oration. *Clin. exp. Derm.* **4**, 1.
6. Sayre, R. M., Marlowe, E., Poh Agin, P., LeVee, G. L. and Rosenberg, E. W. (1979). Performance of Six Sunscreen Formulations on Human Skins. *Archs Derm.* **115**, 46.
7. Kaidbey, K. H. and Kligman, A. M. (1978). Phototoxicity to a sunscreen ingredient Padimate A. *Archs Derm.* **114**, 547.
8. Emmet, E. A., Taphorn, B. R. and Krominsky, J. R. (1977). Phototoxicity occurring during the manufacture of ultraviolet-cured ink. *Archs Derm.* **113**, 770.
9. Emmet, E. A. (1979). Phototoxicity from exogenous agents. *Photochem. Photobiol.* **30**, 429.
10. Mathias, C. G., Maibach, H. L. and Epstein, J. (1978). Allergic contact photodermatitis to para aminobenzoic acid. *Archs Derm.* **114**, 1665.
11. Goldman, T. F., Jr. (1970). Photodermatitis from a sunscreening agent. *Archs Derm.* **10**, 563.
12. Thomson, G., Maibach, H. and Epstein, J. (1977). Allergic contact dermatitis from sunscreen preparations complicating photodermatitis. *Archs Derm.* **113**, 1252.
13. Cronin, Etain (1980). 'Contact Dermatitis', p. 454. Churchill Livingstone, London.
14. Thomson, G., Maibach, H. and Epstein, J. (1977). Allergic contact dermatitis from sunscreen preparations complicating photodermatitis. *Archs Derm.* **110**, 1252.

Contact allergic sensitivity to PABA ester appears to occur much less frequently than to benzocain (ethyl aminobenzoate).[1] Of perhaps more importance, however, is the development of a contact or photocontact allergy to fragrance constituents which have been incorporated in sunscreen preparations; as for example, 6-methylcoumarin.[2,3,4] This fragrance allergy is particularly relevant when perfumed sunscreens are prescribed for subjects with a persistent light reaction and who are prone to contact allergic sensitivity to multiple allergens, including fragrance constituents.[5]

The efficacy of the various sunscreen preparations also depend on their resistance to water, the effect of sweating and of friction, the importance of the necessity for frequent applications. For example, benzophenones require more frequent applications than para-aminobenzoic acid and its esters because the latter are able to build up depot formations.[6]

The use of para-aminobenzoic acid has been questioned in view of the *in vitro* evidence for its photosensitized mutagenic and phototoxic activity.[7,8,9,10] Thus, the theoretical possibility of a carcinogenic potential for PABA must be considered since it is likely to be applied repeatedly to skin exposed to sunlight. However, there is no evidence of an increased skin cancer incidence in experimental animals which have been exposed to UVR and para-aminobenzoic acid: in fact, there was a reduced incidence of malignant tumours due to the UV screening effect of the compound. Also, despite the possible carcinogenic action of PABA, it has

1. Hjorth, N., Wilkinson, D., Magnusson, B., Bandmann, H. J. and Maibach, H. (1978). Glyceryl p-aminobenzoate patch testing in benzocaine-sensitive subjects. *Contact Dermatitis* **4**, 46.
2. Kaidbey, K. H. and Kligman, A. M. (1978). Contact Photoallergy to 6-Methylcoumarin in Proprietary Sunscreens. *Archs Derm.* **114**, 1709.
3. Maurer, X., X., Weiruch, G. and Hess, R. (1980). Evaluation of the photocontact allergic potential of 6-methylcoumarin in the guinea pig. *Contact Dermatitis* **6**, 275.
4. Jackson, R. T., Nesbit, L. E. and DeLeo, V. A. (1980). 6-Methylcoumarin photocontact dermatitis. *J. Am. Acad. Derm.* **2**, 124.
5. Johnson, B. E. and Frain-Bell, W. (1981). Unpublished data.
6. Kaidbey, K. H. and Kligman, A. M. (1978). Laboratory methods for appraising the efficacy of sunscreens. *J. Soc. cosmet. Chem.* **29**, 525.
7. Hodges, N. D., Moss, S. H. and Davies, D. J. (1976). Evidence of increased genetic damage due to the presence of a sunscreening agent para aminobenzoic acid during irradiation with near ultraviolet light (Proceedings). *J. Pharm. Pharmacol.* **28**, Supplement 53P.
8. Hodges, N. D., Moss, S. H. and Davies, D. J. (1977). The sensitizing effect of a sunscreening agent, para aminobenzoic acid, in near UV-induced damage in a repair deficient strain of *Escherischia coli*. *Photochem. Photobiol.* **26**, 493.
9. Hodges, N. D., Moss, S. H. and Davies, D. J. (1977). Elucidation of the nature of genetic damage formed in the presence of a sunscreening agent, para aminobenzoic acid, during irradiation with near UV-light (Proceedings). *J. Pharm. Pharmacol.* **29**, Supplement 72P.
10. Osgood, P. J., Moss, S. H. and Davies, D. J. G. (1982). The sensitization of near-ultraviolet radiation killing of mammalian cells by the sunscreen agent Para-aminobenzoic acid. *J. invest. Derm.* **79**, 354.

been effective in reducing the number of skin tumours in xeroderma pigmentosum,[1] and it is interesting in this respect that PUVA treatment of xeroderma pigmentosum was discontinued on account of the rapid development of skin cancers.[2] However, protective sun preparations which do not have this potential mutagenic are available and are theoretically more acceptable.[3]

B. Systemic Agents

It is perhaps somewhat surprizing that cutaneous photosensitivity is little helped by systemic photoprotective agents. A number of such agents have, however, been used, in particular, beta-carotene, chloroquine and vitamin A.

1. Beta-carotene

The protective action of beta-carotene is complex but appears to be directed primarily against photosensitized oxidation.[4, 5, 6] It may interact directly with free radicals,[7] but it may also alter the excited singlet state oxygen,[8, 9] both forms of highly reactive intermediate being quenched in the process. Being a coloured pigment, it might also act as an optical filter. Beta-carotene inhibits the photohaemolysis induced by protoporphyrin and haematoporphyrin[10, 11] and also haematoporphyrin

1. Goldstein, N. and Hay-Roe, P. (1975). Prevention of skin cancer with a PABA in Alcohol sunscreen in xeroderma pigmentosum. *Cutis* **15**, 61.
2. Reed, W. B., Sugarman, G. I. and Mathis, R. A. (1977). De-Sanctis-Cacchione Syndrome. A case report with autopsy findings. *Archs Derm.* **113**, 1561.
3. Osgood, P. J., Moss, S. H. and Davies, D. J. G. (1982). The sensitization of near-ultraviolet radiation killing of mammalian cells by the sunscreen agent Para-aminobenzoic acid. *J. invest. Derm.* **79**, 354.
4. Matthews, M. M. and Sistrom, W. R. (1959). Function of carotenoid pigments in non-photosynthetic bacteria. *Nature* **184**, 1892.
5. Krinsky, I. (1968). The protective function of carotenoid pigments. *In* 'Photophysiology', Vol. III (Ed. Giese, A. C.), p. 123. Academic Press, London, Orlando and New York.
6. Matthews-Roth, M. M. and Krinsky, N. I. (1970). Carotenoid pigments and the stability of the cell membrane of Sarcina lutea. *Biochim. biophys. Acta* **203**, 357.
7. Fugimori, E. and Tavla, M. (1966). Light-induced electron transfer between chlorophyll and hydroquinone, and the effect of oxygen and beta-carotene. *Photochem. Photobiol.* **5**, 877.
8. Foote, C. S. and Denny, R. W. (1968). Chemistry of singlet oxygen VII. Quenching by beta-carotene. *J. Am. chem. Soc.* **90**, 6233.
9. Foote, C. S., Chang, Y. C. and Denny, R. W. (1970). Chemistry of singlet oxygen, XI. Cis-trans isomerization of carotenoids by singlet excited oxygen and a probable quenching mechanism. *J. Am. chem. Soc.* **92**, 5218.
10. Swanbeck, G. and Wennersten, G. (1973). Effect of beta-carotene on photohaemolysis. *Acta derm-venereol. (Stockholm)* **53**, 283.
11. Moshell, A. N. and Bjornson, L. (1977). Photoprotection in erythropoeitic protoporphyria: mechanisms of photoprotection by beta-carotene. *J. invest. Derm.* **68**, 157.

photosensitized damage to fibroblasts in culture.[1] The lethal effects of haematoporphyrin photosensitization in mice are also prevented by systemically administered beta-carotene.[2, 3]

Despite these studies, the mechanisms involved are still not entirely clear. The action as an optical filter appears unlikely since concentrations of beta-carotene which inhibit photohaemolysis are ineffective when separated from the porphyrin containing red cells;[4] also when it is applied topically it fails to suppress the phototoxic reaction in erythropoietic protoporphyria.[5] Although the excited singlet oxygen pathway is a major part of protoporphyrin phototoxicity and the ability of carotenoids to protect against photosensitization is a function of their ability to quench excited singlet oxygen,[6, 7] it is still not certain that the protective action of beta-carotene against porphyrin phototoxicity is by this mechanism. Free radicals also play a part in protoporphyrin induced photohaemolysis[8] and free radical scavengers, such as tocopherol, do afford some protection in this system.[2]

Beta-carotene has no significant protective effect against sunburn in man,[9] but there is some evidence that it modifies the carcinogenic effect of UVR in experimental animals.[10] Dietary anti-oxidants are effective in reducing the number of lesions and severity of UV-induced squamous cell carcinomas in hairless mice.[11] Glutathione, vitamin A and alpha-tocopherol (vitamin E) all failed to inhibit the acute erythema reaction of mouse skin to UVR, but butylated hydroxytoluene was shown to be

1. Fritsch, P., Gschnait, F., Hönigsmann, H. and Wolff, K. (1976). Protective action of beta-carotene against lethal photosensitization of fibroblasts *in vitro. Br. J. Derm.* **94**, 263.
2. Moshell, A. N. and Bjornson, L. (1977). Photoprotection in erythropoietic protoporphyria: mechanism of photoprotection by beta-carotene. *J. invest. Derm.* **68**, 157.
3. Matthews, M. M. (1964). Protective effect of beta-carotene against lethal photosensitisation by haematoporphyrin. *Nature* **203**, 1092.
4. Swanbeck, G. and Wennersten, G. (1973). Effect of beta carotene on photohaemolysis. *Acta derm-venereol. (Stockholm)* **53**, 283.
5. Matthews-Roth, M. M., Pathak, M. A., Fitzpatrick, T. B., Harber, L. C. and Kass, E. H. (1970). Beta-carotene as a photoprotective agent in erythropoietic protoporphyria. *Trans. Ass. Am. Phys.* **83**, 176.
6. Matthews-Roth, M. M., Wilson, T., Fujimori, B. and Krinsky, N. I. (1974). Carotenoid chromatophore length and protection against photosensitisation. *Photochem. Photobiol.* **19**, 217.
7. Foote, C. S., Chang, Y. C. and Denny, R. W. (1970). Chemistry of singlet excited oxygen X. Carotenoid quenching parallels biological protection. *J. Am. chem. Soc.* **92**, 5216.
8. Goldstein, B. D. and Harber, L. C. (1972). Erythropoietic protoporphyria: lipid peroxidation and red cell membrane damage associated with photohaemolysis. *J. clin. Invest.* **51**, 892.
9. Matthews-Roth, M. M., Pathak, M. A., Parrish, J. A., Fitzpatrick, T. B., Kass, E. H., Toda, K. and Clemens, W. (1972). A clinical trial of the effects of oral beta-carotene on the responses of human skin in solar radiation. *J. invest. Derm.* **59**, 349.
10. Epstein, J. H. (1977). Effects of beta-carotene on ultraviolet induced cancer formation in the hairless mouse. *Photochem. Photobiol.* **25**, 211.
11. Black, H. S. and Chan, J. T. (1975). Suppression of ultraviolet light induced tumour formation by dietary antioxidants. *J. invest. Derm.* **65**, 412.

effective.[1] Beta-carotene has been used in the treatment of many of the photodermatoses, with conflicting results.[2, 3, 4, 5, 6, 7, 8]

2. Chloroquine

Chloroquine has also been used extensively in the treatment of the photodermatoses; in particular, polymorphic light eruption. The clinical impression that it is beneficial in this form of cutaneous photosensitivity is minimally supported by recent studies involving the measurement of exposure to ultraviolet radiation.[9]

As with other synthetic antimalarial compounds, chloroquine has various interactions with biological systems, which might explain such a therapeutic effect in photodermatoses, such as polymorphic light eruption, solar urticaria, and lupus erythematosus. These include anti-inflammatory and antihistamine actions, binding to, and stabilization of, DNA chains and lysosome membranes.

The use of chloroquine in porphyria cutanea tarda is unrelated to any direct suppression of photosensitivity. Here the compound acts to reduce the excess porphyrin levels, particularly in the liver, by binding with the intracellular porphyrin and leading to its increased excretion in the urine.[10]

3. Vitamin A

There has been a clinical impression over the years that systemic vitamin

1. De Rios, G., Chan, J. T., Black, H. S., Rudolph, A. H. and Knox, J. M. (1968). Systemic protection by antioxidants against UVL-induced erythema. *J. invest. Derm.* **70**, 123.
2. Matthews-Roth, M. M., Pathak, M. A., Fitzpatrick, T. B., Harber, L. C. and Kass, E. H. (1974). Beta-carotene as an oral photoprotective agent in erythropoietic protoporphyria. *J. Am. Med. Ass.* **228**, 1004.
3. Zaynoun, S. T., Hunter, J. A. A., Darby, F. J., Zarembski, P., Johnson, B. E. and Frain-Bell, W. (1977). The treatment of erythropoietic protoporphyria. Experience with beta-carotene. *Br. J. Derm.* **97**, 663.
4. Swanbeck, G. and Wennersten, G. (1972). Treatment of polymorphous light eruptions with beta-carotene. *Acta derm-venereol. (Stockholm)* **52**, 462.
5. Jansen, C. T. (1974). Beta-carotene treatment of polymorphous light eruptions. *Dermatologica* **149**, 363.
6. Matthews-Roth, M. M., Pathak, M. A., Fitzpatrick, T. B., Harber, L. H. and Kass, E. H. (1977). Beta-carotene therapy for erythropoietic protoporphyria and other photosensitivity diseases. *Acta derm-venereol.* **113**, 1229.
7. Wennersten, G. (1980). Carotenoid treatment for light sensitivity: a reappraisal and six years' experience. *Acta derm-venereol. (Stockholm)* **60**, 251.
8. Haeger-Aronsen, Birgitta, Krook, C. and Abdulla, M. (1979). Oral carotenoids for photo-sensitivity in patients with erythropoietic protoporphyria, polymorphous light eruptions and lupus erythematosis disorder. *Int. J. Derm.* **18**, 73.
9. Corbett, M. F., Hawk, J. L. M., Herxheimer, A. and Magnus, I. A. (1982). Controlled therapeutic trials in polymorphic light eruption. *Br. J. Derm.* **107**, 571.
10. Scholnick, P. L., Epstein, J. H. and Marver, H. S. (1973). The molecular basis of the action of chloroquine in porphyria cutanea tarda. *J. invest. Derm.* **61**, 226.

A helps to minimize the reaction of normal skin to sunlight.[1] However, attempts to show alterations in sunburn erythema or in the action spectrum for erythema in normal subjects following the administration of vitamin A have failed,[2,3] as have controlled double-blind trials in groups of subjects exposed to variable amounts of sunshine.[4]

1. Cluver, E. H. (1964). Sun Trauma Prevention. *S. Afr. med. J.* **38**, 801.
2. Findlay, G. H. and van der Merwe, R. W. (1965). Epidermal vitamin A and sunburn in man. *Br. J. Derm.* **77**, 622.
3. Anderson, F. E. (1969). Studies in the relationship between serum vitamin A and sun exposure. *Aust. J. Derm.* **10**, 26.
4. Furman, K. I. (1972). Sylvasun and prevention of sun-trauma. *S. Afr. med. J.* 4th November, 1970.

83 | Phototherapy

B. E. JOHNSON

*Department of Dermatology, University of Dundee,
Ninewells Hospital, Dundee, Scotland*

I. INTRODUCTION

Ultraviolet radiation (UVR) is used to treat a variety of skin diseases. It is however only recently that the availability of accurate irradiation equipment has allowed the selection of appropriate wavebands leading to an improved understanding of the effects of UV-B (280–315 nm) and UV-A (315—400 nm) either alone, together, or in combination with photoactive substances such as tar and the psoralens. Certain visible wavelengths beyond the UV (>400 nm) are also now used; for example, blue light (around 460 nm peak) is effective in altering, and thus reducing the harmful amounts of bilirubin in jaundiced newborn children.[1] As early as the beginning of this century the photoactive dye, eosin, was used in association with light because of their combined destructive action on the cells of skin tumours.[2] However, the combination of a photoactive agent with light therapy was not developed further until about 10 years ago, when haematoporphyrin and light were used for the treatment of glioma in the rat,[3] and the same compound was

1. Cremer, R. J. *et al*. (1958). Influence of light on the hyperbilirubinaemia of infants. *Lancet* **i**, 1094.
2. Jesionek, A. and Tappenier, V. (1903). Zur Behandlung der Hautcarcinome mit fluorescirender Stoffen. *Münch. Med. Wochschr.* **47**, 1175.
3. Diamond, I., Granelli, S. G., McDonogh, A. F., Nielsen, S., Wilson, C. B. and Jaenicke, R. (1972). Photodynamic Therapy of Malignant Tumours. *Lancet* **ii**, 1175.

PHYSIOL. PATHOPHYSIOL. OF SKIN Vol. 8
ISBN 0 12 380608 9

used in association with fluorescent light for the control of mouse mammary tumours.[1, 2]

The commonly reported decrease in photosensitivity during the summer in subjects with polymorphic light eruption has led to the suggestion that some form of "desensitization" may occur. This desensitization may be achieved with controlled exposures to UV-B[3, 4, 5] and the photosensitivity of solar urticaria may be decreased in this way also.[6] Although some degree of hyperpigmentation and thickening of the horny layer may result from this treatment, it is not certain that the greater attenuation of incident radiation due to these changes is the sole reason for the decreased photosensitivity. Mediator exhaustion or a direct/indirect effect on the immune system may be more relevant. Photosensitization with 8-methoxypsoralen is also useful as a treatment for various photodermatoses,[7, 8, 9, 10] although, again, it is not clear whether the effect is due to hyperpigmentation or whether some more complex mechanism is involved. Whatever the mechanism, phototherapy appears to be a most useful addition to the prophylaxis available for certain photodermatoses.

II. PSORIASIS

Some psoriatics improve when their skin is exposed to solar radiation, and it is possible that this effect may partly account for the reported decreased

1. Dougherty, T. J., Grindey, G. B., Fiel, R., Weishaupt, K. R. and Boyle, D. G. (1975). Photoradiation therapy II. Cure of animal tumours with haematoporphyrin and light. *J. natn. Cancer Inst.* **55**, 115.
2. Dougherty, T., Boyle, D., Weishaupt, K., Gomer, C., Borcicky, D., Kaufman, J., Goldfarb, A. and Grindey, G. (1977). Phototherapy of Human Tumors. *In* 'Research in photobiology' (Ed. Castellani, Amleto), p. 435. Plenum Press, New York.
3. Van der Leun, J. C. and van Weelden, H. (1975). Light induced tolerance to light in the photodermatoses. *J. invest. Derm.* **64**, 280.
4. Frain-Bell, W. (1979). Dowling Oration. What is that thing called light? *Clin. exp. Derm.* **4**, 1.
5. Morrison, W. L., Momatz, K., Mosher, D. B. and Parrish, J. A. (1982). UV-B phototherapy in the prophylaxis of polymorphous light eruption. *Br. J. Derm.* **106**, 231.
6. Ramsay, C. A. (1977). Solar urticaria treatment by inducing tolerance to artificial irradiation and natural light. *Archs Derm.* **113**, 1122.
7. Gschnait, F., Hönigsman, H., Brenner, W., Fritsch, P. and Wolff, K. (1978). Induction of UV light tolerance by PUVA in patients with polymorphous light eruption. *Br. J. Derm.* **99**, 293.
8. Parrish, J. A., Levine, M. J., Morrison, W. L., Gonzalez, E. and Fitzpatrick, T. B. (1979). Comparison of PUVA and beta-carotene in treatment of polymorphous light eruption. *Br. J. Derm.* **100**, 187.
9. Holzle, E., Hoffman, C. and Plewig, G. (1980). PUVA treatment of solar urticaria and persistent light reaction. *Archs derm. Res.* **269**, 87.
10. Jansen, C. T., Karvonen, J. and Malminharju, T. (1982). PUVA therapy for polymorphous light eruptions: comparison of systemic methoxsalen and topical troxsalen regimens and evaluation of local protective mechanisms. *Acta Derm.* **62**, 317.

incidence of psoriasis as one nears the equator. However, there are psoriatic patients who react badly to the sun's rays and are liable to develop new patches of psoriasis or to show an exacerbation of pre-existing lesions. It would seem that the new psoriatic lesions developing in these circumstances represent a Koebner reaction following the induction of an erythema. Of 14 such cases of photosensitive psoriasis, seven were found to have an abnormal erythema action spectrum in that their minimal erythema dose was less than that for normal subjects using UV-B wavelengths.[1]

Occasionally psoriasis may occur in association with other photodermatoses, although the incidence of these cases (3%) is about the same as that for the frequency of psoriasis in the general population (2%). Of 429 cases with polymorphic light eruption, 12 (2·8%) were found to have psoriasis, and of 197 cases with photosensitivity dermatitis and the actinic reticuloid syndrome, five had psoriasis.[2]

On account of the beneficial action of ultraviolet radiation patients travel from Scandinavia and parts of northern Europe to the Dead Sea where the sunburn portion of the sun's spectrum (290–320 nm) is relatively weak, due to these wavelengths being filtered off by the mist resulting from the evaporation of the inflow of fresh water in to the Dead Sea which has no outlet.[3] The Dead Sea is 1500 feet below sea level and the increased depth of the atmosphere at this point will also presumably contribute to the filtration of these rays. It is suggested that these environmental factors allow prolonged exposures to the less harmful solar rays. The results from this form of therapy are good, but the relapse rate is high, and continued therapy is obviously difficult for those living away from the area.

However, UV-B rays in the range of 290–320 nm from artificial sources are particularly beneficial for psoriatics, whereas the longer UV-A waves are less effective unless given in impractically large doses.[4, 5, 6] It has now become apparent that broad band UV-B has to be given in a sufficient dosage to cause a minimal erythema in order to be effective. This means that each incremental dose has to be as near as possible to the tolerance level for an individual patient.

1. Frain-Bell, W. (1979). Dowling Oration. What is that thing called light? *Clin. exp. Derm.* **4**, 1.
2. Addo, H. A. and Frain-Bell, W. (1980). Unpublished data.
3. Montgomery, B. J. (1979). Bathing psoriasis in the Dead Sea. *J. Am. med. Ass.* **241**, 227.
4. Young, E. and Van der Leun, J. C. (1975). Treatment of psoriasis with long-wave ultraviolet light. *Dermatologica* **150**, 352.
5. Parrish, J. A. (1977). Treatment of psoriasis with longwave ultraviolet light. *Arch. Derm.* **113**, 1525.
6. Le Vine, M. J., White, H. A. D. and Parrish, J. A. (1979). Components of the Goeckerman Regimen. *J. invest. Derm.* **73**, 170.

The longer UV-A wavelengths become effective when the skin has been previously treated with photoactive substances such as tar or psoralens. The former was the supposed basis for the early Goeckerman regime.[1] The light sources originally employed for this treatment emitted both UV-B and UV-A. Thus in this earlier mode of treatment the psoriatic patches were affected by the UV-B rays, by the action of the tar, and by the combined effect of UV-A plus tar.[2] It is possible that the combined action of UV-A with UV-B also had an effect.[3]

There are differing views as to the relative efficacy of the various components of this form of combined therapy.[4] Some believe that UVR has little, if any, effect on psoriasis[5] and that the active agent in these earlier forms of treatment was the tar, or, in the case of the regime used by Ingram, dithranol.[5]

There are a number of possible explanations for these differing views. Thus if one is using tar, inadequate amounts of UV-A may be given because of the limiting effect on UV dosage of the erythema induced by the UV-B portion of the spectrum which was also being emitted from the radiation source.[4] As to whether UVR plus tar is more effective than UVR alone, evidence is now available to suggest that the UVR is the principal agent because if vaseline is substituted for tar there is very little difference in the therapeutic effect.[4] Although tar sensitization with UV-A may be effective, the accompanying phototoxic burning sensations make the treatment unacceptable.[6] Moreover, in the past it has not been appreciated that UV-B therapy has to be pushed to the limits of tolerance if it is to be effective.[7, 8, 9, 10]

1. Goeckermann, W. H. (1925). Treatment of psoriasis. *Northwest Med.* **24**, 229.
2. Fischer, T. (1977). Comparative treatment of psoriasis with UV-light. Trioxsalen plus UV-light and coal tar plus UV-light. *Acta derm-venereol. (Stockholm)* **57**, 345.
3. Stern, W. K. and Kihczak, G. (1974). Photobiology of psoriasis. Wavelength dependence. *Arch. Derm.* **109**, 502.
4. Le Vine, M. J., White, H. A. D. and Parrish, J. A. (1979). Components of the Coeckerman Regimen. *J. invest. Derm.* **73**, 170.
5. Young, E. (1972). Ultraviolet therapy of psoriasis. A critical study. *Br. J. Derm.* **87**, 379.
6. Parrish, J. A., Morison, W. L., Gonazalez, E., Krop, T., White, H. A. D. and Rosario, R. (1978). Therapy of psoriasis by tar photosensitization. *J. invest. Derm.* **70**, 111.
7. Van Weelden, H., Young, E. and Van der Leun, J. C. (1980). Therapy of Psoriasis: Comparison of Photochemotherapy and several Variants of Phototherapy. *Br. J. Derm.* **103**, 1.
8. Kenicer, K. J. A., Lakshmipathi, T., Addo, H. A., Johnson, B. E. and Frain-Bell, W. (1981). An assessment of the effect of conventional and of low irradiation dose photochemotherapy (PUVA) and of UV-B phototherapy in the treatment of psoriasis. Paper read to the Annual General Meeting of the British Association of Dermatologists, London.
9. Tronnier, H. and Heidbuchel, H. (1976). Zur Therapie der Psoriasis Vulgaris met Ultravioletten Strahlen. *Z. HautKrankh.* **51**, 405.
10. Pullmann, H., Wichmann, A. C. and Steigleder, G. K. (1978). Praktische Erfahrungen mit verschiedenen Phototherapieformen der Psoriasis—PUVA-, SUP-, Teer-UV-Therapie-. *Z. HautKrankh.* **53**, 641.

It is possible that the tar will only provide an additional effect to that resulting from the UV-B only when the latter is given in sub-erythema doses. Ingram[1] recommended the application of dithranol as an addition to the Goeckerman regime. In this instance dithranol appears to act in its own right on the proliferating epidermal cells (see page 2618) and not as a photoactive agent. Despite the advent of psoralen photochemotherapy, UV-A and UV-B, either alone or in combination with tar, and the use of topical dithranol, all remain important measures for the routine treatment of psoriasis.

III. CELLULAR MECHANISMS INVOLVED IN THE TREATMENT OF PSORIASIS WITH ULTRAVIOLET RADIATION

The molecular and cellular changes which precede and accompany the clearing of psoriatic lesions during UV-B therapy have not been clearly identified, but more is known concerning such changes in normal skin. However, there is no unequivocally determined causal relationship between them and the acute inflammatory sunburn response, or the premature ageing and tumour formation resulting from repeated exposures.

It is now generally accepted that DNA is the major molecular target for the biological action of shorter wavelength UVR, including UV-B. Because of its central role in the control of cellular, genetic, and metabolic action, any alteration in DNA structure would be expected to give rise to changes in these functions. *In vitro* studies have demonstrated that cellular manifestations of UV-induced damage such as inhibition of DNA synthesis, transformation, mutation, and cell death correlate with the incidence of a DNA specific photochemical lesion producing the thymine containing dimer.[2,3,4] These pyrimidine dimers have been isolated from UV-B irradiated mammalian skin[5] and their UV-induced formation in human epidermis is inferred from evidence of the dimer related, excision

1. Ingram, J. T. (1953). The approach to psoriasis. *Br. med. J.* **2**, 591.
2. Setlow, R. B. and Setlow, J. K. (1962). Evidence that ultraviolet-induced thymine dimers in DNA cause biological damage. *Proc. natn. Acad. Sci.* **48**, 1250.
3. Setlow, R. B., Swenson, P. A. and Carrier, W. L. (1963). Thymine dimers and inhibition of DNA synthesis by ultraviolet irradiation of cell. *Science* **142**, 1464.
4. Hart, R. W. and Setlow, R. B. (1975). Direct evidence that pyrimidine dimers in DNA result in neoplastic transformation. *In* 'Molecular Mechanisms for Repair of DNA', Part B (Eds Hanawalt, P. C. and Setlow, R. B.), p. 719. Plenum Press, New York.
5. Johnson, B. E. (1978). Formation of thymine containing dimers in skin exposed to ultraviolet radiation. *Bull. Cancer* **65**, 283.

repair process detected as unscheduled DNA synthesis following *in vivo*[1] UVR irradiation. The inhibition of normal DNA synthesis is a major feature of the general inhibition of macromolecular synthesis observed in UV-irradiated epidermis.[2] In a disease such as psoriasis, where the most prominent feature of the pathophysiology is seen as gross epidermal hyperproliferation, any treatment which inhibits DNA synthesis should be useful in terms of improving the lesions. Indeed, the ability of topically applied steroids to inhibit DNA synthesis in hairless mouse epidermis correlates well with their efficiency in clearing psoriatic plaques.[3] A comparative study of various treatment regimes, using the same model, confirmed the short-term inhibitory effect of UV-B on epidermal DNA synthesis.[4] It is possible, then, that the molecular and cellular events which form the basis of successful UV-B therapy for psoriasis may be simply defined as the formation of pyrimidine dimers in the DNA of the hyperproliferating cells. The inhibition of DNA synthesis in these cells results directly from this dimer formation and this causes a reduction of cell numbers in the hyperproliferative epidermis. However, such a concept is probably too simple and probably incorrect. There is no evidence of an acute depression in DNA synthesis in the epidermis of UV-B treated psoriatics.[5] The dose required to produce a significant inhibition of DNA synthesis in the epidermis may vary from two to 10 times the minimal erythema dose for normal skin.[4,6] Erythema may accompany the clearing of psoriatic lesions during UV treatment, and whilst the high dose regimen causing such erythema may be beneficial, it is not essential for successful therapy.[7] The skin's reaction which follows an exposure dose necessary to induce a 50% inhibition of epidermal DNA synthesis is that of a severe sunburn. Moreover, even when an initial 70% inhibition is achieved, recovery is evident by 24 h, followed by increased levels of synthesis associated with post UV damage hyperplasia.[1,8]

1. Epstein, W. L., Fukuyama, K. and Epstein, J. H. (1969). Early effects of ultraviolet light on DNA synthesis in human skin *in vivo*. *Archs Derm.* **100**, 84.
2. Epstein, J. H., Fukuyama, K. and Fye, K. (1970). Study of the influence of ultraviolet light on the mitotic cycle and macromolecule synthesis in hairless mouse epidermis. *Photochem. Photobiol.* **12**, 57.
3. Du Vivier, A., Bible, R., Jr, Mikuriya, R. K. and Stoughton, R. B. (1976). An animal model for screening drugs for antipsoriatic properties using hydroxyapatite to isolate DNA rapidly from epidermis. *Br. J. Derm.* **94**, 1.
4. Walter, J. F., Stoughton, R. B. and DeQuoy, P. R. (1978). Suppression of epidermal proliferation by ultraviolet light, coal tar, and anthralin. *Br. J. Derm.* **99**, 89.
5. Hodgson, C. H. and Hell, E. (1972). Ultraviolet radiation and psoriasis. *Archs Derm.* **106**, 498.
6. Johnson, B. E. (1978). Formation of thymine containing dimers in skin exposed to ultraviolet radiation. *Bull. Cancer* **65**, 283.
7. Parrish, J. A. and Jaenicke, K. F. (1981). Action Spectrum for Phototherapy of Psoriasis. *J. invest. Derm.* **76**, 359.
8. Cooke, A. and Johnson, B. E. (1977). Unpublished data.

Actively dividing cells are more sensitive to UVR and it is therefore possible that the hyperproliferative cell population in a psoriatic lesion has an enhanced susceptibility; cell division and DNA synthesis being inhibited at dose levels which would have little effect in normal skin. However, there is no experimental evidence to support such a supposition, and an increased sensitivity of the cells in the lesion could be counteracted by a greater attenuation of the incident UV-B by the abnormal thick horny layer. The direct, short term, inhibition of DNA synthesis induced by single exposures seems unlikely to play a major role in the clearing of psoriasis by UV-B radiation. In fact, the reverse would appear to be the case as UV-B induces raised levels of ornithine decarboxylase and polyamine growth factors[1] which are also characteristic of psoriatic epidermis.[2, 3] Glucocorticoids, however, not only cause inhibition of DNA synthesis and cell proliferation, but also decreased levels of ornithine decarboxylase and polyamines.[4]

The marked parakeratosis of psoriatic epidermis is a clear indication of incomplete autolysis resulting from an abnormality of keratinization which is a primary feature of the disease.[5] A return to more normal keratinization may be brought about by accelerated cell death in the superficial layers of psoriatic epidermis following UV-B induced changes in the nuclear protein of the differentiating cells.

It has been suggested earlier in this work (page 232, Vol. 1) that alteration of lysosomal membranes result in the loss of a coordinated release of hydrolytic enzymes in the region of the granular layer. There is a consequent absence of a granular layer and the formation of a parakeratotic stratum corneum. The action of UV-B on the membranes of the more superficial epidermal cells, like the cellular reaction of vitamin A, could result in release of these enzymes in the upper layers of the epidermis, and this would tend to reform a granular layer[6] (see also Vol. 1, p. 246).

1. Lowe, N., Verma, A. K. and Boutwell, R. K. (1978). Ultraviolet light induces epidermal ornithine decarboxylase activity. *J. invest. Derm.* **71**, 417.
2. Bohlen, P., Grove, J., Baya, M. F., Kock-Weser, J., Henry, M. H. and Grosshans, E. (1978). Skin polyamine levels in psoriasis: the effect of dithranol therapy. *Eur. J. clin. Invest.* **8**, 215.
3. Voorhees, J. J. (1979). Polyamines and psoriasis. *Archs Derm.* **115**, 943.
4. Russell, D. H., Combest, W. L., Duell, E. A., Stavriski, M. A., Anderson, T. F. and Voorhees, J. J. (1978). Glucocorticoid inhibits elevated polyamine biosynthesis in psoriasis. *J. invest. Derm.* **71**, 177.
5. Braun-Falco, O. (1977). The initial psoriatic lesion. *In* 'Psoriasis: Proceedings of the Second International Symposium' (Eds Farber, E. M. and Cox, A. J.), p. 1. Yorke Medical Books, New York.
6. Daniels, F., Jr and Johnson, B. E. (1974). Normal, physiologic and pathologic effects of solar radiation on the skin. *In* 'Sunlight and Man, normal and abnormal photobiologic responses' (Ed. Fitzpatrick, T. B.), p. 117. University of Tokyo Press, Tokyo.

The specific involvement of the cyclic nucleotides, c̄AMP and c̄GMP, in the modulation of normal cell proliferation and that in psoriatic epidermis is at present uncertain. From the available evidence it would seem that the experimentally observed changes of these compounds are secondary, rather than primary, phenomena. The original findings of a lowered cyclic AMP and a raised cyclic GMP in psoriatic epidermis[1] have not been confirmed.[2,3] Also it would appear that in the living animal an increased cell turnover may or may not be associated with increased cyclic AMP levels.[4] Moreover, the hyperplasia of UV-irradiated pig skin is associated with an increased cyclic AMP rather than the earlier induced inhibition of cell division and DNA synthesis.[5]

It has been suggested that the increase in c̄AMP follows the UV-induced synthesis of prostaglandin mediators which also regulate cyclic nucleotide metabolism.[6] In psoriasis increased levels of prostaglandins may result in a reduction of c̄AMP, and this could be due to a reduction of adenylate cyclase activity.[7] Prostaglandins may have a more central role in the pathology and treatment of psoriasis. Horrobin[8] suggests that a failure in prostaglandin E synthesis is the basic defect which leads to a loss of thromboxane A2 feedback control of the inflammatory process. The UV-B induced increase of prostaglandin synthetase activity[9] might counteract this failure of prostaglandin formation.

1. Voorhees, J. J., Kelsey, W., Staviski, M. A., Smith, E., Duell, E. A., Haddox, M. and Goldberg, N. (1973). Increased cyclic GMP and decreased cyclic AMP levels in the rapidly proliferating epithelium of psoriasis. In 'The role of cyclic nucleotides in carcinogenesis' (Eds Shultz, J. and Gretzner, H. G.), Vol. 6, p. 325. Academic Press, Orlando, New York and London.

2. Harkonen, M., Hopsu–Havu, V. K. and Raji, K. (1974). Cyclic adenosine monophosphate, adenyl cyclase and cyclic nucleotide phosphodiesterase in psoriatic epidermis. Acta derm-venereol. **54**, 13.

3. Yoshikawa, K., Adachi, K., Halprin, K. M. and Levine, V. (1975). Is the cyclic AMP in psoriatic epidermis low? Br. J. Derm. **93**, 253.

4. Adachi, K. (1977). Epidermal cyclic AMP system and its possible role in proliferation and differentiation. In 'Biochemistry of Cutaneous Epidermal Differentiation' (Eds Seiji, M. and Bernstein, I. A.), p. 288. University Park Press, Baltimore.

5. Halprin, K. M. (1976). Cyclic nucleotides and epidermal cell proliferation. J. invest. Derm. **66**, 339.

6. Adachi, K., Yoshikawa, K., Halprin, K. M. and Levine, V. (1975). Prostaglandins and cyclic AMP in epidermis. Br. J. Derm. **92**, 381.

7. Aso, K., Orenberg, E. K. and Farber, E. M. (1975). Reduced epidermal cyclic AMP accumulation following prostaglandin stimulation: its possible role in the pathophysiology of psoriasis. J. invest. Derm. **65**, 375.

8. Horrobin, D. F. (1978). 'Prostaglandins: physiology, pharmacology and clinical significance'. Churchill Livingstone, Edinburgh.

9. Black, A. K., Greaves, M. W., Hensby, C. M. and Plummer, N. A. (1978). Increased prostaglandins E$_2$ and F$_2$ in human skin at 6 and 24 h after ultraviolet B irradiation (290–320 nm). Br. J. clin. Pharmac. **5**, 431.

A. T Lymphocyte Changes

The difficulties in defining mechanisms for UV-B therapy are compounded by recent findings of significant changes in the immunological status of mice in UV-B carcinogenesis experiments.[1, 2] A single exposure is sufficient to induce "suppressor" T lymphocyte formation in these animals. Whether or not this kind of lymphocyte behaviour occurs in man exposed to UV-B phototherapy is not known. However, changes in T cell function as indicated by decreased E rosette forming cells in the peripheral blood after a single whole-body erythema-producing exposure have been reported.[3] T cell function is defective in active psoriasis,[4] but appears to approach normal levels following successful treatment. The initial decrease in T cell activity due to UV-B treatment may result in a rebound T cell increase, just as epidermal hyperplasia follows an initial mitotic inhibitory phase. If the immune system should play a major part in the pathogenesis of psoriasis,[5] then UV-B has been shown to be capable of producing significant changes in this system.

IV. COAL TAR DERIVATIVES

The cellular mechanisms involved in the clearing of psoriatic lesions following the topical use of tar preparations are complex. Within 24 h of the topical application of crude coal tar to psoriatic lesions there was a decrease in mitotic activity but this was not associated with any change in the transitional zone.[6] However, after 14 days there was a marked reduction in mitotic activity and evidence of the formation of a granular layer.

The tail scale of the mouse is formed without a granular layer and has features similar to a psoriatic plaque. Following the topical application of crude coal tar fractions Wrench and Britten demonstrated the formation

1. Spellman, C. W. and Danes, R. A. (1977). Modification of immunological potential by ultraviolet radiation. II. Generation of suppressor cells in short-term UV-irradiated mice. *Transplantation* **24**, 120.
2. Kripke, M. L. (1977). Ultraviolet radiation and tumor immunity. *J. reticuloendothel. Soc.* **22**, 217.
3. Morison, W. L., Parrish, J. A., Bloch, K. J. and Krugler, I. (1979). *In vivo* effect of UV-B on lymphocyte function. *Br. J. Derm.* **101**, 513.
4. Glinski, W., Obalek, S., Langner, A., Jablonska, S. and Haftek, M. (1978). Defective function of T lymphocytes in psoriasis. *J. invest. Derm.* **70**, 195.
5. Cormane, R. H., Hunyadi, J. and Hamerlinck, P. (1975). Psoriasis: autoimmune disease. *Z. HautKrankh.* **50**, 971.
6. Fry, L. and McMinn, R. M. H. (1968). The action of themotherapeutic agents on psoriatic epidermis. *Br. J. Derm.* **80**, 373.

of a granular layer and a change in keratinization after 3 weeks' treatment.[1] Normal human skin, either intact or with increased mitotic activity induced by stripping, failed to show the mitotic inhibition[2] reported in psoriatic skin by Fry and McMinn.

In normal hairless mice and in mice that are deficient of essential fatty acids, some depression of epidermal DNA synthesis could be demonstrated within 1 to 4 h after the application of crude coal tar.[3] Also a partially refined tar product produced a reduction in mitotic activity.[4]

The covalent binding of polycyclic hydrocarbons, such as benzpyrene or of their activated metabolites into the DNA of dividing cells may cause an inhibition of cell proliferation.[5] This binding also represents the initial stage of chemical carcinogenesis which is evidenced by the induction of epitheliomata in mice following repeated application of tar[6] and by epidermal proliferation in the hairless hamster.[7]

In the latter animal therefore, tar causes increased mitotic activity and not a reduction. The mutagenicity of coal tar preparations used in the treatment of psoriasis has also been demonstrated.[8]

A. Coal Tar and UVR

The effects of UVR used in conjunction with topical tar are wavelength dependent. In hairless mouse epidermis, inhibition of DNA synthesis by UV-B, and to a lesser extent by UV-C, appears to be additive[4] and due to a synergistic effect. The combination of UV-A and tar significantly increases the inhibition of DNA synthesis and mitotic activity due to tar alone. The UV-A radiation alone has no action on either DNA synthesis

1. Wrench, R. and Britten, A. Z. (1975). Evaluation of coal tar fractions for use in psoriasiform diseases using the mouse tail test. III. High boiling tar oil acids. *Br. J. Derm.* **93**, 67.
2. Fisher, L. B. and Maibach, H. I. (1973). Topical antipsoriatic agents and epidermal mitosis in man. *Archs Derm.* **108**, 374.
3. Stoughton, R. B. De Quoy, P. and Walter, J. F. (1978). Crude coal tar plus near ultraviolet light suppresses DNA synthesis in epidermis. *Archs Derm.* **114**, 43.
4. Walter, J. F., Stoughton, R. B. and De Quoy, P. R. (1978). Suppression of epidermal proliferation by ultraviolet light, coal tar and anthralin. *Br. J. Derm.* **99**, 89.
5. Miller, E. C. and Miller, J. A. (1976). In 'Chemical Carcinogens'. ACS Monograph 173 (Ed. Searle, C. E.), p. 737. American Chemical Society, Washington, D.C.
6. Shabad, L. M., Khesina, A., Jr, Linnik, A. B. and Serkovskaya, G. S. (1970). Possible carcinogenic hazards of several tars and of locacorten-tar ointment (spectro-fluorescent investigations and experiments in animals). *Int. J. Cancer* **6**, 314.
7. Foreman, M. I., Picton, W., Lukowiecki, G. A. and Clark, C. (1979). The effect of topical crude coal tar treatment on unstimulated hairless hamster skin. *Br. J. Derm.* **100**, 707.
8. Saperstein, M. D. and Wheeler, A. D. (1979). Mutagenicity of coal tar preparations used in the treatment of psoriasis. *Toxicol. Letters* **3**, 325.

or mitotic activity,[1, 2] and its action in combination with tar appears to be due to the photosensitizing action of the tar. The photosensitizing components of coal tar include in decreasing order of phototoxic potential, anthracene, fluoranthrene, phenanthrene, benzpyrene and acridine.[3] It is suggested that the antipsoriatic efficacy of various tar products may vary directly with their photosensitizing potential. Anthracene itself does not inhibit DNA synthesis in hairless mouse epidermis.[4]

The mechanism of coal tar photosensitization is not clear. When the organic constituents of the preparations are bound covalently to DNA, the binding may be increased by exposure to UV-A. Cross links would be induced in this manner.[5] Anthracene forms cross links in double stranded DNA when exposed to UV-A[6] and the photosensitized, short-term inhibition of DNA synthesis obtained may be explained by this action. However, in terms of the overall changes in psoriatic epidermis brought about by coal tar and UVR, the concentration of substances such as anthracene within lysosomes and the subsequent release of hydrolytic enzymes by the photosensitized damage to the membranes[7] may be equally, if not more, important.

The carcinogenic action of crude coal tar alone is undoubted, and the combination of crude coal tar and UVR resulted in a marked increase in tumour incidence in mouse ear skin.[8] There is an association between the photodynamic and carcinogenic actions of polycyclic hydrocarbons.[9] However, repeated anthracene photosensitization does not result in tumourogenesis in hairless mouse skin.[10]

1. Walter, J. P., Stoughton, R. B. and De Quoy, P. R. (1978). Suppression of epidermal proliferation by ultraviolet light, coal tar and anthralin. *Br. J. Derm.* **99**, 89.
2. Stoughton, R. B., De Quoy, P. R. and Walter, J. F. (1978). Crude coal tar plus near ultraviolet light suppresses DNA synthesis in epidermis. *Archs Derm.* **114**, 43.
3. Kaidbey, K. H. and Kligman, A. M. (1977). Clinical and histological study of coal tar phototoxicity in humans. *Archs Derm.* **113**, 592.
4. Walter, J. F. and De Quoy, P. R. (1978). Anthracene with near ultraviolet light inhibiting epidermal proliferation. *Archs Derm.* **114**, 1463.
5. Pathak, M. A. and Biswas, R. K. (1977). Skin photosensitization and DNA cross-linking ability of photochemotherapeutic agents. *J. invest. Derm.* **68**, 236.
6. Blackburn, G. M., Buckingham, J., Fenwick, R. G., Taussig, P. E. and Thompson, M. H. (1973). Photochemical binding of anthracene and other aromatic hydrocarbons to deoxyribonucleic acid with attendant loss of tritium. *J. chem. Soc. (PI)* **1**, 2809.
7. Allison, A. C., Magnus, I. A. and Young, M. R. (1966). Role of lysosomes and cell membranes in photosensitization. *Nature* **209**, 874.
8. Urbach, F. (1959). Modification of ultraviolet carcinogenesis by photoactive agents. *J. invest Derm.* **32**, 373.
9. Epstein, S. S., Small, M., Falk, H. L. and Mantel, N. (1964). On the association between photodynamic and carcinogenic activities in polycyclic compounds. *Cancer Res.* **24**, 855.
10. Forbes, P. D., Davies, R. E. and Urbach, F. (1976). Phototoxicity and photocarcinogenesis comparative effects of anthracene and 8-methoxypsoralen in the skin of mice. *Food cosmet. Toxicol.* **14**, 303.

In contradiction to the use of tar alone, there is some evidence for an increased incidence of skin carcinoma in patients with psoriasis treated with topical tar and artificial ultraviolet radiation.[1]

V. ANTHRALIN (DITHRANOL)

The molecular structure and stereochemistry of anthralin and similar polycyclic hydrocarbons are such that they form an intercalated complex with DNA *in vitro*.[2] Such binding causes inhibition of DNA synthesis in guinea-pig epidermis[3] and a decrease in both DNA synthesis and mitotic index in hairless mouse epidermis[4, 5] within hours of topical application.

Anthralin treatment of psoriasis results in a demonstrable decrease in epidermal mitosis[6, 7, 8] and DNA synthesis.[9, 10] However, the rapid changes obtained with experimental animals are not seen in psoriatic lesions treated with anthralin. Anthralin does not induce a granular layer in the parakeratotic scale areas of mouse tail epidermis.[11] Controversy remains concerning the relative importance of changes in respiratory enzyme activity in the region of the regenerating granular layer, the decrease in parakeratosis, and the direct effects of DNA binding on the inhibition of cell proliferation.[12, 13]

1. Stern, R. S., Zieler, S. and Parrish, J. A. (1980). Skin carcinoma in patients with psoriasis treated with topical tar and artificial ultraviolet radiation. *Lancet* **i**, 732.
2. Swanbeck, G. and Thyresson, N. (1965). Interaction between dithranol and nucleic acids. *Acta derm-venereol.* **45**, 344.
3. Swanbeck, G. and Liden, S. (1966). The inhibitory effect of dithranol (anthralin) on DNA synthesis. *Acta derm-venereol.* **46**, 228.
4. Fisher, L. B. and Maibach, H. I. (1975). The effect of anthralin and its derivatives on epidermal cell kinetics. *J. invest. Derm.* **64**, 338.
5. Walter, J. F., Stoughton, R. B. and De Quoy, P. B. (1978). Suppression of epidermal proliferation by ultraviolet light, coal tar, and anthralin. *Br. J. Derm.* **99**, 89.
6. Krebs, A. and Schaltegger, H. (1968). Experimentelle Untersuchungenüber den Wirkungsmechanismus von Chrysarobin and Dithranol bei Psoriasis. *Dermatologica* **131**, 1.
7. Fry, L. and McMinn, R. M. H. (1968). The action of chemotherapeutic agents on psoriatic epidermis. *Br. J. Derm.* **80**, 373.
8. Baxter, D. L. and Stoughton, R. B. (1970). Mitotic index of psoriatic lesions treated with anthralin, glucocorticosteroid and occlusion only. *J. invest. Derm.* **54**, 410.
9. Steigleder, G. K., Schumann, H. and Lennartz, K. J. (1973). Authradiographic *in vitro* examination of psoriatic skin before, during, and after dithranol treatment. *ARCH. Derm. Forsch.* **246**, 231.
10. Liden, S. and Michalsson, G. (1974). Dithranol (anthralin) in psoriasis. The effect on DNA synthesis, granular layer and parakeratosis. *Br. J. Derm.* **91**, 447.
11. Wrench, R. and Britten, A. Z. (1975). Evaluation of dithranol and a 'synthetic tar' as antipsoriatic treatments using the mouse tail test. *Br. J. Derm.* **93**, 75.
12. Braun-Falco, O., Burg, G. and Schoefinius, H. H. (1971). Über die Wirkung von Dithranol (Cignolin) bei Psoriasis Vulgaris. *Arch. Derm. Forsch.* **241**, 217.
13. Cox, A. J. and Watson, W. (1972). Histological variations in lesions of psoriasis. *Archs Derm.* **106**, 503.

Whatever cellular mechanism underlies the therapeutic effect of anthralin, inhibition of epidermal DNA synthesis by this compound is not altered by UV-A, and its effects in conjunction with UV-B are additive rather than due to photosensitization.[1] During complex treatment regimens in which the major therapeutic agent is anthralin, cutaneous polyamine levels are seen to decrease, and it is suggested that this might represent the initial step in the reduction of cellular proliferation.[2]

1. Walter, J. P., Stoughton, R. B. and De Quoy, P. R. (1978). Suppression of epidermal proliferation by ultraviolet light, coal tar, and anthralin. *Br. J. Derm.* **99**, 89.
2. Proctor, M. S., Wilkinson, D. I., Orenberg, E. K. and Farber, E. (1979). Lowered cutaneous and urinary levels of polyamines with clinical improvement in treated psoriasis. *Archs Derm.* **115**, 945.

Photochemotherapy and its Complications

84

B. E. JOHNSON

Department of Dermatology, University of Dundee,
Ninewells Hospital, Dundee, Scotland

I. PHOTOCHEMOTHERAPY OF SKIN DISEASES

A. Psoriasis

The use of plant extracts containing psoralens to repigment leucodermic skin dates back to early times. Reference to the treatment of vitiligo with black seeds from the plant called *Bavachee* or *Vasuchika*, which has now been identified as *Psoralea corylifolia*, can be found in the Ebers Papyrus (c. 1550 BC), the Atharva Veda (c. 1400 BC), and other Indian and

PHYSIOL. PATHOPHYSIOL. OF SKIN Vol. 8
ISBN 0 12 380608 9

Buddhist medical literature (c. AD 200); Chinese manuscripts from the Sung period (c. AD 700) also mention the plant.[1]

Ammi majus, originally called "Aatrillal" is a weed found growing intensively in the Nile Valley and has been used for centuries in Egypt together with sunlight for the treatment of leucoderma. Since about 1947 pharmacological studies of the Aatrillal powder demonstrated that its active components were 8-methoxypsoralen, 8-isoamylenoxypsoralen, and 5-methoxypsoralen.[2,3] They were given the trade names of ammoidin, ammidin, and majudin, and were subsequently found to be identical with previously isolated xanthotoxin, imperatin, and bergapten. The oral and/or topical administration of these psoralens was found to be at least partly effective in the treatment of vitiligo.[4,5,6] Later tripsoralen was synthesized and has proved useful as a topical preparation. During the study of the action of psoralens on the skin in association with UVR it was noted that there was inhibition of cellular DNA synthesis.[7] The possibility that this action could affect the increased epidermal cell proliferation in psoriasis[8] stimulated further work.[9] More recently confirmation was obtained for clinical improvement in psoriasis following the topical application of psoralens plus exposure to UV-A.[10,11,12,13] However, it was not until the psoralen was administered orally that the full potential for psoralen photochemotherapy was appreciated.[14]

1. Benedetto, A. V. (1977). The psoralens. An historical perspective. *Cutis* **20**, 469.
2. Fahmy, I. R. and Abu-Shady, H. (1947). Ammi majus Linn: pharmacognostical study and isolation of crystalline constituent, ammoidin. *G.J. Pharm. Pharmacol.* **20**, 281.
3. Fahmy, I. R. and Abu–Shady, H. (1948). The isolation and properties of ammoidin, ammidin, and majudin and their effect in the treatment of leucoderma. *G.J. Pharm. Pharmacol.* **21**, 449.
4. El Mofty, A. M. (1968). 'Witiligo and Psoralens', p. 1. Pergamon Press, Oxford.
5. Jarrett, A. and Szabo, G. (1956). The pathological varieties of vitiligo and their response to treatment with meladinine. *Br. J. Derm.* **68**, 313.
6. Lerner, A. B., Denton, C. R. and Fitzpatrick, T. B. (1953). Clinical and experimental studies with 8-MOP in vitiligo. *J. invest. Derm.* **20**, 299.
7. Walter, J. F., Voorhees, J. J., Kelsey, W. H. and Duell, E. A. (1973). Psoralen plus black light inhibits epidermal DNA synthesis. *Archs Derm.* **107**, 861.
8. Weinstein, G. C. and Frost, P. (1968). Abnormal cell proliferation in psoriasis. *J. invest. Derm.* **50**, 254.
9. Walter, J. F. and Voorhees, J. J. (1973). Psoriasis improved by psoralen plus black light. *Acta derm-veneriol. (Stockholm)* **53**, 469.
10. Tronnier, H. and Schule, D. (1973). Zur dermatologischen Therapie von Dermatosen mit langwelligen UV nach Photosensibilerung der Haut mit Methoxsalen Erste Ergebnisse bei der Psoriasis Vulgaris. *Z. Haut GeschlechtsKrankh.* **48**, 385.
11. Weber, G. (1973). Technik und Ergebnisse der Blacklight-Bestrahlung bei Psoriatikern, Vortrag 101 Tg. Vereinig Rhein-Westfal. Dermatologen, Wuppertal.
12. Weber, G. (1974). Combined 8-MOP and black light therapy of psoriasis. Technique and Results. *Br. J. Derm.* **90**, 317.
13. Mortazawi, S. A. M. and Oberste–Lehn, H. (1973). Lichtsensibilistoren und ihre therapeutischen Fanigheiten, X. *Z. Haut GeschlechtsKrankh.* **48**, 1.
14. Parrish, J. A. Fitzpatrick, T. B., Tanebaum, K. and Pathak, M. A. (1974). Photochemotherapy of psoriasis with oral methoxsalen and longwave ultraviolet light. *New Engl. J. Med.* **291**, 1207.

The UV-A interactions with psoralens such as 8-methoxypsoralen (8-MOP) in biological materials[1, 2, 3] qualify as a special case which was discussed in some detail in the sections on photosensitization and phototoxicity (see page 2548). Here, we will deal only with major points as they relate specifically to the cellular mechanisms involved in the various forms of psoralen photochemotherapy.

Although an oxygen dependent photo-conjugation of 8-MOP with protein may occur[4, 5] with consequent damage to ribosomes and biomembranes as part of the overall photosensitized reaction,[6, 7] the major photobiologic effects of the psoralens do not require oxygen. They are mediated primarily through the UV-A induced covalent binding to chromosomal DNA producing monofunctional photoadducts and bifunctional interstrand cross links with pyrimidine bases. It would appear that the thymines in the DNA double helix are particularly involved in this process. These photoproducts have been detected in isolated DNA, micro-organisms, mammalian cells in culture, and mammalian epidermis irradiated *in vivo*.[8, 9, 10] At cellular levels the biological consequences of psoralen binding are similar to those of thymine dimer formation by UV-B in that there is an early inhibition of DNA synthesis and cell replication, induction of mutation, and cell death. Although the photochemical lesions may be repaired, the processes involved in human

1. Musajo, L. and Rodighiero, G. (1972). Mode of photosensitizing action of furocoumarins. *In* 'Photophysiology', Vol. VII (Ed. Giese, A.), pp. 115–147. Academic Press, Orlando, New York and London.
2. Scott, B. R., Pathak, M. A. and Mohn, G. R. (1976). Molecular and genetic basis of furocoumarin reactions. *Mutation Res.* **39**, 29.
3. Song, P. A. and Tapley, J. J., Jr (1979). Photochemistry and photobiology of psoralens. *Photochem. Photobiol.* **29**, 1177.
4. Mizuno, N., Tsuneishi, S., Matsuhashi, S., Kimura, S., Fuzimura, Y. and Ushizima, T. (1974). Some aspects on the action mechanism of 8-methoxypsoralen photosensitization. *In* 'Sunlight and Man' (Ed. Fitzpatrick, T. B.), pp. 389–409. University of Tokyo Press, Tokyo.
5. Yoshikawa, K., Mori, N., Sakakibara, S., Mizuno, N. and Song, P. S. (1979). Photo-conjugation of 8-methosypsoralen with proteins. *Photochem. Photobiol.* **29**, 1127.
6. Meffert, H., Diezel, M., Gunther, W. and Sonnichsen, N. (1976). Fotochemotherapie der Psoriasis mit 8-methoxypsoralen und UVA. 11. Bindung des Fotosensibilisators an Protein. *Derm. Mschr.* **162**, 887.
7. Wennersten, G. (1979). Membrane damage caused by 8-MOP and UVA treatment of cultivated cells. *Acta derm-venereol.* **39**, 21.
8. Musajo, L. and Rodighiero, G. (1972). Photo-C,-cyclo-addition reactions to the nucleic acids. *In* 'Research Progress in Organic, Biological and Medicinal Chemistry' (Eds Gallo, U. and Santamaria, L.), Vol. 3, pt 1, pp. 155–182. North Holland Publishing Company, Amsterdam.
9. Pathak, M. A., Kramer, D. M. and Fitzpatrick, T. B. (1974). Photobiology and photochemistry of furocoumarins (psoralens). *In* 'Sunlight and Man' (Ed. Fitzpatrick, T. B.), pp. 335–358. University of Tokyo Press, Tokyo.
10. Pathak, M. A., Fitzpatrick, T. B., Parrish, J. A. and Biswas, R. (1976). Photochemotherapeutic, photobiological and photochemical properties of psoralens. *In* 'Research in Photobiology' (Ed. Castellani, A.), pp. 267–281. Plenum Press, New York.

skin do not appear to include unscheduled DNA synthesis as demonstrated by 3H-thymidine labelling.[1,2]

Attempts to determine the relative contributions of monoadducts and cross links to the various effects observed in bacteria[3,4,5] and mammalian cells[6,7] have produced equivocal results. Psoralens, having a molecular structure which restricts the photochemical products to the monoadduct form, such as angelicin and 3-carbethoxypsoralen and the bifunctional psoralens such as 8-methoxypsoralen, with two stage irradiation, have been used to investigate the relative importance of monoadducts and cross links. It is apparent that both types of lesion contribute to the inhibitory, mutagenic and lethal effects. However, cross linking which constitutes only some 10% of the total photoadduct produced with 8-methoxypsoralen may be the most efficient in causing these changes.

Increased levels of chromosome aberrations may also result from both forms of psoralen photoadduct.[7] Sister chromatid exchange (SCE) appears to be a particularly sensitive indicator of this type of DNA damage.[8,9] Increased levels of SCEs are detected in human lymphocytes exposed *in vitro* to relatively low concentrations of 8-methoxypsoralen $(0.02-20\ \mu g/ml)$ using exposure doses of UV-A in the range of $1\ J/cm^{-2}$. Concentrations of 8-methoxypsoralen in excess of $0.1\ \mu g/ml$ are required to demonstrate a significant photosensitized inhibition of phyto-

1. Bishop, S. C. (1979). DNA repair synthesis in human skin exposed to ultraviolet radiation used in PUVA (psoralen and UV-A) therapy for psoriasis. *Br. J. Derm.* **101**, 399.
2. Bioulac, P., Denechaud, M., Dubuisson, L., Doutre, M. S., Ducassou, D. and Beylot, C. (1980). Unscheduled DNA synthesis in psoriatic skin after ultraviolet irradiation and the effects of a combined treatment with 8-methoxypsoralen and longwave ultraviolet radiation: a clinical study. *Br. J. Derm.* **102**, 285.
3. Seki, T., Nozu, K. and Kondo, S. (1978). Differential causes of mutation and killing in *Escherichia coli*: monoadducts and cross links. *Photochem. Photobiol.* **27**, 19.
4. Bridges, B. A., Mottershead, R. P. and Knowles, A. (1979). Mutation induction and killing of *Escherichia coli* by DNA adducts and cross links: a photobiological study with 8-methoxypsoralen. *Chem. Biol. Interact.* **27**, 221.
5. Dall'Acqua, F., Bordin, F., Vedaldi, D., Becher, M. and Rodighiero, G. (1979). Photochemical interaction between xanthyletine and DNA. *Photochem. Photobiol.* **28**, 283.
6. Coppey, J., Averbeck, D. and Moreno, G. (1979). Herpes virus production in monkey kidney and human skin cells treated with angelicin or 8-methoxypsoralen plus 365 nm light. *Photochem. Photobiol.* **29**, 797.
7. Ashwood-Smith, M. J., Grant, E. L., Heddle, J. A. and Friedman, G. B. (1977). Chromosome damage in Chinese hamster cells sensitized to near ultraviolet light by psoralen and angelicin. *Mut. Res.* **43**, 377.
8. Latt, S. A. (1974). Sister chromatid exchanges, indices of human chromosome damage and repair: detection by fluorescence and induction by Mitomycin. *Proc. nat. Acad. Sci. U.S.A.* **71**, 3162.
9. Mourelatos, D., Faed, M. J. W. and Johnson, B. E. (1977). Sister chromatid exchanges in human lymphocytes exposed to 8-methoxypsoralen and longwave UV radiation prior to incorporation of Bromo-deoxyuridine. *Experientia* **33**, 1091.

haemagglutinin-stimulated DNA synthesis in lymphocytes,[1,2] but there is an inverse relationship between 8-methoxypsoralen concentration (down to $0.02\,\mu g/ml$) and UV-A dose for the inhibition of growing cultures of 373 (Swiss albino) cells.[3] Similar results were obtained with other cell lines such as Ehrlich ascites[4] and Chinese hamster,[5] and also with other psoralens such as trimethylpsoralen.[4] The inhibition of DNA synthesis in human skin fibroblasts by 8-methoxypsoralen photosensitization *in vitro* fits into this general pattern.[6,7,8]

Trimethylpsoralen at a final concentration of $2\,\mu M$ and UV-A at approximately $0.2\,J/cm^{-2}$ produced an average 70% inhibition of DNA synthesis in mouse epidermis within 4 h of *in vitro* irradiation.[9] Topical applications of 1% 8-methoxypsoralen in acetone and exposure to UV-A *in vivo* produced similar results in normal hairless mouse epidermis[10] and a greater degree of inhibition was demonstrated in UV-C induced hyperproliferative epidermis.[11] As with the inhibition of epidermal DNA synthesis by UV-B, there is recovery of activity which probably represents the several hyperproliferative responses when tissue is damaged. The latent period for this delayed stimulation of DNA synthesis varies with the exposure dose, but for a given degree of initial inhibition it appears to be longer in the case of psoralen photosensitization. Unlike the reaction to UV-B, the inhibition of DNA synthesis is not accompanied by an early inhibition of RNA and protein synthesis.[10] In guinea-pigs an

1. Scherer, R., Kern, B. and Braun-Falco, O. (1977). The human peripheral lymphocyte: a model system for studying the combined effect of psoralen plus black light. *Klin. Wschr.* **55**, 137.
2. Kruger, J. P., Christophers, E. and Schlaak, M. (1978). Dose effects of 8-methoxypsoralen and UV-A in cultured human lymphocytes. *Br. J. Derm.* **98**, 141.
3. Pohl, J. and Christophers, E. (1979). Dose effects of 8-methoxypsoralen and long wave UV-light in 3T3 cells: evaluation of a phototoxic index. *Experientia* **35**, 247.
4. Musajo, L., Visentini, P., Baccichetti, F. and Razzi, M. A. (1967). Photoinactivation of Ehrlich ascites tumour cells *in vitro* obtained with skin-photosensitizing furocoumarins. *Experientia* **23**, 335.
5. Ben-Hur, E. and Elkind, M. M. (1973). Psoralen plus near ultraviolet light inactivation of cultured Chinese hamster cells and its relation to DNA cross links. *Mut. Res.* **18**, 315.
6. Baden, H. P., Parrington, J. M., Delhanty, J. D. A. and Pathak, M. A. (1972). DNA synthesis in normal and xeroderma pigmentosum fibroblasts following treatment with 8-methoxypsoralen and long-wave UV light. *Biochim. Biophys. Acta* **262**, 247.
7. Pohl, J. and Christophers, E. (1978). Photoinactivation of cultured skin fibroblasts by sublethal doses of 8-methoxypsoralen and longwave ultraviolet light. *J. invest. Derm.* **71**, 316.
8. Pohl, J. and Christophers, E. (1979). Photoinactivation of skin fibroblasts by fractionated treatment with 8-methoxypsoralen and UVA. *J. invest. Derm.* **73**, 176.
9. Walter, J. F., Voorhees, J. J., Kelsey, W. H. and Duell, E. A. (1973). Psoralen plus black light inhibits epidermal DNA synthesis. *Arch. Derm.* **107**, 861.
10. Epstein, J. H. and Fukuyama, K. (1975). Effects of 8-methoxypsoralen induced phototoxic effects on mammalian epidermal macromolecule synthesis *in vivo*. *Photochem. Photobiol.* **21**, 325.
11. Walter, J. F. and DeQuoy, P. R. (1978). Anthracene with near ultraviolet light inhibiting epidermal proliferation. *Arch. Derm.* **114**, 1463.

average inhibition of DNA synthesis of around 70% is obtained with topical 0·15% 8-methoxypsoralen applied 1 h before exposure to 2·4 or 6 J/cm^{-2} of UV-A.[1]

When hairless mice are treated with sufficient oral 8-methoxypsoralen to elicit a UV-A induced oedematous skin reaction, epidermal DNA synthesis is not inhibited unless the epidermis is previously made hyperproliferative by tape stripping.[2] It is suggested that such an hyperproliferative skin might provide a model for studies of mechanisms involved in PUVA therapy. A similar model is provided by the 8-methoxypsoralen photosensitized inhibition of hair growth in mouse skin stimulated by plucking.[3] However, as with the other treatment modalities, the inhibition of epidermal DNA synthesis by PUVA has not been proven to be the primary mechanisms involved. Metabolic[4, 5] and pharmacokinetic[6, 7, 8, 9, 10] studies of oral 8-methoxypsoralen effects have shown that most of the chemical is excreted in the urine within 12 h as its metabolites, although there is little evidence for its metabolism in the kidney, liver or epidermis. Trimethylpsoralen on the other hand is demonstrably metabolized by liver microsomes,[4] and this may explain why this compound is less effective than 8-methoxypsoralen when given orally but has similar effects if used topically. Depending on the type of preparation, maximum plasma 8-methoxypsoralen levels in the majority of patients are attained 1–2 h after oral administration. The peak of skin photosensitivity appears to coincide with the peak in plasma con-

1. Pullman, H., Galosi, A., Jakobeit, C. and Steigleder, G. K. (1980). Effects of selective ultraviolet phototherapy (SUP) and local PUVA treatment on DNA synthesis in guinea pig skin. *Arch. derm. Res.* **267**, 37.

2. Fritsch, P. O., Gschnait, P., Kaaserer, G., Brenner, W., Chaikittisilpa, S., Ronigsmann, H. and Wolff, K. (1979). PUVA suppresses the proliferative stimulus produced by stripping on hairless mice. *J. invest. Derm.* **73**, 188.

3. Johnson (1981). Unpublished data.

4. Mandula, B. B. and Pathak, M. A. (1978). Metabolic reactions *in vitro* of psoralens with liver and epidermis. *Biochem. Pharmac.* **28**, 127.

5. Stevenson, I. H. (1981). Unpublished data.

6. Thune, P. and Volden, G. (1977). Photochemotherapy of psoriasis with relevance to 8-methoxypsoralen plasma level at low intensity irradiation. *Acta derm-venereol. (Stockholm)* **57**, 351.

7. Steiner, I., Prey, R., Gschnait, F., Washuttl, J. and Greiter, F. (1977). Serum level profiles of 8-methoxypsoralen after oral administration. *Arch. dem. Res.* **259**, 299.

8. Gazith, J., Schalla, W. and Schaefer, H. (1978). 8-methoxypsoralen-gas chromatographic determination and serum kinetics. *Archs derm. Res.* **263**, 215.

9. Hensby, C. N. (1978). The qualitative and quantitative analysis of 8-methoxypsoralen by HPLC-UV and GLC-MS. *Clin. Exp. Derm.* **3**, 355.

10. Stevenson, I. H., Kenicer, K. J. A., Johnson, B. E. and Frain-Bell, W. (1981). Plasma 8-methoxypsoralen concentrations in photochemotherapy of psorias. *Br. J. Derm.* **104**, 47.

centration.[1, 2, 3] The average range of peak plasma level varies from 0·1–0·8 $\mu g/ml$, and the dividing cells of psoriatic epidermis may well be exposed to 8-methoxypsoralen at this concentration at the time of irradiation. The 8-methoxypsoralen concentration and UV-A dose required to inhibit DNA synthesis *in vitro* appear to be attained during PUVA treatment in patients. However, neither I nor other authors have detected an early inhibition of DNA synthesis in PUVA-treated psoriatic epidermis.[4, 5, 6] A significant decrease in the labelling index of psoriatic lesions in PUVA-treated patients may be observed but only after four treatments. This, however, is not a consistent finding.

Histologic and ultrastructural studies of 8-methoxypsoralen or trimethylpsoralen-photosensitized skin have been used to examine the various degrees of phototoxic reaction obtained. The phototoxic reactions are similar to UV-induced changes but features such as the appearance of dyskeratotic (sunburn) cells in the epidermis, hyperkeratosis and glycogen deposition are delayed. Membrane damage to lysosomes and mitochondria was not detected.[7] With the exposure dose used in PUVA treatment, there is little change in either the epidermis or the dermis to indicate in which region of the skin the photobiologic effects first develop. Minimal epidermal intercellular oedema is apparent 24–72 h after exposure[8] but the most significant change is observed in the nuclei of the keratinocytes. Soon after PUVA therapy (24 h after exposure) there are pronounced irregularities in the nuclear envelope enlargement of both nucleus and nucleolus accompanied by a decrease in

1. Kligman, A. M. and Goldstein, F. D. (1973). Oral dosage in methoxsalen phototoxicity. *Archs Derm.* **107**, 548.
2. Pathak, M. A., Kramer, D. M. and Fitzpatrick, T. B. (1974). Photobiology and photochemistry of furocoumarins (psoralens). *In* 'Sunlight and Man' (Ed. Fitzpatrick, T. B.), pp. 335–368. Tokyo University Press, Tokyo.
3. Goldstein, D. P., Carter, D. M., Ljunggren, B. and Burkwolder, J. (1982). Minimal phototoxic doses and 8-MOP plasma levels in PUVA patients. *J. invest. Derm.* **78**, 429.
4. Hell, E., Hodgson, C. and Hanna, V. (1979). Psoralen photochemotherapy of psoriasis. *Br. J. Derm.* **101**, 293.
5. Hofmann, C., Landthaler, M., Plewig, G. and Braun-Falco, O. (1980). *In vivo* autoradiography and planimetry of epidermis in psoriatics under PUVA-therapy. *Archs derm. Res.* **267**, 61.
6. Goldberg, L. H., Cox, A. J. and Abel, E. A. (1980). The mitotic index in Psoriatic Plaques and their response to PUVA therapy. *Br. J. Derm.* **102**, 401.
7. Mizuno, N., Tsuneishi, S., Matsuhashi, S., Kimura, S., Fujimura, Y. and Ushijima, T. (1974). Some aspects on the action mechanism of 8-methoxypsoralen photosensitization. *In* 'Sunlight and Man' (Ed. Fitzpatrick, T. B.), pp. 389–409. Tokyo University Press, Tokyo.
8. Wolff, K., Gschnait, F., Honigsmann, H., Konrad, K. Stingl, G., Wolff-Schreiner, E. and Fritsch, P. (1977). Oral photochemotherapy. Results, follow up and pathology. *In* 'Psoriasis, Proceedings of the Second International Symposium' (Eds Farber, E. M. and Cox, A. J.), p. 300. Yorke Medical Books, New York.

fibrillar structures, and increases in nuclear bodies and heterochromatin. These changes are reported as occurring in cells in the superficial epidermis rather than in the basal cell layer, and were taken as evidence for early stages in the correction of abnormal keratinization.[1,2] A part of the mechanisms involved in PUVA therapy therefore may be the re-establishment of normal keratinization due to a reduction in epidermal mitosis.

Much of the normal skin reaction to psoralen photosensitization is similar to that induced by UV-B. Despite the apparent stimulation of oxygen uptake of arachidonic acid in irradiated 8-methoxypsoralen treated skin,[3] and the possible increase in prostaglandin synthesis[4] as suggested by the presence of Woronoffs rings (perilesional blanching) which occurs around the UV-treated psoriasis lesions, there does not appear to be an activation of the arachidonate–prostaglandin cascade.[5,6] It is therefore unlikely that an increased prostaglandin synthesis with secondary changes in the c̄ AMP concentrations are responsible for the PUVA control of the hyperproliferative psoriatic epidermis.

Repeated exposure to 8-methoxypsoralen photosensitization may result in direct inhibition of DNA synthesis in the hyperproliferative cell compartment of psoriatic epidermis, but this seems unlikely. Also, the success of the treatment in essentially non-hyperproliferative conditions such as mycosis fungoides, atopic eczema, vitiligo and polymorphous light eruption, has led to a search for alternative mechanisms. Cytolysis in leucocytes, both *in vitro* and in the dermal infiltrate in mycosis fungoides and lichen planus exposed to PUVA has led to the inference that the action of PUVA is due to the destruction of proliferating and differentiated lymphocytes in the infiltrate.[7,8] There are transient and eventually established changes in the circulating lymphocytes of PUVA-treated

1. Vukas, A., Velfi, D. and Gligora, M. (1977). Ultrastructural features of psoralen plus black light induced successive changes in psoriatic cell. *Dermatologica* **154**, 277.
2. Tsuji, T., and Cox, A. J. (1978). Ultrastructural changes in nuclei and nucleoli in psoriatic epidermis during and after PUVA therapy. *Acta derm-venereol. (Stockholm)* **58**, 383.
3. Lord, J. T., Ziboh, V. A., Rottier, J., Legget, G. and Penneys, N. S. (1976). The effects of photosensitizers and ultraviolet irradiation on the biosynthesis and metabolism of pro-staglandins. *Br. J. Derm.* **95**, 397.
4. Lowe, N. J. and Bures, F. (1978). Woronoff's rings with PUVA therapy. *Archs Derm.* **114**, 278.
5. Warin, A. P. (1978). The ultraviolet erythemas in man. Comment. *Br. J. Derm.* **98**, 473.
6. Heiligstadt, H., Kassis, W., Weismann, K. and Søndergaard, J. (1978). Prostaglandins in PUVA-treated psoriasis. *Acta derm-venereol. (Stockholm)* **58**, 213.
7. Schmoeckel, C., Scherer, R., Dern, B. and Braun–Falco, O. (1978). The cytolytic effect of PUVA treatment on PHA-stimulated human peripheral lymphocytes. *Acta derm-venereol. (Stockholm)* **58**, 203.
8. Ortonne, J. P., Schmitt, D., Alario, A. and Thivolet, J. (1979). Oral photochemotherapy in Lichen Planus (LP) and Mycosis Fungoides (MF): Ultrastructural modifications of the infiltrating cells. *Acta derm-venereol.* **59**, 211.

psoriatics, in particular in the numbers of identifiable T cells.[1, 2, 3] These changes suggest either a direct effect of PUVA on the lymphocytes, or a response of these cells to some local skin effect. For these reasons it has been suggested that PUVA therapy, like UV-B alone, results in a change in the immunopathology of psoriasis which may be directly involved in the correction of the hyperproliferative state in the epidermis.[4]

The role of polymorphonuclear leucocytes in psoriasis is not clear, but their presence in psoriatic epidermis, and their attraction into the psoriatic horny layer could imply some functional activity. PUVA treatment with 8-methoxypsoralen results in a decrease in the leucotactic factor[5] and also a decrease, but not abolition, of leucocyte chemotaxis.[6]

The treatment regime for psoriasis is now well defined and is based on the oral administration of 8-methoxypsoralen in a dose of 0·6 mg/kg body weight, followed 2 h later by irradiation of the affected skin with long wavelength UV-A. The initial dose of UVR depends on the subject's skin type in relation to its susceptibility to sunburn and its ability to pigment, or on a previously determined minimal phototoxic dose. The subsequent dosage increments are varied in accordance with the clinical response and the degree of phototoxic erythema and pigmentation produced. The object being that the progressively increasing amounts of UVR should be related to the development of protective pigmentation so that adequate amounts of irradiation continue to be available for combination with the 8-methoxypsoralen in the skin and at the same time avoid over-irradiation. The desire for a rapid and where possible complete clearance of the psoriatic lesions has to be balanced against the probable advantage of allowing the patient's protective pigmentation to develop, thus minimizing the unwanted phototoxic reactions of the combined treatment. Treatment is given two to three times a week, the frequency being reduced in parallel with clinical improvement leading to the establishment of a maintenance regime where necessary. Pharmacokinetic studies indicate that certain individuals may require a modification of the regime

1. Morison, W. L., Parrish, J. A., Bloch, K. J. and Krugler, J. I. (1979). Transient impairment of peripheral blood lymphocyte function during PUVA therapy. *Br. J. Derm.* **101**, 391.
2. Ortonne, J. P., Claudy, A., Alario, A. and Thivolet, J. (1978). Impairment of thymus derived rosette forming cells during photochemotherapy (psoralen-UVA). *Archs derm. Res.* **262**, 143.
3. Guihou, J. J., Clot, J., Guillot, B., Andary, M. and Meynadier, J. (1980). Immunological aspects of psoriasis. IV. Presence of circulating immune complexes in patients before and after PUVA therapy: correlations with T-cell markers. *Br. J. Derm.* **102**, 173.
4. Cormane, R. H., Hamerlinck, F. and Siddiqui, A. H. (1979). Immunologic implications of PUVA therapy. *Archs derm. Res.* **265**, 245.
5. Mizuno, N., Enami, H. and Esaki, K. (1979). Effect of 8-methoxypsoralen plus UV-A on psoriasis leukotactic factor. *J. Invest. Derm.* **72**, 64.
6. Langer, A. and Christophers, E. (1977). Leukocyte chemotaxis after *in vitro* treatment with 8-methoxypsoralen and UV-A. *Archs derm. Res.* **260**, 51.

because of variations in psoralen serum levels, its absorption and excretion.[1, 2, 3, 4]

The treatment of a benign, although distressing, skin disease such as psoriasis should be free from unwanted side-effects and therefore criteria have been laid down for the selection of patients. These side-effects, and in particular those of carcinogenesis and mutagenic changes, are referred to later (see page 2642). If eventually it is found that the present method of using oral psoralen photochemotherapy and full body UV-A irradiation has disadvantages, then the use of topical psoralens to restricted areas will become a more commonly used alternative. The topical application of psoralens however has not proved to be as effective as that following oral administration. The amount of improvement is often variable and the associated pigmentation sometimes unsightly and persistent. Along with UV-B phototherapy, tar, and dithranol, psoralen photochemotherapy has become an important mode of treatment for psoriasis. This has led to a reduction in the use of topical corticosteroids and of cytoxic agents such as methotrexate.

it is known that psoralen photochemotherapy, in addition to its action on DNA, affects certain immune mechanisms. It is therefore possible that this aspect of its action may be involved in the response of the skin lesions, not only in psoriasis but also in other disorders such as mycosis fungoides. Good results have been reported in alopecia areata, atopic eczema, lichen planus, pityriasis rubra pilaris, pityriasis lichenoides, and in urticaria pigmentosa (see pages 2636–2640).

1. Wavelength Dependence in PUVA

Although broad band UV-A peaking around 350–370 nm obviously induces the required photosensitization, a definitive action spectrum for the clearing of psoriasis by PUVA has not been determined. Early studies of erythema produced in human and guinea-pig skin by 8-methoxypsoralen photosensitization showed a peak activity at 360 nm.[5, 6] The action

1. Thune, P. (1978). Plasma levels of 8-methoxypsoralen and phototoxicity studies during PUVA treatment of psoriasis with meladinine tablets. *Acta derm-venereol. (Stockholm)* **58**, 149.
2. Wagner, G., Hopmann, C., Busch, U., Schmid, J. and Plewig, G. (1979). 8-MOP plasma levels in PUVA problem cases with psoriasis. *Br. J. Derm.* **101**, 285.
3. Ljunggren, B., Carter, D. M., Albert, J. and Reid, T. (1980). Plasma levels of 8-methoxypsoralen determined by high pressure liquid chromatography in psoriatic patients ingesting drug from two manufacturers. *J. invest. Derm.* **74**, 59.
4. Stevenson, I. H., Kenicer, K. J. A., Johnson, B. E. and Frain-Bell, W. (1981). Plasma 8-methoxypsoralen concentrations in photochemotherapy of psoriasis. *Br. J. Derm.* **104**, 47.
5. Buck, H. W., Magnus, I. A. and Porter, A. D. (1960). The action spectrum of 8-methoxypsoralen for erythema in human skin. Preliminary studies with a monochromator. *Br. J. Derm.* **72**, 249.
6. Pathak, M. A. (1961). Mechanism of psoralen photosensitisation and *in vivo* biological action spectrum of 8-methoxypsoralen. *J. invest. Derm.* **37**, 397.

spectrum for the photoreaction of 8-methoxypsoralen with native DNA however shows a peak at 312 nm,[1] but there is still considerable activity at longer wavelengths. Action spectra obtained for 8-methoxypsoralen induced cell killing of *Candida albicans*,[2] *Escherichia coli*,[3] and *Staphylococcus aureus*[4] show peak activity to be in the 310–330 nm range rather than the longer wavelengths. Similar results obtain for inactivation of herpes virus host capacity in mammalian cells[5] and sunburn cell production in mouse epidermis.[6] More recent studies of erythema production in guinea-pig, rabbit,[2,4] and human[7] skin also showed a greater effect with wavelengths ranging from 310 to 330 nm. Although the cellular mechanisms involved in erythema production compared with those for clearing of psoriatic lesions may well be different, it seems likely that the wavelength of the required radiation is similar.

The action spectrum obtained for the 8-methoxypsoralen photosensitized inhibition of hair growth in mouse skin (used as a model for the *in vivo* inhibition of DNA synthesis and cell replication) also showed a peak activity between 310–330 nm (Fig. 1). The filtration of these shorter wavelengths by psoriatic scale keratin is little different from that for the 350–370 nm range, and thus treatment with PUVA might be made more efficient by using a radiation source whose peak emission was at a shorter wavelength than those currently used.

B. Vitiligo

Although over 1% of the general population has vitiligo, it occurs in a much higher incidence in those patients who also have hyperthyroidism, thyroiditis, adrenal insufficiency, pernicious anaemia, certain types of uveitis including Vogy–Koyanagi and Harad's syndrome and sympathetic ophthalmia. There also seems to be an association between

1. Dall'Acqua, F., Marciani, S. and Rodighiero, G. (1969). The action spectrum of xanthotoxin and bergapten for the photoreaction with native DNA. *Z. Naturforsch.* **24b**, 667.
2. Owens, D. W., Glicksman, J. M., Freeman, R. G. and Carnes, R. (1968). Biologic action spectra of 8-methoxypsoralen determined by monochromatic light. *J. invest. Derm.* **51**, 435.
3. Ashwood–Smith, M. and Grant, E. (1974). Effect of temperature on dose-dependent changes in sedimentation characteristics of bacterial DNA produced *in vivo* by near-ultraviolet irradiation and 8-methoxypsoralen. *Cryobiology* **11**, 160.
4. Nakayama, Y., Morikawa, F., Fukuda, M., Hamano, M., Toda, K. and Pathak, M. A. (1974). Monochromatic radiation and its application. Laboratory studies on the mechanisms of erythema and pigmentation induced by psoralen. *In* 'Sunlight and Man' (Ed. Fitzpatrick, T. B.), pp. 591–611. Tokyo University Press, Tokyo.
5. Coohill, T. P. and James, L. C. (1979). The wavelength dependence of 8-methoxypsoralen photosensitization of host capacity inactivation in a mammalian cell-virus system. *Photochem. Photobiol.* **30**, 243.
6. Young, A. R. and Magnus, I. A. (1981). An action spectrum for 8-MOP induced sunburn cells in mammalian epidermis. *Br. J. Derm.* **104**, 451.
7. Cripps, D. T., Lowe, K. J. and Lerner, A. B. (1982). Action spectra of topical psoralens: a re-evaluation. *Br. J. Derm.* **107**, 77.

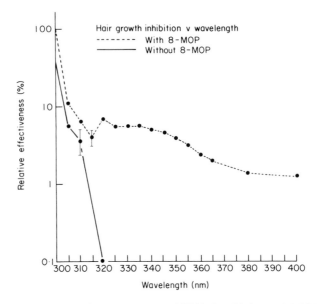

Fig. 1. Action spectra for 8-MOP photosensitized and UV-induced hair growth inhibition in mice.

vitiligo and melanoma.[1] Essentially it is a cosmetic problem but it can cause distress, particularly in racially pigmented subjects. Histologically the pigment-forming melanocytes are absent or greatly reduced in number, and at the border of the patch they are often large with long dentritic processes.

Reference to the treatment of vitiligo by psoralen-containing plants and exposure of sunlight has already been made. This was the first example of the use of photochemotherapy and the more recent and elaborate regimes are all really extensions of this basic concept.

In the photochemotherapy of vitiligo with UV-A irradiation, the psoralen may be applied topically or taken orally. The problem is to minimize the subsequent phototoxic erythema while at the same time maximizing pigment production. Where possible topical application is best avoided so as to reduce the risk of severe phototoxic erythema and blistering. However if a lower topical concentration of psoralen is used, combined with a longer UV-A exposure time, then the severity of the erythema is often reduced.[2] There is some evidence that if 90 mg

1. Lerner, A. B. and Nordlund, J. J. (1978). Vitiligo. What is it? Is it important? *J. Am. med. Assoc.* **239**, 1183.
2. Arora, S. K. (1976). Factors influencing methoxsalen phototoxicity in vitiliginous skin. *Archs Derm.* **112**, 327.

trimethylpsoralen is given orally 2 h before irradiation, pigmentation can occur without prior phototoxic erythema.[1] A smaller dose of 20 mg is incapable of producing the desired pigmentation.[2] Oral trioxsalan in sufficient dosage appears to be as effective as 8-methoxypsoralen and has the added advantage of producing less side-effects.[3] When 8-methoxypsoralen is used it has been suggested that the dose of 20 mg is inadequate and that 40 mg is required to obtain the desired pigmentary response.[4] The advent of equipment able to provide an adequate intensity of UV-A irradiation without excessively prolonged irradiation times means that exposure to sunlight is no longer necessary in the treatment of vitiligo with psoralens.[5]

The repigmentation of vitiligo by long-term PUVA treatment is due to activation of the skin melanocyte population. In normal skin PUVA-induced melanogenesis is due to a delayed tanning effect similar to that produced by UV-B although the intensity of the tan may be greater. Stimulated melanocytes show increased size and a greater number of dendrites. There is an increased migration of melanosomes to the dendrites and their size and number are also increased. The general epidermis shows melanization due to transfer of these melanosomes to keratinocytes.[6, 7] Although topical photosensitization with psoralens may lead to an increased size of melanosome,[8, 9] this does not seem to be a part of the pigmentary action of PUVA.[10] Similarly, although 8-methoxypsoralen and UV-A may induce melanocyte proliferation in normal skin,[7]

1. Kaidbey, K. H. and Kligman, A. M. (1974). Photopigmentation with trioxsalen. *Archs Derm.* **109**, 674.

2. Kligman, A. M. and Goldstein, F. P. (1973). Ineffectiveness of trioxsalen as an oral photosensitizer. *Archs Derm.* **107**, 413.

3. Theodoridis, A., Tsambaos, D., Sivenas, C. and Captanakis, J. (1976). Oral trimethylpsoralen in the treatment of vitiligo. *Acta derm-venereol. (Stockholm)* **56**, 253.

4. Kligman, A. M. and Goldstein, F. P. (1973). Oral dosage in methoxsalen phototoxicity. *Archs Derm.* **107**, 548.

5. Parrish, J. A., Fitzpatrick, R. B., Shea, C. and Pathak, M. A. (1976). Photochemotherapy of vitiligo. Use of orally administered psoralens and a high-intensity long-wave ultraviolet light system. *Archs Derm.* **112**, 1531.

6. Pathak, M. A., Kramer, D. M. and Fitzpatrick, T. B. (1974). Photobiology and photochemistry of furocoumarins (psoralens). *In* 'Sunlight and Man' (Ed. Fitzpatrick, T. B.), p. 335. University of Tokyo Press, Tokyo.

7. Pathak, M. A., Jimbow, K., Szabo, G. and Fitzpatrick, T. B. (1976). Sunlight and melanin pigmentation. *In* 'Photochemical and Photobiological Reviews' (Ed. Smith, K. C.), Vol. 1, p. 211. Plenum Press, New York.

8. Toda, K., Pathak, M. A., Parrish, J. A., Fitzpatrick, T. B. and Quevedo, W. C., Jr (1972). Alteration of racial differences in melanosome distribution in human epidermis after exposure to ultraviolet light. *Nature (New Biol.)* **236**, 143.

9. Zaynoun, S. T., McVittie, E. and Hunter, J. A. A. (1977). Melanosomal pattern in phototoxic pigmentary responses induced by topical psoralens and other photosensitizers. *Clin. exp. Derm.* **2**, 243.

10. Zaynoun, S. T., Konrad, K., Gschnait, F. and Wolff, K. (1977). The pigmentary response to photochemotherapy. *Acta derm-venereol. (Stockholm)* **57**, 431.

similar to that induced by UV-B,[1] this does not occur with the dose schedules usually used in PUVA therapy for psoriasis.[2] The repopulation of amelanotic epidermis with abnormal looking melanocytes after PUVA type treatment often has a patchy distribution[3] and appears to be the result of cell migration from hair follicles.[4] Some epidermal melanocyte proliferation may occur at the periphery of the vitiliginous area also,[5] but this appears to be rare. The latter is possibly a compensating hyper-pigmentation of the normal melanocytes in the border area whilst the former is probably a direct activation of the follicular melanocytes due to PUVA. Increased numbers of nerve endings are present in the epidermis of repeatedly PUVA-treated skin,[6, 7] and these may be related to melanocyte repopulation. Also involvement of the immune system in both the pathology of vitiligo and its treatment by PUVA is a possibility and is, as with psoriasis, an area for investigation.

C. Mycosis Fungoides

Mycosis fungoides is considered to be a T cell lymphoma. Adequate clinical improvement obtained by treating patients with PUVA is mainly confined to those within the earlier plaque and infiltrated stages although some regression of tumours can also occur.[8, 9, 10, 11] However, satisfactory response does not appear to alter the natural history of the condition in that lesions of internal organs still occur despite control of the cutaneous

1. Rosdahl, I. and Szabo, G. (1978). Mitotic activity of epidermal melanocytes in UV-irradiated mouse skin. *J. invest. Derm.* **70**, 143.
2. Rosdahl, I. K. and Swanbeck, G. (1980). Effects of PUVA on the epidermal melanocyte population in psoriasis patients. *Acta derm-venereol. (Stockholm)* **60**, 21.
3. Jarrett, A. and Szabo, G. (1956). The pathological varieties of vitiligo and their response to treatment with meladinine. *Br. J. Derm.* **68**, 313.
4. Ortonne, J. P., MacDonald, D. M., Micoud, A. and Thivolet, J. (1979). PUVA-induced repigmentation of vitiligo: a histochemical (split-DOPA) and ultrastructural study. *Br. J. Derm.* **101**, 1.
5. Africk, J. and Fulton, J. (1971). Treatment of vitiligo with topical trimethylpsoralen and sunlight. *Br. J. Derm.* **84**, 151.
6. Hashimoto, K., Kohda, H., Kumakiri, M., Blender, S. L. and Willis, I. (1978). Psoralen-UVA-treated psoriatic lesions. *Archs Derm.* **114**, 711.
7. Kumakiri, M. and Hashimoto, K. (1978). Cutaneous nerve stimulation by psoralen-ultraviolet A therapy: an ultrastructural study. *J. invest. Derm.* **70**, 163.
8. Gilchrest, Barbara A., Parrish, J. A., Tannenbaum, L., Haynes, H. A. and Fitzpatrick, T. B. (1976). Oral methoxsalen photochemotherapy of mycosis fungoides. *Cancer* **38**, 683.
9. Konrad, K., Gschnait, F., Honigsmann, H., Fritsch, P. and Wolff, K. (1978). Photo-chemotherapie bei Mycosis fungoides. *Hautartz* **29**, 191.
10. Hodge, L., Briffa, D., Vella-Warin, A. P., Gange, R. W. and Bleehen, S. (1977). Photochemo-therapy in mycosis fungoides. *Br. med. J.* **2**, 1257.
11. Lowe, N. J., Cripps, D. J., Dufton, P. A. and Vickers, F. H. (1979). Photochemotherapy for Mycosis fungoides. A clinical and histological study. *Archs Derm.* **115**, 50.

lesions with PUVA.[1] Although there is no proof, the possibility that the generalized extension of the disease could be related to the treatment of the skin should be considered.

The mode of action of PUVA in mycosis fungoides is still uncertain, but it seems unlikely that it is simply due to inhibition of DNA synthesis. A recent evaluation[2] of the effect of PUVA on the immune-mechanism defects in this disease has shown a subsequent improvement in the delayed hypersensitivity responses to various antigens such as *C. albicans* and *Trichophyton* histoplasmin. Despite a reduction in T lymphocyte counts which may be accounted for by the destruction of skin lymphocytes in addition to the action of PUVA on the circulating T cells, treated patients do not appear to have impaired cell mediated immunity reactions.

Clinical improvement with PUVA therapy appears to be related to the disappearance of the dermal infiltrate. Following successful treatment there is disappearance of the proliferating lymphocytes usually seen in mycosis fungoides lesions. Proliferating lymphocytes are more susceptible than resting cells to 8-methoxypsoralen photosensitized damage.[3] However, ultrastructural studies have indicated that both dividing and resting cells are destroyed in patients with mycosis fungoides undergoing systemic PUVA therapy.[4] Therefore, although an indirect effect of PUVA on the immune system may play a part in the successful treatment of mycosis fungoides,[5] a direct phototoxic effect on an abnormal cell population in this disease has been clearly established.

There is the interesting observation that some, although by no means all, patients with mycosis fungoides show cutaneous photosensitivity both clinically and by photosensitivity measurements. The abnormal action spectrum is said to include any part of the UV and light spectrum but particularly the UV-A wavelengths.[6] If, in fact, as has been suggested, mycosis fungoides is a reaction to unidentified antigens,[7] which would

1. Niemi, K. M. (1979). PUVA treatment in Mycosis fungoides. *Dermatologica* **158**, 462.
2. Molin, L., Skogh, M. and Volden, G. (1978). Successful PUVA treatment in the tumour stage of mycosis fungoides. Associated with the appearance of lesions in organs other than the skin. *Acta derm-venereol. (Stockholm)* **58**, 189.
3. Scherer, R., Kern, D. and Braun-Falco, O. (1977). UV-A induced inhibition of proliferation of PHA stimulated lymphocytes from humans treated with 8-methoxypsoralen. *Br. J. Derm.* **97**, 519.
4. Ortonne, J. P., Schmitt, D., Alario, A. and Thivolet, J. (1979). Oral photochemotherapy in Lichen Planus (LP) and Mycosis Fungoides (MF), Ultrastructural modifications of the infiltrating cells. *Acta derm-venereol. (Stockholm)* **59**, 211.
5. Cormane, R. H., Hamerlinck, F. and Siddiqui, A. H. (1979). Immunologic implications of PUVA therapy in psoriasis vulgaris. *Archs derm. Res.* **265**, 245.
6. Volden, G. and Thune, P. O. (1977). Light sensitivity in mycosis fungoides. *Br. J. derm.* **97**, 279.
7. Tan, R. S-H., Butterworth, C. M., McLaughlin, H., Malka, S. and Samman, P. D. (1974). Mycosis fungoides—a disease of antigen persistence. *Br. J. Derm.* **91**, 607.

now appear to be a factor in the photosensitivity dermatitis and actinic reticuloid syndrome,[1] it is perhaps not surprising that cutaneous photosensitivity could be a feature in mycosis fungoides.

D. Atopic Eczema

The effect of psoralen photochemotherapy in atopic eczema is of interest because atopic eczema is not an epidermal proliferative disease like psoriasis and the dermal cells present in atopic eczema are not abnormal like those of mycosis fungoides. It is possible therefore that any beneficial effect of PUVA in atopic eczema occurs as a result of an effect on the immune mechanisms involved. Significant improvement in some patients with atopic eczema is obtained with a PUVA regimen similar to, but with a somewhat longer duration than that used for psoriasis.[2, 3] Moreover it seems necessary for there to be continued maintenance treatment to prevent relapses, although these relapses can be controlled once again when the treatment is restarted.[2, 3] However, this treatment of atopic eczema can result in the development of herpes simplex in 20% of subjects.[4]

E. Lichen Planus

The fact that autoimmune mechanisms may be involved in lichen planus, and that the dermal cellular infiltrate is almost entirely composed of T lymphocytes, and that PUVA is effective in mycosis fungoides (a T cell lymphoma) are some of the reasons which lead one to anticipate the improvement which has been reported in lichen planus following PUVA.[5, 6] The dosage required is double that used to clear psoriasis resulting in histological changes indicating profound alteration of the superficial dermis, and in particular of the elastic fibres. In addition to the disappearance of the dermal infiltrate, photochemotherapy will produce marked changes in the epidermis in the lichen planus lesion, indicating

1. Frain-Bell, W. and Johnson, B. E. (1979). Contact allergic sensitivity to plants and the photosensitivity dermatitis and actinic reticuloid syndrome. *Br. J. Derm.* **101**, 503
2. Morrison, W. L., Parrish, J. A. and Fitzpatrick, T. B. (1979). Oral psoralen photochemotherapy of atopic eczema. *Br. J. Derm.* **98**, 25.
3. Sannwald, C., Ortonne, J. P. and Thivolet, J. (1979). La photochimiotherapie oral de l'eczema atopique. *Dermatologica* **159**, 71.
4. Goldberg, H. C. (1980). The uses of PUVA in atopic dermatitis. *Acta derm-venereol. (Stockholm)* **92**, 119.
5. Ortonne, J. P., Thivolet, J. and Sannwald, C. (1978). Oral photochemotherapy in the treatment of lichen planus (LP). Clinical results, histological and ultrastructural observations. *Br. J. Derm.* **99**, 77.
6. Brenner, W., Gschnait, F., Hönigsmann, H. and Fritsch, P. (1978). Erprobung von PUVA bei verschiedenen Dermatosen. *Hautarzt* **29**, 541.

some degree of atrophy attributable to the possible epidermal origin of lichen planus as well as to the treatment.[1] None the less, as in the treatment of mycosis fungoides by PUVA, the characteristic finding is of nuclear damage in lymphocytes of the superficial infiltrate, subsequent necrosis being restricted to a depth in the dermis at which UV-A is likely to act.[2] The photosensitizing effect of 8-methoxypsoralen is more damaging in dividing than non-dividing cells[3] and although the lymphocytic infiltrate in lichen planus does not have the hyper-proliferative characteristics of that in mycosis fungoides, a number of cells are dividing[4] and may constitute a population which is specifically susceptible to treatments such as PUVA. However, non-dividing cells are killed by PUVA and there is little reason to suppose that this action is any less important in the clearing of the infiltrate in lichen planus than that of killing the few dividing cells only.

Although the aetiology of lichen planus is unknown, it has been suggested that following a change in epidermal cell nucleus of the basal layer during the initial phase of mitosis an antigen situated at this level triggers off a cellular immune response. Ultrastructural studies have suggested that photochemotherapy acts on the two principal factors, i.e. the appearance of a new epidermal antigen and also of the dermal lymphocytic infiltrate.[1]

F. Alopecia Areata

For many years ultraviolet radiation has been prescribed in the treatment of alopecia areata, and although it is not clear whether this treatment is ever clinically effective it has been reported as stimulating regrowth.[5]

It has been postulated that immune mechanisms are involved in the loss of hair in alopecia areata in that antibodies directed to various auto-antigens have been described;[6] also, there is an imbalance between the

1. Ortonne, J. P., Thivolet, J. and Sannwald, C. (1978). Oral photochemotherapy in the treatment of lichen planus (LP). Clinical results, histological and ultrastructural observations. *Br. J. Derm.* **99**, 77.

2. Ortonne, J. P., Schmitt, D., Alario, A. and Thivolet, J. (1979). Oral photochemotherapy in Lichen Planus (LP) and Mycosis Fungoides (MF): Ultrastructural modifications of the infiltrating cells. *Acta derm-venereol. (Stockholm)* **59**, 211.

3. Scherer, R., Kern, D. and Braun-Falco, O. (1977). UVA-induced inhibition of proliferation of PHA stimulated lymphocytes from humans treated with 8-methoxypsoralen. *Br. J. Derm.* **97**, 519.

4. Lachapelle, J. M. and de la Brassine, M. (1973). The proliferation of cells in the dermal infiltrate of lichen planus. *Br. J. Derm.* **89**, 137.

5. Krook, G. (1961). Treatment of alopecia areata with Kromayer's ultraviolet lamp. *Acta derm-venereol. (Stockholm)* **41**, 178.

6. Cunliffe, W., Hall, R., Stevenson, C. J. and Wightman, D. (1969). Alopecia areata, thyroid disease and autoimmunity. *Br. J. Derm.* **81**, 879.

B–T lymphocyte systems and/or between T helper–T suppressor cells, and if the lymphocyte pool is restored by sensitization with DNCB, there is a regrowth of hair.[1]

In mouse skin, hair growth stimulated by plucking may be inhibited by exposure to PUVA treatment with little sign of gross skin damage.[2] The normal response of hair growth to PUVA would therefore seem to be the same as the usual inhibitory effects of photosensitization. However, there is a stimulation of resting follicles into active growth at the periphery of an 8-methoxypsoralen photosensitized skin area; a phenomenon which is probably a non-specific wounding effect. This does not appear to occur in the successful treatment of alopecia areata with PUVA which has been reported.[3, 4, 5] Based on the fact that both *in situ* and circulating lymphocytes may be affected, either directly or indirectly, when the skin is exposed to PUVA therapy,[6] it is suggested that as with psoriasis and vitiligo an immunologic abnormality specific for the disease entity is corrected by the non-specific alteration of lymphocyte behaviour. In the case of alopecia areata, PUVA may act through a non-specific suppressor system directed against the hypothetical hair-associated antigen thought to be responsible for the hair loss.[7]

G. Acne Vulgaris

It is a common belief that some patients with acne are better during the summer and because of this impression artificial UVR has been used for its treatment. The improvement obtained is often short lived, relapses occurring soon after the UVR is stopped. The opposite view has been expressed, i.e. that sunlight in fact can make acne worse and that this may happen in as many as one in five subjects.[8] Also, any summer-time improvement noted may be due to seasonal factors other than UV.[8] Controlled studies of phototherapy (UV-A; UV-B + UV-A) in the

1. Gianetti, A., Di Silverio, A., Castellazi, A. M. and Maccario, R. (1978). Evidence for defective T cell function in patients with alopecia areata. *Br. J. Derm.* **98**, 361.
2. Johnson, B. E. (1981). Unpublished data.
3. Rollier, R. and Warcewski, G. (1974). Le traitement de la pelade par la melandinine. *Bull. Soc. fr. Derm. Syph.* **81**, 97.
4. Weissman, I., Hofmann, Cornelia, Wagner, Gisela, Plewig, G. and Braun-Falco, O. (1978). PUVA-Therapy for Alopecia Areata. *Archs derm. Res.* **262**, 333.
5. Lassus, A., Kianto, U., Johansson, E. and Javakoski, T. (1980). PUVA treatment of alopecia areata. *Dermatologica* **161**, 298.
6. Morrison, W. L., Parrish, J. A. and Epstein, J. H. (1979). Photoimmunology. *Archs Derm.* **115**, 350.
7. Claudy, A. I. and Gagnaire, D. (1980). Photochemotherapy for alopecia areata. *Acta derm-venereol. (Stockholm)* **60**, 171.
8. Mills, O. H. and Kligman, A. M. (1978). Ultraviolet phototherapy and photochemotherapy of Acne Vulgaris. *Archs Derm.* **114**, 221.

treatment of moderately severe papulopustular acne have recorded only moderate improvement with approximately 20% of those treated noticing that the condition had worsened.[1] There is also an acneform eruption, acne aestivalis ("Majorca acne")[2] which appears to be produced *de novo* as a result of excessive sun exposure. Except for the cosmetic improvement provided by the phototoxic pigmentation, PUVA has not been shown to improve acne.[1, 3]

In a small number of subjects receiving PUVA treatment for either psoriasis or vitiligo an acneform eruption has developed.[4, 5] It has been suggested that the mechanisms involved may be similar to those occurring in the tropics where certain forms of acne, especially of the conglabata type, become worse due to increased temperature and humidity in association with exposure to sunshine.[4]

A further study showed that UV-B plus UV-A enhanced the comedogenic effects of human sebum, sulphur, cocoa butter, squalene and coal tar in the external ear canal of rabbits and of coal tar and squalene in man. The possibility therefore exists that in some patients UVR actually enhances the response of the native sebum in a com-edogenic action in follicular epithelium.[6]

H. Urticaria Pigmentosa

As with the other skin diseases for which PUVA is a successful treatment, its ability to eradicate temporarily the wealing and dermographism produced by physical trauma in urticaria pigmentosa and the alleviation of associated "migraine"[7] raises challenging questions as to both the aetiology of the disease and the mode of action of the therapy.

I. Herpes Simplex

It is recognized that recurrent attacks of herpes simplex may be triggered

1. Mills, O. H. and Kligman, A. M. (1978). Ultraviolet phototherapy and photochemotherapy of Acne Vulgaris. *Archs Derm.* **114**, 221.
2. Hjorth, N., Sjolin, K. E., Sylvest, B. *et al.* (1972). Acne aestivales—Mallorca acne. *Acta derm-venereol. (Stockholm)* **52**, 61.
3. Parrish, J. A., Strauss, J. S., Fleming, T. S. and Fitzpatrick, T. B. (1978). Oral Methoxsalen Photochemotherapy for Acne Vulgaris. *Archs Derm.* **114**, 1241.
4. Jones, C. and Bleehen, S. S. (1977). Acne induced by PUVA-treatment. *Br. Med. J.* **11**, 866.
5. Nielsen, E. B. and Thormann, J. (1978). Acne like eruptions induced by PUVA. *Acta derm-venereol. (Stockholm)* **58**, 374.
6. Mills, O. H., Porte, M. and Kligman, A. M. (1978). Enhancement of comedogenic substances by ultraviolet radiation. *Br. J. Derm.* **98**, 145.
7. Christophers, E., Hönigsmann, H., Wolff, K. and Langner, A. (1978). PUVA-treatment of urticaria pigmentosa. *Br. J. Derm.* **98**, 701.

off by exposure to sunshine, although the mechanisms involved in the localization of the reaction are obscure.

As long ago as 1900 Raab demonstrated what is now called the phenomenon of photodynamic inactivation when he showed that low concentrations of acridine which had not had an effect on paramecia, soon destroyed these organisms if also exposed to daylight. Of more recent times, this phenomenon has been allied to the treatment of virus infections and in particular to recurrent herpes simplex infection. It is known that certain heterotricyclene dyes are bound irreversably to the herpes virus *in vitro*, the virus being subsequently inactivated following exposure to fluorescent light; neutral red, proflavine and toluidine blue are the most effective examples of these dyes.[1] Despite the optimism engendered by these *in vitro* findings, the initial impression of clinical efficacy *in vivo* in the human subject[1] has not been borne out.[2] It was also suggested,[3] although subsequently repudiated,[4] that photo-inactivation therapy might have been responsible for the subsequent development of intraepidermal carcinoma of the penis in patients suffering from genital herpes. The basis for this possibility was that the dye will bind with viral DNA and following irradiation will then disrupt the nucleic acid to produce photo-inactivated viral particles which have an increased oncogenic potential.[5] It was subsequently shown that the association between genital herpes and intraepidermal carcinoma occurred in the absence of dye photo-inactivation therapy.[4]

J. Phototherapy of Malignant Tumours[6]

The use of eosin phototoxicity for the treatment of skin tumours[7] showed that photochemotherapy might have a role in the overall treatment of

1. Felber, T. D., Smith, E. B., Knox, J. M., Wallis, C. and Melnick, J. L. (1973). Photodynamic Inactivation of Herpes Simplex. *J. Am. med. Ass.* **233**, 289.
2. Myers, M. G., Oxman, M. N., Clark, Joan E. and Arnot, K. A. (1975). Failure of neutral-red photodynamic inactivation in recurrent herpes simplex virus infections. *New Eng. J. Med.* **293**, 945.
3. Berger, R. S. and Papa, C. M. (1977). Photodye herpes therapy—Cassandra confirmed. *J. Am. med. Ass.* **238**, 133.
4. Kopf, A. W., Ackerman, A. B., Wade, T. and Bart, R. S. (1978). Photodye Herpes Therapy. *J. Am. med. Ass.* **239**, 615.
5. Rapp, F., Li, J. H. and Jerkofsky, M. (1973). Transformation of mammalian cells by DNA-containing viruses following photodynamic inactivation. *Virology* **55**, 339.
6. Dougherty, T., Boyle, D., Weishaupt, K., Gomer, C., Borcicky, D., Kaufman, J., Goldfarb, A. and Grindey, G. (1978). Phototherapy of human tumours. *In* 'Research in Photobiology' (Ed. Castellani, A.), pp. 435–446. Plenum Press, New York.
7. Jesionek, A. and Tappeiner, V. (1903). Zur Behandlung der Hautcarcinome mit fluorescirender Stoffen. *Münch. Med. Wochschr.* **47**, 2042.

cancers, especially of the superficial type. Certain photosensitizing substances, particularly haematoporphyrin and its derivatives, appear to concentrate and accumulate in the cells of neoplastic tissue.[1, 2, 3, 4] There is, therefore, the possibility that phototoxic lethal effects may be induced in tumours while the surrounding, normal tissues are relatively unaffected. A degree of destruction of glioma cells transplanted into rats was obtained with haematoporphyrin and visible radiation while fluorescein and 488 nm radiation retarded the growth of mammary tumours transplanted into mice.[5] Better results, in terms of curing spontaneous or transplanted mammary tumours in rats and mice, were obtained with an acetic acid–sulphuric acid haematoporphyrin derivative[6] and red light.[5] Acridine orange phototoxicity, induced by argon laser irradiation, has been used to destroy transplanted epithelial tumours in mice,[7] and these more recent reports have indicated the possible use of photochemotherapy for human cancer.

Further studies on human bladder cancer, treated with haematoporphyrin derivative and red light, either transplanted to mice[8] or *in situ*[9, 10] have shown that in certain cancer types, photochemotherapy is successful. Moreover, promising preliminary results have been obtained using a haematoporphyrin derivative (2·5–5 mg/kg body weight by intravenous injection) and red light (620–640 nm: 5–15 mW/cm² for 20–120 min) in the treatment of metastasis from carcinoma of the breast and the colon and rectum. Also metastatic melanoma and superficial squamous and

1. Auler, H. and Banger, G. (1942). Untersuchungen über die Rolle der Porphyrine bei geschwulstkranken Menschen und Tieren. *Z. Krebsforsch.* **53**, 65.
2. Figge, F. H. J., Weiland, G. S. and Manganiello, O. J. (1948). Cancer detection and therapy. Affinity of neoplastic, embryonic and traumatized tissues for porphyrins and metalloporphyrins. *Proc. Soc. exp. Biol. Med.* **68**, 640.
3. Lipson, R. L., Baldes, E. J. and Olsen, A. M. (1961). The use of a derivative of haematoporphyrin in tumor detection. *J. nat. Cancer Inst.* **26**, 2.
4. Lipson, R. L., Baldes, E. J. and Olsen, A. M. (1961). Haematoporphyrin derivative: a new aid for endoscopic detection of malignant disease. *J. thorac. cardiovasc. Surg.* **42**, 623.
5. Diamond, I., Granelli, S. G., McDonogh, A. F., Nielsen, S., Wilson, C. B. and Jaenicke, R. (1972). Photodynamic therapy for malignant tumours. *Lancet* **ii**, 1175.
6. Dougherty, T. J. (1974). Activated dyes as antitumor agents. *J. nat. Cancer Inst.* **52**, 1333.
7. Tomson, S. H., Emmett, E. A. and Fox, S. H. (1974). Photodestruction of mouse epithelial tumors after oral acridine orange and argon lasor. *Cancer Res.* **38**, 3124.
8. Kelly, J. F., Snell, M. E. and Berenbaum, M. C. (1975). Photodynamic destruction of human bladder carcinoma. *Br. J. Cancer* **31**, 237.
9. Kelly, J. F. and Snell, M. E. (1976). Haematoporphyrin derivative: a possible aid in the diagnosis and therapy of carcinoma of the bladder. *J. Urol.* **115**, 150.
10. Snell, M. E. (1978). Irradiation of tumours with light. *In* 'Ultraviolet radiation and its medical applications'. The Hospital Physicists' Association Conference Report Series **28**, 30 (London).

basal cell carcinomata have been reported to have responded to this treatment.[1]

Further progress in this aspect of phototherapy appears to depend on the defining of optimal conditions of haematoporphyrin derivative concentration and the finding of a more efficient photosensitizer. Maximum irradiation conditions in terms of wavelength dependence and exposure dose, and the development of apparatus by which the light is efficiently delivered to the target area, are also necessary before this can become an effective form of therapy.

II. COMPLICATIONS OF PUVA THERAPY

A. Nail Changes (Photo-oncholysis)

Discolouration and separation of the distal part of one or more finger nails has been described in association with a number of photocontact reactions such as those associated with tetracycline and porphyria.[2, 3] More recently, PUVA has also been implicated as a cause of nail changes.[4, 5, 6, 7, 8, 9]

Similar nail changes may occur in patients with hydroa vacciniforme, one of the photodermatoses where the action spectrum for erythema is frequently found to be normal, and these changes have also been observed in actinic reticuloid.[10] The long wavelength UV radiation (UV-A) is thought to be able to penetrate the nail plate and cause the pathological changes.

1. Dougherty, T., Boyle, D., Weishaupt, K., Gomer, C., Borcicky, D., Kaufman, J., Goldfarb, A. and Grindey, C. (1978). Phototherapy of human tumours. *In* 'Research in Photobiology' (Ed. Castellani, A.), pp. 435–446. Plenum Press, New York.
2. Orentreich, N., Harber, L. A. and Trohoutich, T. A. (1961). Photosensitivity and photopnycholysis due to demethylchlortetracycline. *Archs Derm.* **83**, 68.
3. Marsden, R. A. and Dawber, R. P. R. (1977). Erythropoietic protoporphyria with onycholysis. *Proc. R. Soc. Med.* **70**, 572.
4. Zala, L., Omar, A. and Krebs, A. (1977). Photo-onycholysis caused by 8-methoxypsoralen. *Dermatologica* **154**, 203.
5. Raw, R. C., Flowers, F. P. and Barrett, J. L. (1978). Photo-onycholysis secondary to psoralen use. *Archs Derm.* **114**, 448.
6. Dawber, R. P. R. (1978). Photo-onycholysis. *Archs Derm.* **114**, 1715.
7. Ortonne, J. P. and Baran, R. (1978). Photo-onycholysis inducté par la photochimiotherapie orale. *Ann. Derm. vener. (Paris)* **105**, 1715.
8. Mackie, Rona M. (1979). Onycholysis occurring during PUVA therapy. *Clin. exp. Derm.* **4**, 111.
9. Naik, R. P. C. and Singh, G. (1979). Nail pigmentation due to oral 8-methoxypsoralen, *Br. J. Derm.* **100**, 229.
10. Frain-Bell, W. (1981). Personal communication.

B. Pigmentation

Apart from the patchy hyperpigmentation associated with localized topical photochemotherapy, a nevus spilus-like hyperpigmentation occurring in the psoriatic lesions during treatment with PUVA has been described.[1, 2]

C. Severe Skin Pain after PUVA Treatment

First referred to by Tegner[3] and found by her in eight out of 210 patients treated with PUVA. Often severe, it is burning and stinging in character and is easily differentiated by the sufferer from itch. It is often worse at night and disturbs the patient's sleep. The explanation for this symptom is unknown but an associated abnormality is a failure to exhibit the axon-flare response following the intradermal injection of histamine into the affected area.[4] The flare response returns to normal about 3 months after PUVA is stopped.

D. Lupus Erythematosus

Some patients receiving PUVA therapy have anti-nuclear antibodies, although antibodies to native DNA have not been found.[5] In addition, the development of both cutaneous discoid lupus erythematosus[6] and systemic lupus erythematosus[7] have been described in psoriatic patients during PUVA therapy. Whether the development of lupus erythe-matosus is coincidental is uncertain, the possibility of PUVA leading to a collagenosis has to be considered, especially in view of the fact that sunlight is known to aggravate or precipitate such conditions. Reference has also been made to the relationship between lupus erythematosus and exposure to artificial UV, particularly UV-B, with associated antigenic changes to DNA. It is also known that antibodies to UV-irradiated DNA

1. Hofmann, Cornelia, Plewig, G. and Braun-Falco, G. (1977). Ungewohnliche Nebenwirkun-gen bei oraler Photochemotherapie (PUVA-Therapie) der Psoriasis. *Hautarzt* **28**, 583.
2. Helland, S. and Bang, G. (1980). Nevus Spilus-like Hyperpigmentation in psoriatic lesions during PUVA therapy. *Acta derm-venereol. (Stockholm)* **60**, 81.
3. Tegner, E. (1979). Severe skin pain after PUVA treatment. *Acta derm-venereol. (Stockholm)* **59**, 467.
4. Jordan, W. P. (1979). PUVA, pruritus, and the loss of the axon flare. *Archs Derm.* **115**, 636.
5. Bjellerup, M., Rbuz, M., Forsgren, A., Krook, G. and Ljunggren, B. (1979). Antinuclear antibodies during PUVA therapy. *Acta derm-venereol. (Stockholm)* **59**, 73.
6. Domke, H. F., Ludwigsen, E. and Thormann, A. (1979). Discoid lupus erythematosus possibly due to photochemotherapy. *Archs Derm.* **115**, 642.
7. Eyanson, S., Greist, Marcy C., Brandt, K. D. and Skinner, B. (1979). Systemic lupus erythematosus associated with psoralen-Ultraviolet-A treatment of psoriasis. *Archs Derm.* **115**, 54.

may crossreact with native non-irradiated DNA.[1] Moreover a specific antiserum directed against DNA-8-methoxypsoralen photoadduct has been described.[2] Ultraviolet radiation, in addition to causing DNA changes, can also alter RNA and cellular proteins. It is thus possible to produce antibodies against PUVA-altered DNA and cellular proteins, and these may play a part in the subsequent development of lupus erythematosus in a predisposed individual.

E. Bullous Pemphigoid

It is not clear why some patients treated with PUVA develop bullae,[3] although the association between exposure to UV-B irradiation and the development of pemphigus or pemphigoid has been recognized.[4] Whether in fact it is simply a non-specific phototoxic reaction or the triggering off of a latent bullous pemphigoid response is not clear. In one of five such patients direct and indirect immunofluorescence supported the diagnosis of PUVA-induced bullous pemphigoid.[5]

Acral bullous eruptions similar to those seen in PUVA treated patients occur in association with the administration of naladixic acid and with frusemide in which a phototoxic reaction is thought to be involved.

F. Eye Complications

Studies of the effects of psoralen photosensitization on the eyes of experimental animals have been comprehensively reviewed.[6, 7]

Long-term treatment of mice, rats, and guinea-pigs, with high doses of 8-methoxypsoralen and UV-A gives rise to damage of the cornea and iris, clouding of the anterior chamber, lens opacities with anterior cortical cataract, and in albino animals there is some evidence of retinal damage.

The majority of UV-B wavelengths below 310 nm are absorbed by the

1. Teen Veen, J. H. and Lucas, C. J. (1970). Induction of antinuclear antibodies by ultraviolet irradiation. *Ann. rheum. Dis.* **29**, 556.
2. Zarebska, Z., Jarzabek-Chorzelska, M., Rzesa, G. and Chorzelski, T. (1978). Antigenicity of DNA induced by photoaddition of 8-methoxypsoralen. *Photochem. Photobiol.* **27**, 37.
3. Robinson, June K., Baughman, R. D. and Provost, T. T. (1978). Bullous pemphigoid induced by PUVA therapy. *Br. J. Derm.* **99**, 709.
4. Thomsen, K. and Schmidt, H. (1976). PUVA-induced bullous pemphigoid. *Br. J. Derm.* **95**, 568.
5. Cram, D. L. and Fukuyama, K. (1972). Immunohistochemistry of ultraviolet-induced pemphigus and pemphigoid lesions. *Archs Derm.* **106**, 819.
6. Parrish, J. A., Anderson, R. R., Urbach, F. and Pitts, D. (1978). 'UV-A. Biological Effects of Ultraviolet Radiation with Emphasis on Human Responses to Longwave Ultraviolet', p. 212. Plenum Press, New York.
7. Parrish, J. A., Chylack, L. T., Woehler, M. E., Cheng, H-M., Pathak, M. A., Morison, W. L., Krugler, J. and Nelson, W. F. (1979). Dermatologic and ocular examinations in rabbits chronically photosensitized and methoxsalen. *J. invest. Derm.* **73**, 256.

cornea, but the longer UV-A waves penetrate the aqueous humour: most are absorbed in the lens, but about 5% reach the retina. It is thought that the incidence of cataract in man is related to lifetime exposure to UVR.[1] It is obvious that subjects are at risk who are receiving psoralen photochemotherapy and do not have a lens. The same problem arises with long-term treatment with chlorpromazine.[2]

The majority of 8-methoxypsoralen is cleared from the lens within 12 h of oral administration. However, if the lens is exposed to UV-A before this period has elapsed, photoaddition products are formed in the lens components including binding to the aromatic amino acid residues, such as tryptophan.[3] Similar reactions with tryptophan, and with prolonged exposure to UV-A alone, are thought to result in increased pigmentation and protein aggregation in the lens producing cataract.[4]

It is important therefore to avoid exposure to ambient light for 12 h or longer after ingestion of the drug so that all the free 8-methoxypsoralen has diffused out of the lens.[5]

There are no reports of eye damage in human subjects treated with psoralens and UVR, and recent follow-up studies of patients with vitiligo who did not use protective glasses while under the long-term treatment with 8-methoxypsoralen and sunlight showed no evidence of eye changes 2 to 3 years after commencement of treatment.[6]

G. Allergic Reactions

It is perhaps not surprising that a few cases of a contact phototoxic type of reaction to 8-methoxypsoralen would, in time, be described in persons handling the drug.[7] Contact allergic sensitivity is rare but has been reported during treatment for alopecia areata with topically applied 8-methoxypsoralen. Confirmation of the sensitization was obtained by positive closed patch test reactions.[8] Photoallergic reactions are also rare,

1. Hiller, Rita, Giacometti, L. and Yuen, Karen (1977). Sunlight and cataract: an epidemiologic investigation. *Am J. epidemiol.* **105**, 450.
2. Bond, W. S. and Yee, G. C. (1980). Occular and cutaneous effects of chronic phenothiazine therapy. *Am. J. Hosp. Pharm.* **37**, 74.
3. Lerman, S. (1980). Potential ocular complications of psoralen UV-A therapy. *Dermatosen in Beruf und Umwelt* **28**, 5.
4. Zigman, S. (1977). Near UV light and cataracts. *Photochem. Photobiol.* **26**, 437.
5. Lerman, S., Megaw, Judith and Willis, I. (1980). Potential ocular complications from PUVA therapy and their prevention. *J. invest. Derm.* **74**, 197.
6. Back, O., Hollstrom, E., Liden, S. and Thorburn, W. (1980). Absence of cataract ten years after treatment with 8-methoxypsoralen. *Acta derm-venereol. (Stockholm)* **60**, 79.
7. de Koning, G. A. J., Notowicz, A. and Stolz, E. (1979). Phototoxische Reaktion auf 8-Methoxypsoralen als Berufsdermatose. *Hautartzt* **30**, 27.
8. Weissmann, I., Wagner, G. and Plewig, G. (1980). Contact allergy to 8-methoxypsoralen. *Br. J. Derm.* **102**, 113.

but the descriptions of their occurrence are consistent with cell mediated immunologic reactions to the combination of 8-methoxypsoralen and UV-A. In five out of 106 patients, a marked erythema followed by eczema developed in areas of vitiligo some 3 to 8 weeks after topical treatment with 8-methoxypsoralen.[1] Three further cases associated with topical 8-methoxypsoralen treatment were confirmed by positive allergic photopatch test reactions: controls were negative.[2] The possibility of delayed hypersensitivity reactions, specific to particular psoralens in combination with UV-A, is confirmed in reports of photoallergic reactions to contact with umbelliferous plants and their psoralen constituents.[3, 4] A further case of a patient undergoing PUVA therapy in which both topical and systemic 8-methoxypsoralen was involved, showed a positive photoallergic type reaction with 8-methoxypsoralen and UV-A combined. However, negative results were obtained with UV-A alone, 8-methoxypsoralen alone, UV-B, UV-C, and with a combination of trimethylpsoralen and UV-A.[5]

H. Skin Malignancy and PUVA treatment

Histological and ultrastructural studies of psoriatic skin repeatedly exposed to 8-MOP and UV-A during PUVA treatment have shown that the re-establishment of a normal stratum granulosum precedes other changes. The return to normal of the horny layer and the partial suppression of acanthosis occur later. This picture is similar to that seen with other methods of treatment and it is difficult to determine which changes are specific to PUVA and which represent the natural sequence of events in the clearing of psoriasis. A major early change in the dermis is the decrease in the cellular infiltrate, though whether this is a direct, cytolytic effect of PUVA as in mycosis fungoides, or a secondary effect

1. Sidi, E. and Bourgeois-Gavardin, J. (1953). Mise au point du traitement du vitiligo par l'Ammi majus. *Presse Médicale* **61**, 436.
2. Fulton, J. E., Jr and Willis, I. (1968). Photoallergy to methoxsalen. *Archs Derm.* **98**, 445.
3. Llungren, B. (1977). Psoralen photoallergy caused by plant contact. *Contact Dermatitis* **3**, 85.
4. Kavli, G., Volden, G. and Raa, J. (1982). Accidental induction of photocontact allergy to Meracheum lociniatum. *Acta derm.* **62**, 435.
5. Plewig, G., Hofmann, Cornelia and Braun-Falco, O. (1978). Photoallergic dermatitis from 8-methoxypsoralen. *Archs derm. Res.* **261**, 201.

following the correction of epidermal abnormalities is not certain.[1, 2, 3]

There is general agreement that over a period of 2 to 3 years PUVA treatment, premature ageing, or premalignant changes, are rarely seen. Superficial dermal changes with disruption of elastic fibres and the development of a generalized perivascular coating of homogeneous material,[2] with the deposition of acid mucopolysaccharide[4] and rarely amyloid[5] have been reported. Bizarre giant cells, probably of fibroblast origin, may also persist in the superficial dermis.[2, 6] An increase in melanocyte size and activity can also persist throughout treatment, resulting in heavy melaninization of the epidermal keratinocytes.[2] However, reversion to normal size and activity of the melanocytes generally occurs on cessation of therapy.[7]

The occasional "sunburn cell" observed early in treatment is not usually present at the later stages. However, in the non-lesioned skin of some patients, patches of epidermal hypertrophy are a prominent feature of the clearing phase of the treatment and may persist for at least a year.[8] Whether these rare, keratosis-like lesions are derived from particularly vigorous PUVA therapy or from over-exposure to the UV-B component of the radiation source is not clear.[8] Patients previously treated with oncogenic agents such as arsenic[1] are at obvious risk. Whatever the exact mechanism involved, the appearance of these lesions draws renewed attention to the data concerning the interactions of 8-MOP and other psoralens with chromosomal DNA and the possible long-term complications of these interactions.

It seems that photochemotherapy is an acceptable and cost effective

1. Braun-Falco, O., Hoffmann, C. and Plewig, G. (1977). Feingewebliche Veränderungen unter Photochemotherapie der psoriasis: Eine histologische und histochemische Studie. *Archs derm. Res.* **257**, 307.
2. Hashimoto, K., Kohda, H., Kumakiri, M., Blender, L. and Willis, I. (1978). Psoralen-UVA-treated psoriatic lesions. Ultrastructural changes. *Archs Derm.* **114**, 711.
3. Wolff, K., Gschnait, F., Hönigsmann, H., Konrad, K., Stingl, G., Wolff–Schreiner, E. and Fritsch, P. (1977). Oral photochemotherapy. Results, follow up, and pathology. *In* 'Psoriasis', Proceedings of the second International Symposium (Eds Farber, E. M. and Cox, A. J.), p. 300. York Medical Books, New York.
4. Bergfeld, W. F. (1977). Histopathologic changes in skin after photochemotherapy. *Cutis* **20**, 504.
5. Greene, I. and Cox, A. J. (1979). Amyloid deposition after psoriasis therapy with psoralen and long-wave ultraviolet light. *Archs Derm.* **115**, 1200.
6. Omar, A., Weismann, U. N. and Krebs, A. (1977). Induction of multinucleate cells by 8-MOP and UV treatment *in vitro* and *in vivo*. *Dermatologica* **155**, 65.
7. Zaynoun, S., Konrad, K., Gschnait, F. and Wolff, K. (1977). The pigmentary response to photochemotherapy. *Acta derm-venereol.* **57**, 431.
8. Cox, A. J. and Abel, E. A. (1979). Epidermal dystrophy. Occurrence after psoriasis therapy with psoralen and long-wave ultraviolet light. *Archs Derm.* **115**, 567.

treatment for psoriasis but before its use is extended, data regarding the possible risks involved should be continually collected and evaluated.[1]

The evidence so far suggests that there may be an increased risk of cutaneous malignancy in certain subjects treated with PUVA.[2] Where tumours have developed during treatment, squamous cell carcinomata, rather than the more usual basal cell type, have predominated and they have appeared in normally covered sites. The chance of this occurring is greater if the PUVA treatment is given to subjects previously exposed to arsenic, X-rays or methotrexate and also if there is a past history of skin malignancy.[2, 3, 4, 5, 6, 7, 8] In fact, the tumour incidence in psoriatic subjects treated with PUVA may be no higher than in those who have received more conventional forms of treatment.[9, 10]

Psoralen photochemotherapy has in the past been used as a prophylactic to reduce the incidence of solar-induced skin cancer in Texas and in Australia.[11, 12] No effect was noted in either of these two studies, although in both the period of observation was relatively short. 8-Methoxypsoralen appeared to be more effective in reducing the incidence of malignant skin change in xeroderma pigmentosum where there is impaired repair of UV damage to DNA.[13] However, others have reported skin tumours developing within a very short time after starting treatment in patients with this disease.[14, 15]

1. Shuster, S. (1979). Photochemotherapy for psoriasis. *Lancet* **i**, 1146.
2. Stern, R. S., Thibodeau, L. A., Kleinerman, R. A., Parrish, J. A. and Fitzpatrick, T. B. and 22 participating investigators (1980). Risk of cutaneous carcinoma in patients treated with oral methoxsalen photochemotherapy for psoriasis. *New Engl. J. Med.* **300**, 809.
3. Moller, R. and Howitz, J. (1978). Methoxsalen and multiple basal cell carcinoma. *Archs Derm.* **112**, 1613.
4. Hoffmann, C., Plewig, G. and Braun-Falco, O. (1979). Bowenoid lesions, Bowen's disease and keratoacanthomas in long-term PUVA treated patients. *Br. J. Derm.* **101**, 685.
5. Verlich, J. (1979). Squamous cell carcinoma. *Archs Derm.* **115**, 1338.
6. Tam, D. W., Van Scott, E. J. and Urbach, F. (1979). Bowen's disease and squamous cell carcinoma. *Archs Derm.* **115**, 203.
7. Hönigsmann, H., Wolff, K., Gschnait, F., Brenner, W. and Jaschke, E. (1980). Keratoses and non-melanoma skin tumours in long term photochemotherapy (PUVA). *J. Am. Acad. Derm.* **3**, 406.
8. Lassus, A., Reunala, T., Idänpää-Heikkila, J., Juvakoski, T. and Salo, O. (1981). PUVA treatment and skin cancer: a follow up study. *Acta Derm.* **61**, 141.
9. Halprin, K. M. (1980). Psoriasis, skin cancer and PUVA. *J. Am. Acad. Derm.* **2**, 334.
10. Halprin, K. M., Comerford, M. and Taylor, J. R. (1982). Cancer in patients with psoriasis. *J. Am. Acad. Derm.* **7**, 633.
11. MacDonald, E. J., Griffin, A. C., Hopkins, C. E., Smith, L., Garrett, H. and Black, G. I. (1963). Psoralen prophylaxis against skin cancer: report of clinical trial 1. *J. invest. Derm.* **41**, 213.
12. Hopkins, C. E., Belisario, J. C., MacDonald, Eleanor J. and Davis, Charlotte T. (1963). Psoralen prophylaxis against skin cancer: report of clinical trial 11. *J. invest. Derm.* **41**, 219.
13. Noojin, R. O. (1965). Xeroderma Pigmentosum treated with oral methoxsalen. *Archs Derm.* **92**, 422.
14 Reed, W. B. (1977). De Sanctis–Cassione Syndrome. A case report with autopsy findings. *Archs Derm.* **113**, 1561.
15. Reed, W. B. (1976). Treatment of psoriasis with oral psoralens and long-wave ultraviolet light. *Acta derm-venereol. (Stockholm)* **56**, 315.

Photosensitization of human lymphocytes with 8-MOP *in vitro* may result in permanent damage to the nuclear DNA of surviving cells, as demonstrated by increased numbers of chromosome aberrations.[1] With greater sensitivity, increased levels of sister chromatid exchanges[2, 3, 4, 5] occur. Known mutagenic and carcinogenic agents increase the sister chromatid exchange levels in Chinese hamster cells[6] and human leukocytes,[7] and it is suggested that these DNA lesions result from aberrations in the post replication repair processes[8, 9] which ultimately lead to mutation.[10] The potential for somatic mutation, malignant transformation and carcinogenesis would therefore seem to be present in cells treated with 8-MOP and UV-A. The estimated 8-MOP concentration and UV-A dose to which psoriatic keratinocytes are exposed during PUVA therapy is about the same as is required to cause these changes in the nuclei of cultured cells.

The mutagenic action of 8-MOP photosensitization has been demonstrated in Drosophila,[11] various micro-organisms,[12, 13, 14, 15, 16] and

1. Swanbeck, G., Thyresson-Hök, M., Bredberg, A. and Lambert, B. (1975). Treatment of psoriasis with oral psoralens and longwave ultraviolet light. Therapeutic results and cytogenetic hazards. *Acta derm-venereol. (Stockholm)* **55**, 367.

2. Carter, D. M., Wolff, K. and Schneid, W. (1976). 8-methoxypsoralen and UV-A promote sister chromatic exchanges. *J. invest. Derm.* **67**, 548.

3. Mourelatos, D., Faed, M. J. W. and Johnson, B. E. (1976). Sister chromatid exchanges in human lymphocytes exposed to 8-methoxy-psoralen and long-wave UV radiation prior to incorporation of bromodeoxyuridine. *Experientia* **33**, 1091.

4. Latt, S. A. and Loveday, K. S. (1978). Characterization of sister chromatid exchange induction by 8-methoxypsoralen plus UV light. *Cytogenet. Cell Genet.* **21**, 184.

5. Lambert, B., Morad, M., Bredberg, A., Swanbeck, G. and Thyresson-Hök, M. (1978). Sister chromatid exchanges in lymphocytes from psoriasis patients treated with 8-methoxypsoralen and long-wave ultraviolet light. *Acta derm-venereol. (Stockholm)* **58**, 13.

6. Perry, P. and Evans, H. J. (1975). Cytological detection of mutagen carcinogen exposure by sister chromatid exchanges. *Nature* **258**, 121.

7. Beek, B. and Obe, G. (1975). The human leukocyte test system. VI. The use of sister chromatid exchanges as possible indicators for mutagenic activities. *Human Genet.* **29**, 127.

8. Kato, H. (1973). Induction of sister chromatid exchanges by UV light and its inhibition by caffeine. *Exp. Cell Res.* **82**, 383.

9. Wolff, S., Bodycote, J. and Painter, R. B. (1974). Sister chromatid exchanges induced in Chinese hamster cells by UV irradiation at different stages of the cell cycle: the necessity for cells to pass through. *S. Mutat. Res.* **25**, 73.

10. Day, R. S. (1977). III. Inductible error-prone repair and cellular senescence. *In* 'DNA Repair Processes: Cellular Senescence and Somatic Cell Genetics' (Eds Nichols, W. W. and Murphy, D. G.), p. 217. Symposium Specialists, Miami.

11. Altenburge, E. (1956). Studies of the enhancement of mutation rate by carcinogens. *Tex. Rep. Biol. Med.* **14**, 481.

12. Igali, S., Bridges, B. A., Ashwood-Smith, M. J. and Scott, B. R. (1970). Mutagenesis in *E. Coli*. IV. Photosensitization to near ultraviolet light by 8-methoxypsoralen. *Mutation Res.* **9**, 21.

13. Igali, S. and Gazso, L. (1971). Photosensitizing, lethal and mutagenic action of 8-methoxypsoralen and near UV light in *Escherichia coli*. *Stud. Biophys.* **229**, 45.

14. Mathews, M. M. (1963). Comparative study of the lethal photosensitization of Sarcina lutea by 8-methoxypsoralen and toluidine blue. *J. Bacteriol.* **85**, 322.

15. Averbeck, D., Chandra, P. and Biswas, R. F. (1975). Structural specificity in the lethal and mutagenic activity of furocoumarins in yeast cells. *Radiat. environ. biophys.* **12**, 241.

16. Townsend, M. E., Hopwood, D. A. and Wright, H. M. (1970). Efficient mutagenesis by near UV in the presence of 8-methoxypsoralen in Streptomyces. *John Innes Inst. Ann. Rep.* **61**, 56.

cultured mammalian cells,[1,2] including human skin fibroblasts.[3] The finding of increased numbers of lymphocyte variants which are 6-thioguanine resistant in the peripheral blood is taken to be a marker for somatic mutation. Their presence in patients undergoing PUVA therapy is confused as there is an increase in the cell type in psoriatics generally.[4] Moreover, the estimated mutation induction in dividing keratinocytes over a lifetime of PUVA therapy amounts to only 2–5% of the total treated cell population.[2] Therefore, although there is no doubt that repeated 8-MOP photosensitization leads to skin cancer in experimental animals,[5,6,7] it is not clear that any skin tumour development in PUVA treated patients is due to this complete carcinogenic action of 8-MOP and UV-A. Where PUVA related skin cancer has been reported, some predisposing factor, either genetic as in the case of xeroderma pigmentosum, or previous treatment with X-rays or arsenic, appears to have been involved. The action of 8-MOP photosensitization in these cases may be that of tumour promotion in an already abnormal tissue. Cell mediated delayed hypersensitivity reactions in guinea-pigs may be inhibited by 8-MOP and UV-A,[8] and impairment of T cell function may be detected in psoriatic patients during PUVA therapy.[9,10,11] However, greater significance may be attached to the observation that (like UV-B) 8-methoxypsoralen and UV-A may induce the development of suppressor T cells in mice, leading to the acceptance and development of strongly antigenic UV-induced tumour cells.[12] PUVA therapy may

1. Arlett, C. F. (1973). Mutagenesis in cultured mammalian cells. *Stud. Biophys.* **36-37**, 139.
2. Burger, P. M. and Simons, J. W. I. M. (1979). Mutagenicity of 8-methoxypsoralen and long-wave ultraviolet irradiation in V-79 Chinese hamster cells. A first approach to a risk estimate in photochemotherapy. *Mutation Res.* **60**, 381.
3. Burger, P. M. and Simons, J. W. I. M. (1979). Mutagenicity and carcinogenicity of 8-MOP/UVA in cell cultures. *Bull. Cancer (Paris)* **65**, 281.
4. Strauss, G. H., Albertini, R. J. Krusinski, P. A. and Baughman, R. D. (1979). 6-thioguanine resistant peripheral blood lymphocytes in humans following psoralen long-wave ultraviolet light (PUVA) therapy. *J. invest. Derm.* **73**, 211.
5. Griffin, A. C. (1959). Methoxsalen in ultraviolet carcinogenesis in the mouse. *J. invest. Derm.* **32**, 367.
6. Forbes, P. D., Davies, R. E. and Urbach, F. (1976). Phototoxicity and photocarcinogenesis: comparative effect of anthracene and 8-methoxypsoralen in the skin of mice. *Food cosmet. Toxicol.* **14**, 303.
7. Grube, D. D., Ley, R. D. and Fry, R. J. M. (1977). Photosensitizing effects of 8-methoxypsoralen on the skin of hairless mice. II. Strain and spectral differences for tumorogenesis. *Photochem. Photobiol.* **25**, 269.
8. Morison, W. L., Woehler, M. E. and Parrish, J. A. (1979). PUVA and systemic immunosuppression in guinea pigs (Abstract). *J. invest. Derm.* **72**, 273.
9. Ortonne, J. P., Claudy, A. L., Alario, A. and Thivolet, J. (1977). Decreased circulating E rosette forming cells in psoralen-UVA treated patients. *Archs derm. Res.* **258**, 305.
10. Cormane, R. H., Hamerlinck, F. and Siddiqui, A. H. (1979). Immunologic implications of PUVA therapy in psoriasis vulgaris. *Archs derm. Res.* **268**, 245.
11. Haftek, M., Glinski, W., Jablonska, S. and Obalek, S. (1979). T lymphocyte E rosette function following photochemotherapy (PUVA) of psoriasis. *J. invest. Derm.* **72**, 214.
12. Roberts, L. K., Schmitt, M. and Daynes, R. A. (1979). Tumor-susceptibility generated in mice treated with subcarcinogenic doses of 8-methoxypsoralen and long-wave ultraviolet light. *J. invest. Derm.* **72**, 306.

therefore interfere with the immune surveillance mechanism which could exist with respect to squamous cell carcinoma.

Although the importance of the mutagenic effects of PUVA therapy would not appear to be great, it remains desirable to seek a variation in the treatment in which satisfactory clearing of psoriatic lesions would be obtained with reduced mutagenic potential. The relative importance of psoralen mono-adducts and cross links in mutagenic induction and cell killing may be studied by comparing the effects of cross linking compounds, such as 8-methoxypsoralen with those of the monofunctional angelicin, or the end group blocked compounds such as 3-carbethoxy-psoralen and 3-(a,a,-dimethylally)-psoralen.[1, 2, 3, 4, 5, 6] Most studies have shown that cross linking is more effective but that all types of DNA lesions give rise to both mutation and cell killing. However, as determined by survival of yeast cells, the monofunctional psoralens, 3-carbethoxypsoralen and 5,7-dimethoxycoumarin caused much less mutation than 8-methoxypsoralen or psoralen.[7] Preliminary studies have demonstrated the successful use of 3-carbethoxypsoralen in topical photochemotherapy for psoriasis, and there was no evidence of photosensitized carcinogenesis in mice.[8]

To date the possibility of PUVA induced skin malignancy remains a theoretical risk, but until we have sound proof that this form of treatment is safe it will continue to be used for selected patients only.[9]

1. Ashwood-Smith, M. J., Grant, E. L., Heddle, J. A. and Friedman, G. B. (1977). Chromosome damage in Chinese hamster cells sensitized to near-ultraviolet light by psoralen and angelicin. *Mutation Res.* **43**, 377.

2. Seki, T., Nozu, K. and Kondo, S. (1978). Differential causes of mutation and killing in *Escherichia coli* after psoralen plus light treatment: monoadducts and cross-links. *Photochem. Photobiol.* **27**, 19.

3. Averbeck, D., Moustacci, E., and Bisagni, E. (1978). Biological effects and repair of damage photo-induced by a derivative of psoralen substituted at the 3,4 reaction site. Photoreactivity of this compound and lethal effect in yeast. *Biochim. biophys. Acta* **518**, 464.

4. Bridges, B. A., Mottershead, R. P. and Knowles, A. (1979). Mutation induction and killing of *Escherichia coli* by DNA adducts and crosslinks: a photobiology study with 8-methoxypsoralen. *Chem. biol. Interact.* **27**, 221.

5. Coppey, J., Averbeck, D. and Moreno, G. (1979). Herpes virus production in monkey kidney and human skin cells treated with angelicin or 8-methoxypsoralen plus 363 nm light. *Photochem. Photobiol.* **29**, 797.

6. Vedaldi, D., dall'Acqua, F., Caffieri, S. and Rodighiero, G. (1979). 3-(a,a-dimethylally)-psoralen: a linear furocoumarin forming mainly 4'5'-monofunctional adducts with DNA. *Photochem. Photobiol.* **29**, 277.

7. Averbeck, D. and Moustacci, E. (1980). Decreased photoinduced mutagenicity of monofunctional as opposed to bi-functional furocoumarins in yeast. *Photochem. Photobiol.* **31**, 475.

8. Dubertret, L., Averbeck, D., Zajdela, F., Bisagni, E., Moustacci, E., Touraine, R. and Latarjet, R. (1978). Photochemotherapy (PUVA) of psoriasis using 3-carbethoxypsoralen, a non-carcinogenic compound in mice. *Br. J. Derm.* **101**, 379.

9. Bridges, B. A. and Strauss, G. H. (1980). Possible hazards of photochemotherapy for psoriasis. *Nature* **283**, 523.

85 | Lasers and the Skin

J. A. COTTERILL

Department of Dermatology,
The General Infirmary at Leeds, England

I. INTRODUCTION

Although Einstein, in 1917, first developed the theoretical concept of stimulated emission, the logical development of this idea only evolved many years later when the laser was produced simultaneously in Russia and the United States. The laser is essentially a powerful light beam whose name is an acronym for "Light Amplification by Stimulated

PHYSIOL. PATHOPHYSIOL. OF SKIN Vol. 8
ISBN 0 12 380608 9

Emission of Radiation". Medical applications became possible when Maiman[1] constructed the first ruby laser in 1960 for the Hughes Research Laboratory. Subsequently many different types of lasers have been produced by using gas, liquid or solids as media. Lasers of dermatological interest include the ruby laser, the argon laser, the CO_2 laser and the tunable dye laser.

II. THE PHYSICS OF LASER PRODUCTION

Atoms and molecules are able to interact with light in three different ways; by absorption, by spontaneous emission, and by stimulated emission. Thus, a molecule or atom at a lower energy level can absorb a photon of energy and make a transition to an upper energy level provided the photon has the correct amount of energy (Fig. 1). Such a process is called absorption.

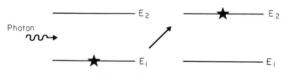

Fig. 1. Absorption.

Also, an atom or a molecule may make a transition to a lower energy level by emitting a photon. This process is termed spontaneous emission (Fig. 2). Furthermore, a photon interacting with a molecule or atom may stimulate the emission of a second photon, having the following properties. The emitted photon has the same direction of propagation and the same frequency as the incoming photon and the associated wave of the emitted photon is in phase with the wave of the incoming photon.

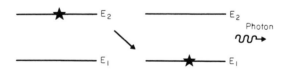

Fig. 2. Spontaneous emission.

1. Maiman, T. H. (1960). Stimulated optical radiation in ruby. *Nature* **187**, 493.

This stimulated emission is equivalent to light amplification and forms the physical basis for the production of laser beam (Fig. 3).

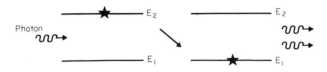

Fig. 3. Stimulated emission.

A. Laser Design

All laser generators consist of three basic elements, namely a lasing medium, a pumping system, and an optical cavity (Fig. 4). The gain, amplifying or lasing medium may be a solid such as a ruby, a gas such as carbon dioxide, or a liquid as for example organic dye lasers. This amplifying medium is placed between two mirrors facing each other, which forms a resonant cavity and this is excited by the pumping system. The mirrors ensure a degree of optical feedback enabling a significant proportion of emitted photons to remain within the system and thus provoke more stimulated emissions. The mirrors are usually selected so that one reflects 100% of the desired wavelength, but the other transmits a fraction of the radiation incident upon it and forms the output of the laser. For this reason the partially transmitting mirror is also sometimes called the output coupler mirror.

The laser system must also create a population inversion as such a state is necessary for the laser to operate. In an unstimulated medium the

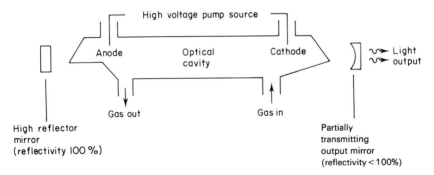

Fig. 4. Basic elements of a laser.

number of atoms at energy level zero (N_0) is greater than those at the higher level N_1: and those at N_1 is greater than those at N_2 and so on until N_{i-1} is greater than N_i, where N_i is the number of atoms at energy level "i". In the population inversion state N_i is greater than N_{i-1}, and it is only in these circumstances that stimulated emission can occur. This population inversion is achieved by raising the atoms to a high energy state, and although these decay rapidly to a lower level they are nevertheless at higher energy levels than unstimulated atoms in their ground state. If their further decay down to the ground state is slower than the rate of providing fresh stimulated atoms, then there is an accumulation of atoms at a raised level and finally a state of population inversion is reached. This raising of the excited state until N_i is greater than N_{i-1} is made by a process of "pumping" the atoms to high energy states. The pumping system or power supply may take the form of optical pumping using a xenon flash tube or another laser. Alternatively, electrical collision pumping may be used. Finally, chemical pumping can be utilized, whereby energy is released by the making and disrupting of chemical bonds, as for instance, in some hydrogen fluoride lasers.

The pumping system energy is stored in electrons, producing a population inversion and spontaneous decay of some electrons to low energy levels initiates a chain reaction. Spontaneously emitted photons impinge on other atoms, but these are not absorbed and they therefore stimulate the electrons of the other atoms to emit photons of identical wavelength, phase and direction. This sequence has been termed stimulated emission.

B. Characteristics of the Light Output

In theory a beam of laser light has three basic properties. It should be collimated or parallel, and coherent in that it is predictable in time and space, and it should be monochromatic. In practice, however, the outputs are known to deviate from these theoretical perfect characteristics in several ways. Thus, medical laser beams may not be exactly parallel, but for practical purposes, the small divergence can usually be disregarded. Whilst the output beam is highly coherent, the laser does not produce strictly monochromatic light and if examined by a spectrophotometer a number of discrete lines may be seen. For instance, the argon laser has at least six different wavelengths but more than 80% of its energy output is at 488 and 514 nm.

C. Power and Power Density

The power of a laser beam is expressed in watts and milliwatts, power density or irradiance being related to the irradiated area and is derived by dividing the total available power by the area of the beam. Power densities vary inversely with the square of the beam diameter. Thus, a relatively small decrease in beam diameter can lead to a correspondingly great increase in power density.

A Q-switched pulse laser system releases energy in extremely short bursts of high energy which can produce great damage to surrounding healthy tissue. Because of this property the use of Q-switched pulse lasers has largely been abandoned in dermatological practice. Pulse lasers in modern medical use have their output controlled by a timer which is preset by the operator, varying from 0·1 up to a few seconds or more. However, there is no general agreement when a pulse laser becomes a continuous wave laser.

D. The Interaction of Laser Light and Living Tissue

The effects of laser light on living tissue depend not only on the intensity, duration and wavelengths of the incident light, but also on the nature of the tissue itself. A spectrum of effects ranging from biostimulative to thermal occur depending on the density of the laser light.

E. Biostimulative Effects

It has been claimed that low intensity laser light may be biostimulative.[1] Mester and his colleagues claimed that repeated pulses of the order of 1 J cm^{-2} of ruby laser radiation was able to stimulate hair growth in depilated mice. The same group of workers also claimed that low power argon and helium–neon laser light was able to stimulate collagen synthesis and capillary growth in healing wounds, and varicose ulcers were said to benefit from this treatment. However, untreated ulcers in the same patient also improved and in the writer's opinion this work needs to be viewed with scepticism.

F. Inhibitory Biological Effects

Increasing the beam intensity produces inhibitory biological effects. A cytotoxic action followed later by a thermal effect are seen with increasing beam intensity. The initial thermal change is one of shrinkage followed by death and finally vapourization of the entire tissue. Such changes are seen when the beam intensity of a CO_2 laser source is increased.

It is the thermal effects of lasers that are at present utilized in medical practice rather than their potential low intensity applications. However,

1. Mester, E. (1981). The biostimulative effect of laser beams, 'Laser Tokyo' 81. Fourth Congress of the International Society for Laser Surgery. (Eds Tsumi, K. and Nimsakul, M.).

the recent use of photosensitizing agents such as haematoporphyrin derivatives may in the future lead to much more selective treatments.

III. PHOTOSENSITIZING AGENTS AND LASER TREATMENT[1, 2]

It is known that malignant tumours may selectively retain photosensitizing drugs, and haematoporphyrin derivative in particular has been used as such an agent. Haematoporphyrin derivative has an absorption peak in the red end of the spectrum at 624 nm. Tumour tissue which has absorbed this drug can then be irradiated using a tunable dye laser at 624 nm, and the selective absorption of the radiant energy by the tumour tissue compared with the surrounding normal tissue results in its selective destruction. The photoactivation of haematoporphyrin derivatives converts triplet oxygen to singlet oxygen, which is cytotoxic. This is a non-thermal effect and so the laser power required is relatively low (200–1000 mW). This power can be developed in conjunction with fibre optic endoscopes and may in the future form the basis of a useful treatment for malignancy.

The treatment of portwine stains by the tunable dye laser (see below) utilizes the natural endogenous pigment, haemoglobin. The portwine stain is irradiated at 577 nm, the principal absorption peak of the haemoglobin molecule. Such irradiation produces a selective vasculitis rather than the necrosis that occurs with conventional argon laser treatment.[3, 4]

A. Selective Melanosome Rupture

Melanin absorbs ultraviolet and visible light in a broad band maximal in the UV region and to a less extent in the visible light portion of the spectrum (Fig. 5). Parrish[5] has recently shown, using the XEF Excimer

1. Dougherty, T. J., Grindey, G. B., Fiel, R., Weishaupt, M. R. and Boyle, D. G. (1975). Photoradiation Therapy II: Cure of animal tumours with haematoporphyrin and light. *J. nat. Cancer Inst.* **54**, 115.
2. Kato, H., Konaka, C., Ono, J., Matsushima, J., Nishimiya, K., Hakoshima, A. and Hayata, Y. (1981). Laser photo radiation with haematoporphyrin derivative in lung cancer. Proc. 4th Congress of the International Society for Laser Surgery, Tokyo. Int. Group. Corp. Japan 14.
3. Anderson, R. R. and Parrish, J. A. (1981). Microvasculature can be selectively damaged using dye lasers in a basic theory and experimental evidence in human skin. *Lasers Med. Surg.* **1**, 263.
4. Greenwald, J., Rosen, S., Anderson, R. R., Harrist, T., MacFarland, F., Noe, J. M. and Parrish, J. A. Comparative histological studies of the tunable dye (at 577 nm) laser and argon laser: the specific vascular effects of the dye laser. *J. invest. Derm.* **77**, 305.
5. Parrish, J. A. (1982). Selective alterations of specific structures within skin with lasers. Paper given at the American Academy of Dermatology, New Orleans.

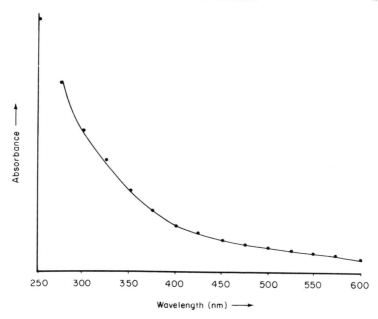

Fig. 5. Absorption spectrum of melanin in 5% KOH solution.

laser emitting at 351 nm, that it is possible to produce melanosome rupture followed by necrosis of the basal cell layer in treated skin. Electron micrographs suggest explosive rupture of the melanosomes in an otherwise intact melanocyte. This observation demonstrates that specific damage can be confined to an organelle within a cell and Parrish concludes that such selective photochemical and thermal effects will probably be increasingly explored for new developments in laser therapy.

IV. THERMAL EFFECTS

Thermal reactions are influenced by the intensity of the source of photons, the duration of exposure, and the power levels attained. To produce clinically useful effects (10–100 W) they have to be much higher than those required to produce the photosensitized reaction described above. The degree of thermal damage depends not only on the maximum temperature achieved, but also on the rate of temperature change. Thermal effects may also vary with the pulse width, as in the case of Q-switch lasers; the degree of penetration being determined by wavelength selection. The optical properties of the target tissue may also help to determine the selected wavelength in order to attain a high absorption.

Absorbance by the target and the duration of exposure also influences the thermal effects. Long exposures allow time for the heat to diffuse away from the target area and this could produce tissue damage at a distance from the target.

A. Other Thermal Effects

With tissue shrinkage small vessels within the treated area may become closed. The ND YAG laser can seal vessels up to 1·5 mm in diameter and the argon laser up to 1 mm in diameter. The localized thermal effect of the CO_2 laser makes it very suitable as a laser knife and, although incisions made with this laser heal more slowly than those made with a conventional scalpel, healing is faster than that following diathermy.

V. TYPES OF LASER

The lasers in medical use, together with their physical properties, are given in Table 1.

Table 1

Lasers of dermatological interest

Type of laser	Colour	Wavelength (nm)
Ruby	Red	694
Argon	Blue–Green	488–514
Tunable dye	Orange	577
Helium–Neon	Pink	633
Neodynium YAG	Near infra-red	1060
Carbon dioxide	Far infra-red	10600
XeF excimer	Ultraviolet	351

A. The Ruby Laser

It was Dr Leon Goldman who first introduced the ruby laser into dermatology[1] following its initial use by ophthalmic surgeons, and he recognized the potential of laser technology in skin disease and the ready accessibility of the skin with its disorders were a distinct advantage.

1. Goldman, L. (1973). Effects of new laser systems on the skin. *Archs Derm.* **108**, 385–390.

However, the argon laser soon superseded the ruby laser for the treatment of skin diseases, particularly those of the vasculature.

B. The Argon Laser

The argon laser provided a dependable method for delivering intense focussable thermal energy to the dermal vascular network. It has therefore been used for the treatment of portwine stains. It is known that haemoglobin has three absorption peaks at 415, 542 and 577 nm (Fig. 6) and that although the argon laser has six different wavelengths, more

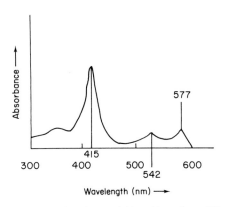

Fig. 6. Absorption spectrum of oxyhaemoglobin with peaks at 415, 542 and 577 nm.

than 80% of its energy output is at 488 and 514 nm which is absorbed to some extent by haemoglobin. The haemoglobin, having absorbed the blue–green laser light, transforms the radiant energy into heat which causes coagulation of blood vessels up to 0·5 mm in diameter. Adjacent skin appendages remain relatively undamaged and are able to take part in the subsequent reconstruction of epidermis. Following argon laser treatment there is rapid healing, leaving an essentially normal epidermis and a diffuse mild subepidermal fibrosis. These changes are known to be permanent and stable over at least a 7-year follow-up period. Malignant neoplasia has not been shown to occur following laser therapy after more than 20 years of clinical experience.

1. Portwine Stains

There are more data on the use of the argon laser for the treatment of portwine stains than on any other vascular lesions.[1-7] Patient selection for optimum results are important. It is generally agreed that the older the lesion, and therefore the older the patient, the better it is likely to respond to argon laser treatment. This is because in the older portwine stains there is an increase in both vessel number and vascular ectasia with an associated colour shift from pink to purple. The purple lesion absorbs the blue–green light much more avidly than the pink lesion, thus giving better clinical results. Pink lesions generally respond unfavourably in that there is either no response or hypertrophic scarring is produced.

It has been shown in patients below the age of 37 years who have portwine stains that a biopsy may be of help in predicting the outcome of laser therapy.[8] In this group the factors favouring a satisfactory result include a histological evaluation of the portion of the dermis occupied by blood vessels, and this should be greater than 5%. The mean vessel area should be greater than 2500 μm^2 and the proportion of vessels containing erythrocytes should be greater than 15%. Adverse factors in the prognosis include age below 17 years, a vascular area below 2%, a mean vessel area less than 1500 μm^2, and the number of vessels containing erythrocytes less than 3%. Thus it is clear that the argon laser is more likely to be effective in patients with purple lesions which are found most often in older patients, and individuals under the age of 17 years should probably not be treated with the argon laser.

This is rather unsatisfactory as almost all parents of children born with portwine stains look for an effective treatment early in life. Of possible help in this situation is the observation of Gilchrest and her colleagues[9] who have shown that cooling the skin deepens the colour of the lesion, and thus may minimize the epidermal injury caused by the argon laser. Therefore lowering the temperature of the skin prior to laser radiation

1. Apfelburg, D. B., Maser, M. R. and Lash, H. (1976). Argon lasers and management of cutaneous vascular deformities. *West J. Med.* **124**, 99.
2. Apfelburg, D. B., Maser, M. R. and Lash, H. (1978). Argon laser treatment of cutaneous vascular abnormalities. *Ann. Plast. Surg.* **1**, 14.
3. Apfelburg, D. B., Maser, M. R. and Lash, H. (1979). Extended clinical use of the argon laser for cutaneous lesions. *Archs Derm.* **115**, 719.
4. Goldman, L. (1976). Treatment of portwine marks by an argon laser. *J. derm. Surg. Oncol.* **2**, 385.
5. Cosman, B. (1980). Clinical experiences from the laser therapy of portwine stains. *Lasers Surg. Med.* **1**, 133.
6. Apfelburg, D. B., Maser, M. R., Lash, H. and Rivers, J. L. (1981). The argon laser for cutaneous lesions. *J. Am. med. Ass.* **235**, 1073.
7. Carruth, J. A. S. (1982). The argon laser in the treatment of vascular naevi. *Br. J. Derm.* **107**, 365.
8. Noe, J. M., Barsky, S. H., Geer, D. E. and Rosen, S. (1980). Portwine stains—the response to argon laser therapy: successful treatment and the predictive role of colour, age and biopsy. *Plast. reconstr. Surg.* **65**, 130.
9. Gilchrest, B. A., Rosen, S. and Noe, J. M. (1982). Chilling portwine stains improves the response to argon laser therapy. *Plast. reconstr. Surg.* **69**, 278.

may enable earlier treatment of these lesions. Scarring after laser therapy is less on the face than on other areas, and in facial lesions this may occur in between 2 and 8% of treated patients.

A wide variety of other vascular lesions have been treated, including spider naevi, telangiectasia, clinical variants of rosaces including ectactic vessels and post-rhinoplasty red nose, adenoma sebaceum, and strawberry naevi. Pyogenic granulomas are also said to respond. Lesions on the head and neck do better than lesions on the lower limbs and superficial varices or sunburst veins often respond very poorly.

C. The Tunable Dye Laser

1. Introduction

It is thought that the colour of the classical portwine stain is determined largely by its haemoglobin content. Studies of the absorption spectra of haemoglobin show three absorption peaks with a maximum peak at 415 nm and lesser peaks at 542 and 577 nm (Fig. 6). However, radiation at 415 nm does not penetrate well through the epidermis, but light at 542 and 577 nm is well transmitted. Recently Anderson and Parrish[1] investigated the possibility of treating patients with portwine stains by irradiating them with the tunable dye laser emitting light at 577 nm.

The dye laser (Fig. 7) consists of an active medium which is usually an organic compound in solution. Light from an argon or krypton ion laser is

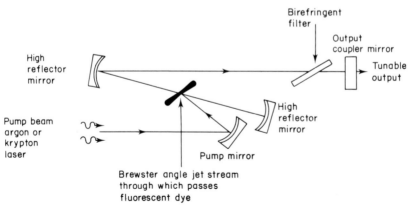

Fig. 7. Diagram of dye laser.

1. Anderson, R. R. and Parrish, J. A. (1981). Microvasculature can be selectively damaged using dye lasers in a basic theory and experimental evidence in human skin. *Lasers Med. Surg.* **1**, 263.

then used to pump the dye optically to the excited singlet state. The molecules subsequently decay to lower vibrational levels, establishing a population inversion. Subsequently, there is a return to the ground electronic state with an emission of radiation. By varying the organic compound employed and/or the optical pumping system, very broad lasing regions can be obtained, covering a spectrum from 400 nm to 1 μm (Fig. 8). If a rhodamine dye mixture is used it is possible to tune the argon laser to a wavelength of 577 nm.

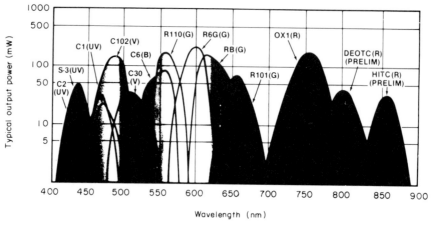

Fig. 8. Typical single frequency Tunning Curve (by courtesy of Coherent (UK) Ltd).

The treatment of portwine stains using the tunable dye laser at 577 nm was compared with conventional treatment using an argon laser.[1] The dye laser was found to be much more selective in its effects, causing specific damage to the cutaneous vascular plexus, in contrast to the greater damage following the use of the argon laser. With the latter there was diffuse nonspecific epidermal and upper dermal necrosis with cell death and a neutrophil response within 48 h: the degree of damage correlated well with the energy applied.

The effect of the dye laser, on the other hand, is to produce a vasculitis with initial red cell aggregation and subsequent vessel rupture and haemorrhage. After 48 h there is a characteristic acute vasculitis in the upper dermis with a prominent perivascular neutrophilic response in the

1. Greenwald, J., Rosen, S., Anderson, R. R., Harrist, T., MacFarland, F., Noe, J. M. and Parrish, J. S. (1981). Comparative histological studies of the tunable dye (at 577 nm) laser and argon laser: the specific vascular effects of the dye laser. *J. invest. Derm.* **77**, 305.

mid-dermis. Focal epidermal necrosis occurs but it is minimal and there is good preservation of skin appendages and collagen. The energy needed to produce these changes is of the order of 3 J cm^{-2} and is much less than that needed with the argon laser. Thus, the tunable dye laser at 577 nm specifically damages vascular structures rather than producing a wide non-specific diffuse coagulative necrosis as seen with either the argon or ruby lasers. It may be possible using the tunable dye laser to treat patients with portwine stains at less than 17 years of age. The author is currently investigating the possibility with the tunable dye laser. Also the future use of the tunable dye laser in conjunction with fluorescent dyes taken up selectively by malignant tissue is likely to offer very sophisticated treatment for tumours involving the skin and its appendages.[1]

D. The Carbon Dioxide Laser

The carbon dioxide laser produces infra-red coherent light at 10 600 nm which is well absorbed by water. As body tissues consist largely of water this laser modality may be used as a high precision bloodless light scalpel. However, when used as a knife it must be remembered that the cosmetic results are no better than if an incision had been made by a conventional scalpel.

It is now becoming apparent that the carbon dioxide laser may have an important part to play in the treatment of portwine stains.[2] Portwine stains which are pale and light pink in colour do better with the carbon dioxide laser than with the argon laser. Moreover, if the lesion blanches well on pressure, the CO_2 laser is more likely to be helpful than the argon laser. Furthermore, if skin biopsy shows few ectatic vessels and little blood content, the CO_2 laser will perform better than the argon laser.

The mechanism of action of the carbon dioxide laser in the treatment of portwine stains is quite different from that of the tunable dye laser or the argon laser. Vapourization of the skin surface is produced with sealing of the superficial plexus of ectatic blood vessels. As these ectatic blood vessels are greatest in number in the immediate subepidermal area[3] a relatively good cosmetic result ensues.

The carbon dioxide laser has also proved useful in a laser modification

1. Kato, H., Konaka, C., Ono, J., Matsushima, Y., Nishimiya, K., Hakoshima, A. and Hayata, Y. (1981). Laser photo radiation with haematoporphyrin derivative in lung cancer. Proc. 4th Congress of the International Society for Laser Surgery, Tokyo. Int. Group Corp. Japan, p. 14.
2. Bailin, P. L. (1982). Treatment of portwine stains with the CO_2 laser: early results. Paper presented at American Academy of Dermatology, New Orleans.
3. Barsky, S. H., Rosen, S., Geer, D. E. and Noe, J. M. (1980). The nature and evolution of portwine stains: a computer-assisted study. *J. invest. Derm.* **74**, 154.

of Moh's surgery.[1] The CO_2 laser modality ensures sterility, haemostasis and seals lymphatics. There is limited postoperative pain, probably because nerve-endings are also sealed. The tissue removed is well conserved and can therefore be used for histological examination. Even bone can be removed using the CO_2 laser and any bleeding vessels can be sealed by defocussing the CO_2 beam: also a very thin section can be removed for histology. The CO_2 laser, therefore, lends itself very well to the fresh tissue Moh's surgery technique.

1. Warts

It has also become apparent that the CO_2 carbon dioxide laser is very effective in the treatment of extensive or recalcitrant warts, particularly of the hands and feet.[2, 3] Eighty-one per cent of treated patients following a single laser treatment suffered no immediate recurrence and were still free of lesions after a 6-month follow-up.[2] Fifteen per cent of patients required a second treatment and four per cent required a third treatment. A disadvantage of the CO_2 laser, besides expense, is that postoperative scarring can occasionally occur, particularly with warts on the hand. Postoperative pain is minimal and postoperative sepsis was not observed. It is easy to differentiate between normal and warty tissue using the operating microscope. Genital warts also do well. Some perilesional swelling may be seen following treatment but this is not infective in nature.

2. Vascular Lesions

Vascular lesions that can be treated include telangiectasia, angiomata, pyogenic granulomata, lymphangiomas and epidermal naevi. The carbon dioxide laser may be preferable to the argon laser for the treatment of postrosacea venules of the face and nose as it can seal the affected vessel at each end.

3. Skin Tumours

It has been claimed that the CO_2 laser is effective in the treatment of keloids.[4] Once the keloid has been destroyed by the laser the area is

1. Bailin, P. L. (1982). Lasers in dermatology. Paper presented at American Academy of Dermatology, New Orleans.
2. McBurney, E. I. (1982). Carbon dioxide laser treatment of verrucae vulgaris. Paper presented at American Academy of Dermatology, New Orleans.
3. Mueller, T. J., Carlson, B. A. and Lindy, M. P. (1980). The use of the carbon dioxide surgical laser for the treatment of verrucae. *J. Am. pod. Assoc.* **70**, 136.
4. Bailin, P. L. (1982). Treatment of portwine stains with the CO_2 laser: early results. Paper presented at American Academy of Dermatology, New Orleans.

infiltrated with triamcinolone. The resultant scar, although it may be prominent, does not become keloidal.

A wide variety of tumours have been treated with the CO_2 laser.[1,2] Walker and Padilla[2] have treated 25 basal cell epitheliomas using the CO_2 laser attached to an operating microscope. Postoperative discomfort was noted but rapid healing occurred within 10 days to 3 weeks. Long-term follow-up will obviously be needed to assess results, but it appears that basal cell epitheliomas can be treated accurately and with good cosmetic results.

A wide variety of other tumours have been treated with the CO_2 laser, including intraepidermal carcinoma, squamous cell carcinoma and Kaposi's sarcoma.

E. The Neodynium–Yttrium Aluminium Garnet (YAG) Laser

The neodynium YAG laser, which emits at 1060 nm in the near infra-red, has at present a limited place in dermatological treatment. However, it has been shown that portwine stains may be successfully treated with this laser.[3,4,5]

1. Treatment of Tattoos

Almost any laser modality can be used to treat tattoos and the ruby laser and neodynium YAG laser, which emit at 694 and 1060 nm respectively have both been used. In addition, both the argon[6] and the CO_2 lasers[7,8,9] are effective. It is likely, therefore, that non-specific tissue destruction rather than specific light absorption is the most important mechanism for tattoo destruction. Ghosting of pigment, particularly

1. Bailin, P. L. (1982). Treatment of portwine stains with the CO_2 laser: early results. Paper presented at American Academy of Dermatology, New Orleans.
2. Walker, N. P. J. and Padilla, R. S. (1982). The carbon dioxide laser in dermatology. Paper presented at 1st British Conference on Lasers in Medicine and Surgery, London.
3. Li, E. S. (1981). A clinical report on the Nd YAG CW laser treatment of 800 cases of haemangioma of the soft tissue and investigation of its mechanism. Laser Tokyo '81 IVth Congress of the International Society for Laser Surgery. (Eds Atsumi, K. and Nimsakul, N.).
4. Wakamatsu, S., Hirayama, T. and Sakirie, H. (1981). YAG treatment of human naevi. Laser Tokyo '81. IVth Congress of the International Society for Laser Surgery. (Eds Atsumi, K. and Nimsakul, N.), p. 24.
5. Lee, T. K., Cho, B. C. and Park, M. (1981). An ultrastructural study of the cutaneous pigmented and vascular lesions treated by the Nd YAG laser. Laser Tokyo '81. IVth Congress of the International Society for Laser Surgery. (Eds Atsumi, K. and Nimsakul, N.), p. 24.
6. Apfelburg, D. B., Maser, M. R. and Lash, M. (1979). Extended clinical use of the argon laser for cutaneous lesions. Archs Derm. 115, 719.
7. Levine, H. L. and Bailin, P. L. (1982). Carbon dioxide laser treatment of cutaneous haemangiomas and tattoos. Archs Otolaryngol. 108, 236.
8. Bailin, P. L., Ratz, J. L. and Levine, H. L. (1980). Removal of tattoos by CO_2 laser. J. derm. Surg. Oncol. 6, 997.
9. Arndt, K. A. and Noe, J. M. (1982). Lasers in Dermatology. Archs Derm. 118, 293.

Indian ink, is common after treatment and so is an atrophic white scar. It is claimed that ghosting is less with the carbon dioxide laser than with the argon laser. When the latter is employed some ghosting may be present in up to 70% of treated patients. It must also be remembered that hypertrophic keloid scarring may occur following carbon dioxide or argon laser treatment of tattoos, particularly in those areas of skin which keloid easily, such as the deltoid area, shoulders and presternal skin.

F. The Helium Neon Laser

The helium neon laser, emitting at 2 mW, has been used for noninvasive measurement of cutaneous blood flow.[1-8] The technique of laser–Doppler flowmetry depends on the fact that laser light is back-scattered from moving red cells with resultant Doppler shifted frequencies which may be converted to flow signals by photo-detectors.

However, there appears to be a poor correlation between the results obtained by laser–Doppler flowmetry and many other methods used to measure skin blood flow. It is thought that the laser–Doppler flowmeter measures blood flowing in both capillaries and in arteriovenous anastomoses, whilst other methods such as the atraumatic epicutaneous[133] Xenon (^{133}Xe) technique, probably measures only capillary blood flow. Thus it is unlikely that there will be a significant correlation between the two methods in areas of skin which have arteriovenous anastomoses. However, the two methods correlate quite well in measurements of blood flow made during episodes of venous stasis, reactive hyperaemia and during orthostatic pressure changes. It is likely that laser–Doppler flowmetry utilizing the red light emitted by a helium neon laser will prove

1. Stern, M. D. (1975). *In vivo* evaluation of microcirculation by coherent light scattering. *Nature* **254**, 56.
2. Holloway, G. A. and Watkins, D. W. (1977). Laser–Doppler measurement of cutaneous blood flow. *J. invest. Derm.* **69**, 306.
3. Stern, M. D., Lappe, D. L., Bowen, P. D., Chimosky, J. E., Holloway, G. A., Keiser, H. R. and Bowman, R. L. (1977). Continuous measurement of tissue blood flow by laser–Doppler spectroscopy. *Am. J. Physiol.* **232**, 441.
4. Powers, E. D. and Frayer, W. W. (1978). Laser–Doppler measurement of blood flow in the microcirculation. *Plast. reconstruct. Surg.* **61**, 250.
5. Watkins, D. W. and Holloway, G. A. (1978). An instrument to measure cutaneous blood flow using the Doppler shift of laser light. *IEEE Trans. biomed. Eng.* **25**, 28.
6. Nilsson, G. E., Tenland, R. and Öberg, P. Å. (1980). A new instrument for continuous measurement of tissue blood flow by light beating spectroscopy. *IEEE Trans. biomed. Eng.* **27**, 12.
7. Nilsson, G. E., Tenland, T. and Öberg, P. Å. (1980). Evaluation of a laser–Doppler flowmeter for measurement of tissue blood flow. *IEEE Trans. biomed. Eng.* **27**, 597.
8. Engelhart, M. and Kristensen, J. K. (1983). Evaluation of cutaneous blood flow responses by 133 Xenon washout and a laser–Doppler flowmeter. *J. invest. Derm.* **80**, 12.

useful in assessing cutaneous blood flow and may supplement other methods such as the atraumatic epicutaneous ^{133}Xe technique.

The helium neon laser has been advocated by beauticians as a way of treating wrinkles. It has a low beam power of 0·5–3 mW and emits red light at 633 nm. It is very doubtful whether this modality does anything to help the ageing skin; only the operator is likely to gain. The same laser is sometimes used as a laser torch during lectures, and also as a focussing beam for other lasers.

VI. LONG-TERM HAZARDS FOLLOWING EXPOSURE TO LASER RADIATION

There are no known carcinogenic effects following laser radiation such as those seen after exposure to UVR or X-rays. Experimental animal work and human skin exposure which included chronic exposure to laser energy failed to induce any mitotic changes.[1] Moreover, histological examination of tissues following laser exposure showed none of the changes seen following x-radiation such as endarteritis, the presence of abnormal fibroblasts and telangiectasis.

VII. ASSESSMENT OF RESULTS

Papers on laser treatment for a wide variety of disorders, including dermatological conditions, are being published in ever-increasing numbers. This explosion of data has led to considerable difficulties in comparing results between different groups of workers because of the lack of standardized nomenclature regarding laser energy.[2] These workers suggested that all future studies should give details of the irradiance (laser flux density) at the irradiated surface in watts cm^{-2}, laser beam cross sectional area, and the shape of the irradiated surface, laser pulse durations of exposure time in seconds, also the pulse repetition rate, pulses per second in the case of pulsed lasers, treatment times and intervals between treatment, the total treated skin area (cm^2), the total number of applied laser pulses or exposures and the type of laser used together with its full spectral distribution.

Improved methods of assessment of results are also important and

1. Goldman, L., Rockwell, R. J., Jr and Richfield, F. (1971). Long-term laser exposure of a senile freckle. *Arch. environ. Health* **22**, 401.
2. Arndt, K. A., Noe, J. M., Northam, D. B. C. and Itzkan, I. (1981). Laser therapy: basic concepts and nomenclature. *J. Am. Acad. Derm.* **5**, 649.

reflectance spectrophotometry may have an important role here,[1, 2] as this modality will define accurately the absorption spectrum of the lesion in question. It may then be possible to irradiate the lesion at the most appropriate wavelength to effect its destruction.

VIII. THE FUTURE OF LASER DERMATOLOGY

It is likely that the carbon dioxide laser, the argon laser and the tunable dye laser will all have an important part to play in the treatment not only of vascular lesions, but also of benign and malignant tumours. Selective destruction, not only of tumours, but also of intra-cellular structures, seems possible. The copper vapour laser emitting at 510–578 nm may also find use in the field of dermatology. Instruments combining the CO_2 laser and argon laser modality are already available and may be useful in the treatment of portwine stains. Ultimately it may be possible to tune a laser the full length of the spectrum from microwaves to X-ray. New advances in fibre-optics permitting the transfer of CO_2 laser light will greatly increase the flexibility of the CO_2 laser. Goldman[3] divided laser surgery in dermatology into three basic categories: (1) where it is obligatory, (2) where it is preferred, and (3) where it should not be used at all. It is likely that the first two categories will increase whilst the third will become smaller. Thus, it is not beyond the bounds of possibility that malignant melanomas may be selectively and effectively treated in future by specific laser techniques.

Laser technology is also open to exploitation by untrained and unqualified persons and for this reason it is important for the medical profession to maintain a control over its future development and use.

1. Ohmori, S. and Huang, C. (1981). Recent progress in the treatment of portwine stains by argon laser: some observations on the prognostic value of relative spectroreflectance (RSR) and the histological classification of the lesions. *Br. J. plast. Surg.* **34**, 249.
2. Dawson, J. B., Barker, D. J. and Ellis, D. J. (1980). A theoretical and experimental study of light absorption and scattering by *in vivo* skin. *Physics Med. Biol.* **25**, 695.
3. Goldman, L. (1982). The future of laser dermatology in medicine and surgery. Paper presented at American Academy of Dermatology, New Orleans.

Author Index

Foerster, H. R., 2573
Foix, C., 2521
Foote, C. S., 2544, 2603, 2604
Forbes, P. D., 2417, 2491, 2569, 2617, 2650
Foreman, M. I., 2616
Forest, I. S., 2571
Fornace, A. J., 2527, 2529
Forsgren, A., 2643
Forsythe, W. E., 2427
Fortner, J. G., 2489
Fosnaugh, R. P., 2592
Fowlks, W. L., 2557, 2565
Fox, S. H., 2641
Frain-Bell, W., 2384, 2391, 2392, 2424, 2493, 2494, 2495, 2496, 2506, 2509, 2510, 2514, 2515, 2518, 2539, 2566, 2567, 2574, 2578, 2582, 2594, 2597, 2600, 2601, 2602, 2605, 2608, 2609, 2610, 2626, 2630, 2636, 2642
Frank, S. B., 2581
Frayer, W. W., 2668
Freeman, R. G., 2392, 2424, 2453, 2473, 2484, 2488, 2515, 2560, 2564, 2581, 2631
Fregert, S., 2596
Frenk, E., 2417
Freund, E., 2557, 2577
Friedberg, E. C., 2446, 2529, 2530, 2532
Friedman, G. B., 2624, 2651
Frisk-Homberg, M., 2584
Fritsch, P., 2564, 2604, 2608, 2627, 2634, 2636, 2647
Fritsch, P. D., 2626
Frost, P., 2580, 2622
Frumkin, A., 2592
Fry, L., 2615, 2618
Fry, R. J. M., 2449, 2451, 2650
Fugimori, E., 2603, 2604
Fuhrman, D. L., 2580
Fujimara, Y., 2529, 2531
Fujimori, B., 2604
Fujimori, E., 2460, 2484
Fujimura, Y., 2627
Fujita, H., 2567, 2583
Fujita, M., 2497
Fukuda, M., 2426, 2551, 2569, 2597, 2598, 2631
Fukuma, M., 2507
Fukuyama, K., 2435, 2446, 2447, 2457,
2460, 2469, 2472, 2473, 2520, 2527, 2534, 2539, 2612, 2625, 2644
Fulton, J., 2634
Fulton, J. E., Jr, 2551, 2646
Furuyama, J-I., 2529
Fusaro, R. M., 2600
Fuselier, C. O., 2532
Fuzimura, Y., 2623
Fye, K., 2435, 2457, 2460, 2612

G

Gabriel, R., 2550, 2566
Gagnaire, D., 2638
Galosi, A., 2626
Gallo, U., 2542
Gandhi, V. M., 2478
Ganesan, A. K., 2446
Gange, R. W., 2634
Gardiner, J. S., 2574
Garraz, G., 2567, 2568
Garrett, H., 2648
Garretts, M., 2585, 2587
Gates, F. L., 2439
Gaylor, J. R., 2404, 2474
Gazith, J., 2626
Gazso, L., 2648
Geer, D. E., 2662, 2665
Gell, P. G. H., 2504
German, J., 2527, 2535, 2536
Gerstein, W., 2488
Gervais, A., 2593, 2595
Giacometti, L., 2645
Giannelli, F., 2500, 2526, 2527, 2529, 2531, 2532, 2533, 2534, 2536
Gianetti, A., 2638
Gibson, J. B., 2522
Giese, A. C., 2375, 2439, 2458
Gilchrest, B. A., 2634, 2662
Gillman, T., 2486
Giovizaao, V. J., 2597
Girrotti, A., 2561
Glass, B., 2375
Gleiser, C. A., 2569
Glew, W. B., 2566
Gligora, M., 2628
Glinski, W., 2615, 2650
Glisksman, J. M., 2631

Subject Index